Clinical Applications of Functional MRI

Editor

JAY J. PILLAI

NEUROIMAGING CLINICS OF NORTH AMERICA

www.neuroimaging.theclinics.com

Consulting Editor
SURESH K. MUKHERJI

November 2014 • Volume 24 • Number 4

ELSEVIER

1600 John F. Kennedy Boulevard • Suite 1800 • Philadelphia, Pennsylvania, 19103-2899

http://www.neuroimaging.theclinics.com

NEUROIMAGING CLINICS OF NORTH AMERICA Volume 24, Number 4
November 2014 ISSN 1052-5149, ISBN 13: 978-0-323-32383-3

Editor: John Vassallo (j.vassallo@elsevier.com)
Developmental Editor: Donald Mumford

Neuroimaging Clinics of North America (ISSN 1052-5149) is published quarterly by Elsevier Inc., 360 Park Avenue South, New York, NY 10010-1710. Months of issue are February, May, August, and November. Business and editorial offices: 1600 John F. Kennedy Blvd., Suite 1800, Philadelphia, PA 19103-2899. Business and editorial offices: 6277 Sea Harbor Drive, Orlando, FL 32887-4800. Periodicals postage paid at New York, NY, and additional mailing offices. Subscription prices are USD 360 per year for US individuals, USD 514 per year for US institutions, USD 180 per year for US students and residents, USD 415 per year for Canadian individuals, USD 655 per year for Canadian institutions, USD 525 per year for international individuals, USD 655 per year for international institutions and USD 260 per year for Canadian and foreign students and residents. To receive student/resident rate, orders must be accompanied by name of affiliated institution, date of term, and the *signature* of program/residency coordinator on institution letterhead. Orders will be billed at individual rate until proof of status is received. Foreign air speed delivery is included in all *Clinics* subscription prices. All prices are subject to change without notice. POSTMASTER: Send address changes to *Neuroimaging Clinics of North America*, Elsevier Health Sciences Division, Subscription Customer Service, 3251 Riverport Lane, Maryland Heights, MO 63043. Telephone: 1-800-654-2452 (U.S. and Canada); 314-447-8871 (outside U.S. and Canada). Fax: 314-447-8029. E-mail: journalscustomerservice-usa@elsevier.com (for print support); journalsonlinesupport-usa@elsevier.com (for online support).

Reprints. For copies of 100 or more of articles in this publication, please contact the Commercial Reprints Department, Elsevier Inc., 360 Park Avenue South, New York, NY 10010-1710. Tel.: 212-633-3874; Fax: 212-633-3820; E-mail: reprints@elsevier.com.

Neuroimaging Clinics of North America is covered by *Excerpta Medical/EMBASE,* the RSNA Index of Imaging Literature, *MEDLINE/PubMed (Index Medicus),* MEDLINE/MEDLARS, SciSearch, Research Alert, and Neuroscience Citation Index.

PROGRAM OBJECTIVE

The goal of *Neuroimaging Clinics of North America* is to keep practicing radiologists and radiology residents up to date with current clinical practice in radiology by providing timely articles reviewing the state of the art in patient care.

TARGET AUDIENCE

Practicing radiologists, radiology residents, and other healthcare professionals who utilize neuroimaging findings to provide patient care.

LEARNING OBJECTIVES

Upon completion of this activity, participants will be able to:
1. Review diffusion tensor imaging in patients with brain tumors, brain malformations and epilepsy.
2. Discuss the application of bold fMRI in motor systems, visual mapping, and presurgical planning.
3. Describe pediatric fMRI for pretherapeutic planning.

ACCREDITATION

The Elsevier Office of Continuing Medical Education (EOCME) is accredited by the Accreditation Council for Continuing Medical Education (ACCME) to provide continuing medical education for physicians.

The EOCME designates this enduring material for a maximum of 15 *AMA PRA Category 1 Credit*(s)™. Physicians should claim only the credit commensurate with the extent of their participation in the activity.

All other health care professionals requesting continuing education credit for this enduring material will be issued a certificate of participation.

DISCLOSURE OF CONFLICTS OF INTEREST

The EOCME assesses conflict of interest with its instructors, faculty, planners, and other individuals who are in a position to control the content of CME activities. All relevant conflicts of interest that are identified are thoroughly vetted by EOCME for fair balance, scientific objectivity, and patient care recommendations. EOCME is committed to providing its learners with CME activities that promote improvements or quality in healthcare and not a specific proprietary business or a commercial interest.

The planning committee, staff, authors and editors listed below have identified no financial relationships or relationships to products or devices they or their spouse/life partner have with commercial interest related to the content of this CME activity:

Shruti Agarwal, PhD; Monica G. Allen, PhD; Thangamadhan Bosemani, MD; Nicole P. Brennan; Umair J. Chaudhary, MBBS, MSc, PhD; Catherine Chiron, MD, PhD; Chris J. Conklin, MS; John S. Duncan, MA, DM, FRCP, FMedSci; Scott H. Faro, MD; Meredith Gabriel, MA; Sachin K. Gujar, MD; Carl D. Hacker, MD, PhD; Kristen Helm; Lucie Hertz-Pannier, MD, PhD; Thierry A.G.M. Huisman, MD; Brynne Hunter; Mudassar Kamran, MBBS; Andrew P. Klein, MD; Sandy Lavery; Eric C. Leuthardt, MD; Leighton P. Mark, MD; Mary Pat McAndrews, PhD; Jill McNair; Timothy J. Mitchell, PhD; Feroze B. Mohamed, PhD; Wade M. Mueller, MD; Suresh K. Mukherji, MD, MBA, FACR; Marion Noulhiane, PhD; Kyung K. Peck, PhD; Jay J. Pillai, MD; Andrea Poretti, MD; Ryan V. Raut; Sebastian Rodrigo, MD, PhD; Haris I. Sair, MD; Joshua S. Shimony, MD, PhD; Abraham Z. Snyder, MD, PhD; Karthikeyan Subramaniam; John Vassallo; David M. Yousem, MD, MBA; Domenico Zacà, PhD.

The planning committee, staff, authors and editors listed below have identified financial relationships or relationships to products or devices they or their spouse/life partner have with commercial interest related to the content of this CME activity:

Edgar A. DeYoe, PhD is a consultant for, has stock ownership in, and has a research grant from Prism Clinical Imaging.
Andrei I. Holodny, MD has stock ownership in fMRI Consultants.
Jay J. Pillai, MD is a consultant/advisor for Prism Clinical Imaging; has a research grant from Siemens Healthcare USA and has royalties/patents with Springer Science+Business Media.
John L. Ulmer, MD is a consultant/advisor and has stock ownership in Prism Clinical Imaging.

UNAPPROVED/OFF-LABEL USE DISCLOSURE

The EOCME requires CME faculty to disclose to the participants:
1. When products or procedures being discussed are off-label, unlabelled, experimental, and/or investigational (not US Food and Drug Administration (FDA) approved); and
2. Any limitations on the information presented, such as data that are preliminary or that represent ongoing research, interim analyses, and/or unsupported opinions. Faculty may discuss information about pharmaceutical agents that is outside of FDA-approved labelling. This information is intended solely for CME and is not intended to promote off-label use of these medications. If you have any questions, contact the medical affairs department of the manufacturer for the most recent prescribing information.

TO ENROLL

To enroll in the *Neuroimaging Clinics of North America* Continuing Medical Education program, call customer service at 1-800-654-2452 or sign up online at http://www.theclinics.com/home/cme. The CME program is available to subscribers for an additional annual fee of $235 USD.

METHOD OF PARTICIPATION

In order to claim credit, participants must complete the following:

1. Complete enrolment as indicated above.
2. Read the activity.
3. Complete the CME Test and Evaluation. Participants must achieve a score of 70% on the test. All CME Tests and Evaluations must be completed online.

CME INQUIRIES/SPECIAL NEEDS

For all CME inquiries or special needs, please contact elsevierCME@elsevier.com.

NEUROIMAGING CLINICS OF NORTH AMERICA

NOW AVAILABLE FOR YOUR iPhone and iPad

Contributors

CONSULTING EDITOR

SURESH K. MUKHERJI, MD, MBA, FACR
Professor and Chairman, W.F. Patenge
Endowed Chair, Department of Radiology,
Michigan State University, East Lansing,
Michigan

EDITOR

JAY J. PILLAI, MD
Associate Professor and Director of Functional
MRI, Neuroradiology Division, Russell H.
Morgan Department of Radiology and
Radiological Science, The Johns Hopkins
University School of Medicine, The Johns
Hopkins Hospital, Baltimore, Maryland

AUTHORS

SHRUTI AGARWAL, PhD
Postdoctoral Fellow, Division of
Neuroradiology, Russell H. Morgan
Department of Radiology and Radiological
Science, The Johns Hopkins Hospital, Johns
Hopkins University School of Medicine,
Baltimore, Maryland

MONICA G. ALLEN, PhD
Department of Neurological Surgery,
Mallinckrodt Institute of Radiology,
Washington University School of Medicine,
St Louis, Missouri

THANGAMADHAN BOSEMANI, MD
Section of Pediatric Neuroradiology, Russell H.
Morgan Department of Radiology and
Radiological Science, Charlotte R. Bloomberg
Children's Center, The Johns Hopkins University
School of Medicine, Baltimore, Maryland

NICOLE P. BRENNAN, BA
Functional MRI Laboratory, Department of
Radiology, Memorial Sloan-Kettering Cancer
Center, New York, New York

UMAIR J. CHAUDHARY, MBBS, MSc, PhD
Clinical Research Associate, Department of
Clinical and Experimental Epilepsy, UCL
Institute of Neurology, London; MRI Unit,
Epilepsy Society, Buckinghamshire,
United Kingdom

CATHERINE CHIRON, MD, PhD
UMR 1129, INSERM, Paris Descartes
University, CEA-Saclay; UNIACT/Neurospin,
I2BM, DSV, CEA-Saclay, Gif sur Yvette,
France

CHRIS J. CONKLIN, MS
Research Associate, Department of
Electrical Engineering and Radiology, Temple
University Magnetic Resonance Imaging
Center, Temple University, Philadelphia,
Pennsylvania

EDGAR A. DeYOE, PhD
Professor, Department of Radiology,
Medical College of Wisconsin, Milwaukee,
Wisconsin

JOHN S. DUNCAN, MA, DM, FRCP, FMedSci
Professor of Neurology, Department of Clinical
and Experimental Epilepsy, UCL Institute of
Neurology, London; MRI Unit, Epilepsy
Society, Buckinghamshire; Clinical Director,
Queen Square Division, UCLH NHS
Foundation Trust, London, United Kingdom

SCOTT H. FARO, MD
Professor, Department of Radiology,
Bioengineering and Electrical Engineering,
Temple University Magnetic Resonance
Imaging Center, Temple University,
Philadelphia, Pennsylvania

MEREDITH GABRIEL, BA
Functional MRI Laboratory, Department of
Radiology, Memorial Sloan-Kettering Cancer
Center, New York, New York

SACHIN K. GUJAR, MBBS
Assistant Professor, Division of
Neuroradiology, Russell H. Morgan
Department of Radiology and Radiological
Science, The Johns Hopkins Hospital, Johns
Hopkins University School of Medicine,
Baltimore, Maryland

CARL D. HACKER, BA
Medical Student Training Program,
Washington University School of Medicine,
St Louis, Missouri

LUCIE HERTZ-PANNIER, MD, PhD
UMR 1129, INSERM, Paris Descartes
University, CEA-Saclay; UNIACT/Neurospin,
I2BM, DSV, CEA-Saclay, Gif sur Yvette,
France

ANDREI I. HOLODNY, MD
Chief of the Neuroradiology Service; Director of
the Functional MRI Laboratory; Professor,
Department of Radiology, Memorial Sloan-
Kettering Cancer Center, Weill Medical College
of Cornell University, New York, New York

THIERRY A.G.M. HUISMAN, MD
Section of Pediatric Neuroradiology, Russell H.
Morgan Department of Radiology and
Radiological Science, Charlotte R. Bloomberg
Children's Center, The Johns Hopkins
University School of Medicine, Baltimore,
Maryland

MUDASSAR KAMRAN, MD, PhD
Mallinckrodt Institute of Radiology,
Washington University School of Medicine,
St Louis, Missouri

ANDREW P. KLEIN, MD
Assistant Professor, Department of Radiology,
Medical College of Wisconsin, Milwaukee,
Wisconsin

ERIC C. LEUTHARDT, MD
Department of Neurological Surgery,
Washington University School of Medicine,
St Louis, Missouri

LEIGHTON P. MARK, MD
Professor, Department of Radiology, Medical
College of Wisconsin, Milwaukee, Wisconsin

MARY PAT McANDREWS, PhD
Krembil Neuroscience Centre, Toronto
Western Research Institute, University Health
Network; Department of Psychology,
University of Toronto, Toronto, Ontario,
Canada

TIMOTHY J. MITCHELL, PhD
Department of Neurological Surgery,
Mallinckrodt Institute of Radiology,
Washington University School of Medicine,
St Louis, Missouri

FEROZE B. MOHAMED, PhD
Associate Director, Temple University
Magnetic Resonance Imaging Center;
Professor, Department of Radiology,
Neuroscience, Bioengineering and Electrical
Engineering, Temple University, Philadelphia,
Pennsylvania

WADE M. MUELLER, MD
Professor, Department of Neurosurgery,
Medical College of Wisconsin, Milwaukee,
Wisconsin

MARION NOULHIANE, PhD
UMR 1129, INSERM, Paris Descartes
University, CEA-Saclay; UNIACT/Neurospin,
I2BM, DSV, CEA-Saclay, Gif sur Yvette, France

KYUNG K. PECK, PhD
Functional MRI Laboratory, Department of
Radiology, Memorial Sloan-Kettering Cancer
Center, New York, New York

JAY J. PILLAI, MD
Associate Professor and Director of Functional MRI, Division of Neuroradiology, Russell H. Morgan Department of Radiology and Radiological Science, The Johns Hopkins Hospital, Johns Hopkins University School of Medicine, Baltimore, Maryland

ANDREA PORETTI, MD
Section of Pediatric Neuroradiology, Russell H. Morgan Department of Radiology and Radiological Science, Charlotte R. Bloomberg Children's Center, The Johns Hopkins University School of Medicine, Baltimore, Maryland

RYAN V. RAUT
Department of Radiology, University of Wisconsin-Madison, Madison, Wisconsin

SEBASTIAN RODRIGO, MD, PhD
UMR 1129, INSERM, Paris Descartes University, CEA-Saclay; UNIACT/Neurospin, I2BM, DSV, CEA-Saclay, Gif sur Yvette, France

HARIS I. SAIR, MD
Assistant Professor, Division of Neuroradiology, Russell H. Morgan Department of Radiology and Radiological Science, The Johns Hopkins Hospital, Johns Hopkins University School of Medicine, Maryland

JOSHUA S. SHIMONY, MD, PhD
Mallinckrodt Institute of Radiology, Washington University School of Medicine, St Louis, Missouri

ABRAHAM Z. SNYDER, MD, PhD
Department of Neurology, Mallinckrodt Institute of Radiology, Washington University School of Medicine, St Louis, Missouri

JOHN L. ULMER, MD
Professor, Department of Radiology, Medical College of Wisconsin, Milwaukee, Wisconsin

DAVID M. YOUSEM, MD, MBA
Director of Neuroradiology; Associate Dean of Professional Development, The Russell H. Morgan Department of Radiology and Radiological Science, Johns Hopkins Medical Institution, Baltimore, Maryland

DOMENICO ZACÀ, PhD
Center for Mind/Brain Sciences, University of Trento, Italy; Division of Neuroradiology, Russell H. Morgan Department of Radiology and Radiological Science, The Johns Hopkins Hospital, Johns Hopkins University School of Medicine, Baltimore, Maryland

Contents

> Functional magnetic resonance imaging (fMRI) has become a common tool for pre-surgical sensorimotor mapping, and is a significant preoperative asset for tumors located adjacent to the central sulcus. fMRI has changed surgical options for many patients. This noninvasive tool allows for easy display and integration with other neuroimaging techniques. Although fMRI is a useful preoperative tool, it is not perfect. Tumors that affect the normal vascular coupling of neuronal activity will affect fMRI measurements. This article discusses the usefulness of blood oxygen level dependent (BOLD) fMRI with regard to preoperative motor mapping.

> Functional magnetic resonance imaging (fMRI) is used clinically to map the visual cortex before brain surgery or other invasive treatments to achieve an optimal balance between therapeutic effect and the avoidance of postoperative vision deficits. Clinically optimized stimuli, behavioral task, analysis, and displays permit identification of cortical subregions supporting high-acuity central vision that is critical for reading and other essential visual functions. Emerging techniques such as resting-state fMRI may facilitate the use of fMRI–based vision mapping in a broader range of patients.

> The use of functional magnetic resonance imaging to map language and sensori-motor regions in the brain is rapidly becoming a clinical standard in neurosurgical centers. Despite a wealth of cognitive neuroscience data showing focal medial temporal activation elicited by memory encoding and retrieval tasks in controls, translating such findings to generate reliable metrics for clinical use has been slow. The current review documents some of the successes that have been achieved, using both activation and resting-state functional connectivity in the clinical context of temporal lobe epilepsy, and discusses some of the challenges that remain to be addressed.

Preoperative mapping has revolutionized neurosurgical care for brain tumor patients. Maximizing resections has improved diagnosis, optimized treatment algorithms, and decreased potentially devastating postoperative deficits. Although mapping has multiple steps and complimentary localization sources, diffusion tensor imaging (DTI) excels in its essential role in depicting white matter tracts. A thorough understanding of DTI, data visualization methods, and limitations with mastery of functional and dysfunctional white matter anatomy is necessary to realize the potential of DTI. By establishing spatial relationships between lesion borders and functional networks preoperatively and intraoperatively, DTI is central to high-risk neurosurgical resections and becoming the standard of care.

In this article, the basics of diffusion-weighted imaging/diffusion tensor imaging (DTI) are discussed, including a short historical perspective on the fiber dissection technique, followed by a review of selected brain malformations in which DTI and tractography have contributed to a better understanding of the malformations, and by a clinical case in which DTI showed a disorder of the internal neuroarchitecture that could not be correctly appreciated by conventional anatomic magnetic resonance imaging.

In this article, some specificities of functional magnetic resonance imaging (fMRI) in children (eg, blood-oxygen-level-dependent response and brain maturation, paradigm design, technical issues, feasibility, data analysis) are reviewed, the main knowledge on presurgical cortical mapping in children (motor, language, reading, memory) is summarized, and the emergence of resting state fMRI in presurgical cortical mapping is discussed.

Resting-state functional MR imaging (rsfMR imaging) measures spontaneous fluctuations in the blood oxygen level–dependent (BOLD) signal and can be used to elucidate the brain's functional organization. It is used to simultaneously assess multiple distributed resting-state networks. Unlike task-based functional MR imaging, rsfMR imaging does not require task performance. This article presents a brief introduction of rsfMR imaging processing methods followed by a detailed discussion on the use of rsfMR imaging in presurgical planning. Example cases are provided to highlight the strengths and limitations of the technique.

The lifetime prevalence of epilepsy ranges from 2.7 to 12.4 per 1000 in Western countries. Around 30% of patients with epilepsy remain refractory to antiepileptic drugs and continue to have seizures. Noninvasive imaging techniques such as functional magnetic resonance imaging (fMRI) and diffusion tensor imaging (DTI) have helped to better understand mechanisms of seizure generation and propagation, and to localize epileptic, eloquent, and cognitive networks. In this review, the clinical applications of fMRI and DTI are discussed, for mapping cognitive and epileptic networks and organization of white matter tracts in individuals with epilepsy.

Clinical application of functional magnetic resonance imaging (fMRI) based on blood oxygenation level–dependent (BOLD) effect has increased over the past decade because of its ability to map regional blood flow in response to brain stimulation. This mapping is primarily achieved by exploiting the BOLD effect precipitated by changes in the magnetic properties of hemoglobin. BOLD fMRI has utility in neurosurgical planning and mapping neuronal functional connectivity. Conventional echo planar imaging techniques are used to acquire stimulus-driven fMR imaging BOLD data. This article highlights technical aspects of fMRI data analysis to make it more accessible in clinical settings.

In this review, limitations affecting the results of presurgical mapping with blood-oxygen-level-dependent (BOLD) functional magnetic resonance imaging (fMRI) are discussed. There is a great need to standardize fMRI acquisition and analysis methods and establish guidelines to address quality control issues. Several national and international organizations are formulating guidelines and standards for both clinical and research applications of BOLD fMRI. Consensus regarding management of these issues will likely both improve the clinical standard of care and enhance future research applications of fMRI.

It is difficult to justify maintaining a clinical functional magnetic resonance imaging (fMRI) program based solely on revenue generation. The use of fMRI is, therefore, based mostly in patient care considerations, leading to better outcomes. The high costs of the top-of-the-line equipment, hardware, and software needed for state-of-the-art fMRI and the time commitment by multiple professionals are not adequately reimbursed at a representative rate by current payor schemes for the Current Procedure Terminology codes assigned.

Foreword

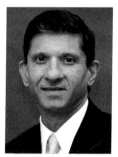

Suresh K. Mukherji, MD, MBA, FACR
Consulting Editor

First, I would like to thank Dr Jay Pillai for creating this important issue. This issue of *Neuroimaging Clinics* addresses the current clinical state-of-the-art in functional brain magnetic resonance imaging. Functional imaging has arguably changed the standard of care for patients undergoing surgical resection of brain tumors, epileptogenic tissue, and other structural brain lesions. This issue explores applications of BOLD and DTI to presurgical and other pretherapeutic planning and includes articles that focus on the motor, language, memory, and visual systems. The economic issues relating to the actual running of a clinical BOLD fMRI service has its own separate article with a description of current procedural terminology codes used for billing. This article should be especially helpful for those practices considering initiating their own service. I would also like to thank the authors for their wonderful contributions. This is a comprehensive, yet practical, monograph that should benefit numerous disciplines interested in learning more about functional brain imaging.

Suresh K. Mukherji, MD, MBA, FACR
Department of Radiology
Michigan State University
846 Service Road
East Lansing, MI 48824, USA

E-mail address:
mukherji@rad.msu.edu

Neuroimag Clin N Am 24 (2014) xv
http://dx.doi.org/10.1016/j.nic.2014.09.001
1052-5149/14/$ – see front matter © 2014 Elsevier Inc. All rights reserved.

neuroimaging.theclinics.com

Preface
Clinical Applications of Functional MRI

This issue of *Neuroimaging Clinics* addresses the current clinical state-of-the-art in functional brain magnetic resonance imaging. Although other "functional" imaging modalities such as MR spectroscopy and MR perfusion imaging have been deliberately omitted in favor of an emphasis on blood-oxygen level-dependent (BOLD) fMRI and diffusion tensor imaging (DTI), this is largely due to the ever-increasing breadth and depth of current clinical applications of the latter. Functional imaging has arguably changed the standard of care for patients undergoing surgical resection of brain tumors, epileptogenic tissue, and other structural brain lesions. In addition, BOLD fMRI and DTI have been useful for increasing our scientific understanding of different functional networks in the brain and how such networks and their connectivity may be disrupted in disease states. This issue explores applications of BOLD and DTI to presurgical and other pretherapeutic planning and includes articles with focus on the motor, language, memory, and visual systems, often in the context of pretherapeutic planning or specific diseases or patient populations. In particular, applications to epilepsy and pediatric neuroimaging are included, as well as both technical and practical aspects of clinical use of these imaging methods. In addition to conventional task-based BOLD imaging, resting state BOLD imaging is also discussed. Last, economic/business issues relating to the actual running of a clinical BOLD fMRI service are considered, with description of current procedural terminology codes used for billing. Many high-quality color illustrations are included throughout this issue to display important eloquent cortex and white matter tracts in the brain, and an extensive list of references is included for each article in this issue. I hope that this compendium of clinically relevant articles will serve as a broad overview of different functional imaging techniques and applications that will prove to be useful to neuroradiologists, neurologists, and neurosurgeons as well as those who are in training in these respective fields.

Jay J. Pillai, MD
Associate Professor
Director of Functional MRI
Neuroradiology Division
Russell H. Morgan Department of Radiology and
Radiological Science
The Johns Hopkins University School of Medicine
& The Johns Hopkins Hospital
1800 Orleans Street
Baltimore, MD 21287, USA

E-mail address:
jpillai1@jhmi.edu

Neuroimag Clin N Am 24 (2014) xvii
http://dx.doi.org/10.1016/j.nic.2014.09.002
1052-5149/14/$ – see front matter © 2014 Elsevier Inc. All rights reserved.

Blood Oxygen Level Dependent Functional Magnetic Resonance Imaging for Presurgical Planning

Meredith Gabriel, BA, Nicole P. Brennan, BA,
Kyung K. Peck, PhD, Andrei I. Holodny, MD*

KEYWORDS

- fMRI sensorimotor mapping • Intraoperative motor mapping • BOLD fMRI

KEY POINTS

- Functional magnetic resonance imaging (fMRI) has become a common tool for presurgical sensorimotor mapping.
- fMRI is a significant preoperative asset for tumors located adjacent to the central sulcus.
- fMRI has changed surgical options for many patients. This noninvasive tool allows for easy display and integration with other neuroimaging techniques.
- Although fMRI is a useful preoperative tool, it is not perfect. Tumors that affect the normal vascular coupling of neuronal activity will affect fMRI measurement.

INTRODUCTION

In the early 1990s, functional magnetic resonance imaging (fMRI) entered neuroimaging as a unique resource in the arsenal of preoperative planning tools for patients with brain tumors. fMRI is a technique that takes advantage of the differences in magnetic susceptibility between oxyhemoglobin and deoxyhemoglobin. It is a less invasive neuroimaging method than its positron emission tomography (PET) predecessor, given that the contrast agent is endogenous.[1] fMRI is possible because oxyhemoglobin has a magnetic resonance (MR) signal different from that of than deoxyhemoglobin. When a task is performed, oxygenated blood in excess of the amount needed (termed luxury perfusion) is delivered to the active area. The difference in magnetic susceptibility between deoxyhemoglobin concentrations and oxyhemoglobin concentrations creates the signal in functional imaging. This effect is termed the blood oxygen level dependent (BOLD) signal. fMRI provides good spatial localization (as low as 1 mm) and temporal acquisition resolution (as low as 1 second) but is limited by the resolution of the hemodynamic response (8–30 seconds). The superior spatial resolution is particularly advantageous for mapping peritumoral eloquent areas for treatment planning.[2]

fMRI can effectively map the sensory and motor areas. The motor gyrus is somatotopically organized, with all body parts represented in a way that is preserved across different people. fMRI can provide a multidimensional map in a single mapping session. Such maps of sensorimotor function help the surgeon to assess the risks of surgery and guide intraoperative mapping techniques.[2,3] The primary motor and sensory areas in fMRI are of particular interest for surgical planning, because iatrogenic damage to these areas can cause permanent neurologic deficits. As a result the precise localization of various motor

Functional MRI Laboratory, Department of Radiology, Memorial Sloan-Kettering Cancer Center, 1275 York Avenue, New York, NY 10065, USA
* Corresponding author.
E-mail address: holodnya@mskcc.org

Neuroimag Clin N Am 24 (2014) 557–571
http://dx.doi.org/10.1016/j.nic.2014.07.003
1052-5149/14/$ – see front matter © 2014 Elsevier Inc. All rights reserved.

and sensory areas is useful, particularly in the setting of a space-occupying lesion.

Primary motor and sensory cortices are distinct in the functions they subserve. However, as a result of significant neuronal reciprocity in the region, injury to either can result in a mixed motor/sensory deficit. For example, injury to the primary motor gyrus usually leads to a permanent, largely irreversible paresis.[4] Injury to the sensory cortex, while producing the expected sensory perceptual deficits, can also lead to a similar type of paresis seen with injury to the motor strip as a result of the lack of proprioceptive information. A variety of other deficits is seen with injury to the postcentral gyrus, depending on whether the left or right hemisphere is damaged. Some of these include 2-point discrimination, astereognosis (inability to discern objects by feeling them), and agraphism (inability to write). This article discusses the usefulness of BOLD fMRI with regard to preoperative motor mapping.

ANATOMIC ORGANIZATION OF THE SENSORIMOTOR SYSTEM

The 4 main regions that subserve motor control that are of interest to neurosurgeons are the primary motor cortex, the primary sensory cortex, the premotor cortex, and the supplementary motor area (SMA). The motor and sensory gyri taken together are often referred to as one larger area termed the primary sensorimotor cortex.[5]

The Primary Sensorimotor Cortex

The primary motor cortex, located in the precentral gyrus, is responsible for executing movement (**Fig. 1**). Its position delineates the frontal from the parietal lobes. The motor gyrus marks the posterior limit of the frontal lobe and the sensory gyrus marks the start of the parietal lobe. The motor gyrus is somatotopically mapped; different body regions are distinctly represented in cortical space in a common (but not steadfast) pattern medially to laterally. Historically, the motor gyrus has been localized using anatomic markers. The most salient anatomic marker of the motor gyrus is the reverse omega portion of the central sulcus (see **Fig. 1**). This reverse omega typically demarcates the location of the hand motor region of the motor homunculus.[6] However, the presence of this marker is occasionally unreliable. **Fig. 2** shows a case whereby a reverse omega sign would have incorrectly indicated the position of the motor gyrus. Although cases like this are rare, they do occur. Furthermore, lesions can obscure traditional anatomic markers, making difficult their identification based on visual inspection of MR images alone. **Fig. 3** shows a case in which anatomic markers have been obscured by tumor, making anatomic prediction of the location of the motor gyrus impossible without a technique such as fMRI.

The face/tongue region of the primary motor gyrus is located on the lateral/inferior aspect of

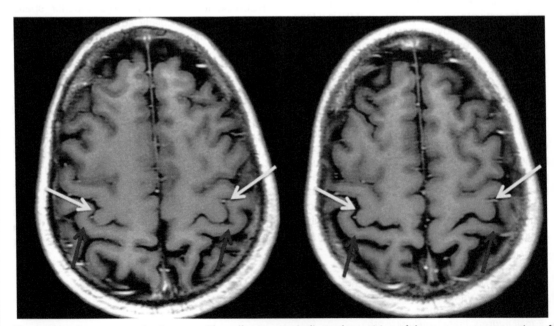

Fig. 1. The primary sensory/motor gyrus: The yellow arrows indicate the position of the reverse omega portion of the primary motor gyrus in the posterior frontal lobe. The red arrows show the position of the sensory gyrus.

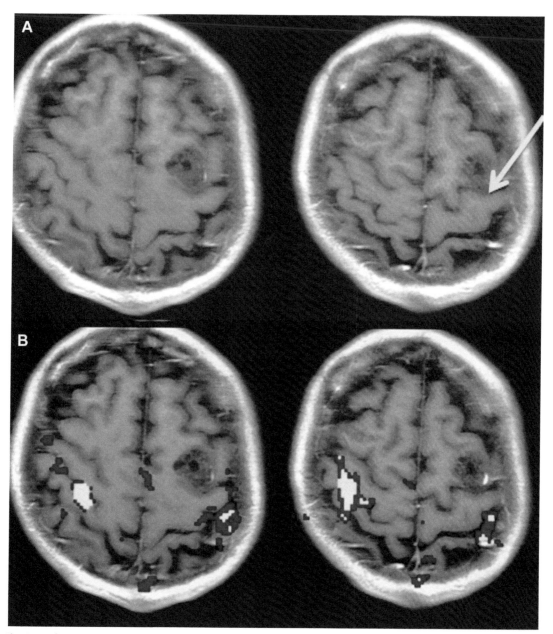

Fig. 2. Ambiguous anatomy. In rare instances the reverse omega (*yellow arrow*) does not indicate the position of the central sulcus. Without fMRI (*A*), this lesion would have been assumed to be in the motor gyrus (*B*).

the motor gyrus. This region is anatomically just posterior to the area of Broca in the inferior frontal gyrus. **Fig. 4** shows an fMRI map of both hand and tongue motor movements acquired simultaneously from an intact patient. Of note, finding the tongue motor region by "pulling down" the sulcus, whereby one first locates the more cephalad component of the central sulcus/reverse omega and follows the sulcus inferiorly, can be misleading and inaccurate. The inferior aspect of the central sulcus moves anteriorly as it is traced inferiorly

and shortens, making precise localization of the inferior aspect of the motor gyrus particularly difficult to be discerned anatomically alone. For this reason, fMRI is particularly useful for localizing the face/lips/tongue portion of the motor gyrus at its inferior aspect.

Another way in which fMRI contributes significantly to motor gyrus localization is in the foot motor region. The foot motor region is located most medially just over the interhemispheric fissure. This region is often localized medial and slightly posterior

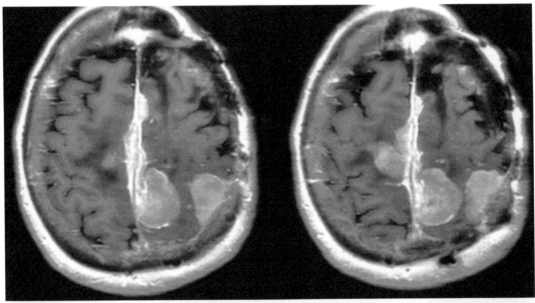

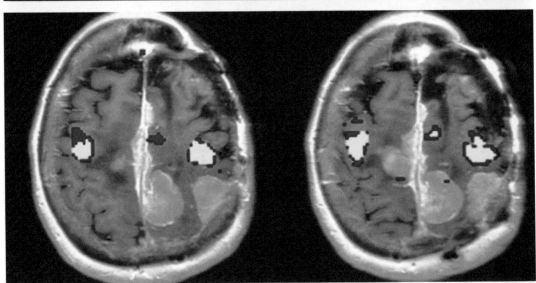

Fig. 3. Where is the motor gyrus? fMRI is particularly useful in cases where tumor has obscured normal anatomy. In this case multiple extra-axial lesions make the motor gyrus localization impossible without a technique such as fMRI.

to the hand motor region in the axial plane (**Fig. 5**). Direct cortical stimulation (the surgeon's intraoperative gold standard for functional mapping) of this region is difficult because the sagittal sinus makes the cortex difficult to access. Therefore, fMRI localization of the foot motor region is valuable for presurgical planning.

fMRI typically maps these 3 main motor areas (foot, hand, and face/tongue) for neurosurgical planning, partly because these 3 areas span the gyrus medially to laterally and partly because tasks involving these areas are easily amenable to functional paradigms.

The primary sensory gyrus (also known as the postcentral gyrus) is located just posterior to the precentral gyrus, from which it is divided by the central sulcus. Like the primary motor gyrus, the organization of the sensory gyrus is also somatotopically organized (see **Fig. 1**).

Secondary Motor Areas

Although the primary motor and sensory areas are the main focus of most neurosurgical planning targets, damage to secondary motor areas also carries a risk of morbidity.[7–10] As a result, their

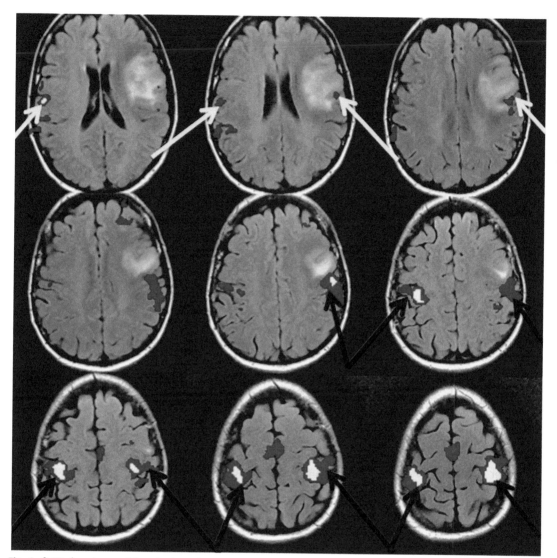

Fig. 4. fMRI showing positions in the primary motor gyrus of the hand (*blue arrows*) and tongue (*yellow arrows*) signals.

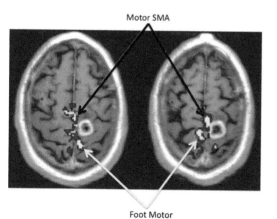

Fig. 5. Foot motor and supplementary motor (SMA) regions of the primary motor gyrus.

precise localization is becoming increasingly important during fMRI examinations. The most common secondary motor areas of interest for neurosurgical planning are the SMA and the premotor area. To study the secondary areas, paradigms often focus on a unilateral volitional movement contrasted with rest.[11]

Supplementary Motor Area

The SMA is located in the superior frontal gyrus just medial to the superior frontal sulcus (**Fig. 6**). Although it is an expansive area with ill-defined anterior borders, the posterior border of the SMA is the foot motor region of the primary motor gyrus. The SMA is made up of an anterior portion (pre-SMA), more active on fMRI during language tasks,

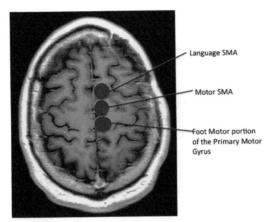

Language SMA

Motor SMA

Foot Motor portion of the Primary Motor Gyrus

Fig. 6. Supplementary motor area (SMA). The SMA is located in the superior frontal gyrus, and is functionally segregated into motor (posterior) and speech (anterior) components.

and a posterior portion, more active on fMRI during motor tasks. The boundary between the pre-SMA and SMA proper has been delineated using a VCA (vertical commissure anterior) line or a line drawn vertically from the AC/PC (anterior/posterior commissure) line.[12]

Recent studies suggest that the motor portion of the SMA is, like the primary motor gyrus, also somatotopically arranged. In lower animals, it has been shown that the hind limb is located in caudal sites, whereas the forelimb and facial movements are closer to the pre-SMA, the more anterior, language-related portion of the SMA, and are thus more rostral.[13–17] Although somatotopic organization is more commonly associated with the primary motor cortex, the 3 main motor areas (hand, foot, and face/tongue) may also be somatotopically mapped along the more rostral axis of the SMA.[18,19]

The SMA is broadly responsible for motor planning and activates temporally before the primary motor gyrus.[20–22] Furthermore, it is active when movements are both internally and externally cued.[20] The SMA is best known for being associated with voluntary movement but will also activate on fMRI during passive tasks.[23] The posterior portion of the SMA is more involved in finger-movement tasks, whereas the anterior part of the SMA is active during cognitive and language processing.[24] A centralized region of the SMA that is active during both language and motor tasks suggests a region that may be essential. Further investigation is needed to determine whether insult to this centralized region carries an increased incidence or degree of postoperative deficit.

More recent work suggests a role for the SMA in cortical compensation. BOLD fMRI can be used

preoperatively to look at the patterns of activation as a tumor invades either the primary motor area or the supplementary motor area.[25] The SMA has been shown to be involved in temporal planning and organization of motor movements before execution, in addition to sequencing multiple movements.[26] Peck and colleagues[25,27] characterized the role of the SMA in patients with high-grade gliomas and their role in cortical reorganization. The study used fMRI to look at the BOLD hemodynamic responses in the primary motor and SMA of tumor patients. Here, block paradigms were used to assess latency differences so that the more sensitive hemodynamic response would be isolated. This work concluded that patients with glial tumors located within the primary motor cortex experienced lesion-induced compensation in the BOLD magnitude and firing pattern in both the primary motor cortex and the SMA. Cortical reorganization was visibly demonstrated, with the SMA's role assuming functions for which the primary motor cortex was likely previously responsible.

WHY FUNCTIONAL MR IMAGING?

fMRI is especially useful for locating the primary sensorimotor cortex if normal sulci and/or gyral patterns are distorted, or in rare cases when reorganization has occurred secondary to an invasive tumor.[28] fMRI, as a preoperative neuroimaging tool to localize the sensory/motor system, is popular for a variety of reasons. This method is minimally invasive and easily repeatable. Moreover, given that patients with brain tumors are often impaired, fMRI of sensorimotor regions can be acquired with a variety of paradigms that are both volitional and passive. Patients undergo preoperative motor mapping for a multitude of reasons; mostly when anatomic landmarks cannot be identified with certainty by traditional anatomic means. fMRI is also being investigated as a tool to predict deficits.[6] Lastly, fMRI can be used to interrogate cortical reorganization in the motor system, the clinical utility of which is still under investigation.[25]

Several studies over the past decade provide evidence for the usefulness of fMRI for preoperative sensorimotor mapping. In a 2007 study by Pujol and colleagues,[29] patients were examined to identify the sensory motor cortex over a 5-year period. Subjects performed a hand-motion paradigm (opening and closing). The fMRI map correctly identified the location of the sensorimotor cortex in 96% of the cases (141 of 147 patients examined). The 4% that could not be identified displayed head motion greater than 2 mm. Although both conventional MR and fMRI were used and compared in this study, fMRI significantly increased the confidence of the identification of motor gyrus.

Studies investigating the outcomes of fMRI for preoperative identification of eloquent areas are ongoing. An important step in this direction was published by Petrella and colleagues,[30] who investigated presurgical fMRI in 39 patients who were candidates for tumor resection. Two paradigms were used to map sensorimotor areas. Treatment plans following inspection of the fMRI results were altered in 49% of patients. In this study, fMRI sufficiently changed treatment options, offering patients who would have otherwise been deemed inoperable the chance for surgical resection. In addition, in 9 patients for whom surgery was not originally offered, 5 were reconsidered for a craniotomy with intraoperative mapping. In cases where the course of treatment continued as planned, fMRI provided the neurosurgeons with further confidence in their surgical decision making. In a 2003 study by Wilkinson and colleagues,[2] preoperative maps created through fMRI data were essential to safe resection by way of allowing for gross total resections and no postoperative deficits in 17 patients mapped with fMRI. Identifying the eloquent areas to prevent damage during tumor removal is of the utmost importance during mapping.[31] Tumors initially believed to be at too high risk for safe resections were now possible to resect because anatomic locations were available through preoperative fMRI. In this study, no patients displayed permanent neurologic damage after surgery.

PARADIGMS

fMRI localization depends on the paradigm used to elicit the activation. In the motor system, these paradigms are relatively straightforward. Common paradigms for the motor area are finger tapping, tongue motion, and foot motion. Finger tapping most commonly involves having patients tap their fingers while in the scanner, while simultaneously avoiding movement of the arms or shoulders. During the tongue-motion paradigm, patients are asked to keep teeth closed to avoid head-motion artifacts and sweep their tongue against the back of their teeth. Motor foot localization consists of repetitive flexion and extension of the toes without moving the ankles. In most cases, small movements of the foot, hand, or tongue provide a significant signal, particularly when head motion is absent.[11]

A variety of ways is used to perform motor paradigms with patients. Some methods are designed to localize the motor gyrus in both hemispheres simultaneously with bilateral finger tapping (to asses motor gyrus displacement), and in some cases patients can be asked to both move their tongue while tapping their fingers to localize both hand and tongue in a single experimental run. Yet another design involves no rest; that is, instead of alternating between a single motor task and rest, patients are instead asked to alternate between finger tapping and tongue motion. In all cases, careful attention should be paid to minimizing head motion. Short scanning time and clear instruction helps to minimize artifacts.

fMRI examinations of motor function, like any fMR examination, can be performed using a block design or an event-related design. In many fMRI examinations there are 2 states that are statistically contrasted in postprocessing analysis. In an event-related design the patient performs one event (eg, a finger tap), which is followed by rest. This type of paradigm allows for detailed estimation of the hemodynamic response.[32] Event-related designs, though possible in patient populations, are arguably preferred in basic science fMRI, as more precise neuroanatomic parameters can be extracted from single events. However, this type of design requires many repetitions because the change from baseline for any one event is small (on the order of about 2%–6%). Accordingly, event-related designs tend to be longer than block designs given the need for many repetitions for adequate statistical power. This approach can be problematic for patients with brain tumors who, in the authors' experience, can have trouble keeping still and following complicated instructions with rapid alternations in task demand.

Block designs, by contrast, average the signal from many of the same types of events over a single epoch.[23] For example, a typical block-designed motor task would have the patient resting for 5 images and finger tapping for 5 images. This alternating cycle of rest and task would repeat 5 or 6 times and last approximately 5 minutes, depending on the time to repeat of the images.[31,33–35] The advantage of the block design is that the task-related images and the rest-related images are signal averaged. Therefore the block design maximizes detection of the signal, whereas the event-related design maximizes estimation of the signal.[32,36] That being said, there is a role for event-related motor paradigms. Marquart and colleagues[37] indicated that for finger-movement tasks whereby head-motion artifacts are less likely to occur, a block trial is preferred because of greater activation seen within the sensorimotor cortex and/or the SMA. However, for toe- and tongue-movement tasks that are more susceptible to movement artifacts, event-related or single-event paradigms adequately localize the foot motor areas.

There are also many special considerations when using fMRI maps for clinical use. For example, in patients with brain tumor it is helpful to have a shorter task or paradigm duration, as patients have a more difficult time than normal controls in keeping their head still. Whereas fMRI data are often acquired using an event-related design in healthy control subjects, patients with brain tumors often benefit from the signal averaging afforded by block designs. Furthermore, areas can be activated that are associated with the task being investigated but are not essential for the task. Of course, this is an important consideration for BOLD fMRI mapping for neurosurgical planning, the goal of which is to isolate essential eloquent areas. That being said, fMRI is commonly used to map eloquent areas presurgically and has been shown to be sufficiently accurate, particularly in motor areas, for neurosurgical planning in a multitude of studies.[2,23]

PARESIS

Paresis or weakness often occurs when the primary motor gyrus is injured or infiltrated by tumor or edema.[5] Paradigms for patients with paresis or weakness should be altered on a case-by-case basis. For example, sequential finger tapping can be modified to hand clenching for patients with partial hand paralysis.[5] In patients with complete paralysis, sensory stimulation of the hand (such as brushing, stroking, or rubbing) often elicits motor activation and sensory activation as a result of significant reciprocity between the sensory motor systems (**Fig. 7**).[5] The same can be done for the face and foot. Instead of asking the patient to move the affected area, the examiner strokes or scrubs the paretic region. Although this fMRI map is biased toward the sensory gyrus, strong motor signals are often still seen.[5,11] Extra caution in interpretation must be exercised when dealing with preoperative scanning of patients with paresis. In the authors' experience scans on paretic patients tend to have more head motion as they struggle to move the affected limb during the fMRI examination.[38]

Artifacts

Artifacts during fMR scans are common in patients with brain tumors.[39] Artifacts can be motion related or can result from anything that disrupts the T2* signal (ie, susceptibility artifact). Motion-related artifacts can be periodic (arising from heartbeat or breathing) or random, as is often the case with head motion. Modern statistical analyses can easily remove periodic artifacts as long as they vary with a frequency different from that of the stimulus presentation. Trend (motion that occurs in a linear fashion) is also fairly straightforward to correct because it looks different from the cycling BOLD signal. Stimulus-correlated motion (eg, nodding the head concurrently while performing a finger-tapping paradigm), however, can look so similar to a real oscillating signal that it can be difficult to remove with standard motion correction algorithms and may, in turn, adversely affect the study. Other artifacts such as signal dropout can be caused by dental work, blood products, hemosiderin from a previous surgery, or infarct, and can also be a source of false-negative function (**Fig. 8**). Dropout artifacts from the air-tissue interface at the base of the brain are also common in the patient population with brain tumors.[23] As a result, T2* source images should be routinely inspected.

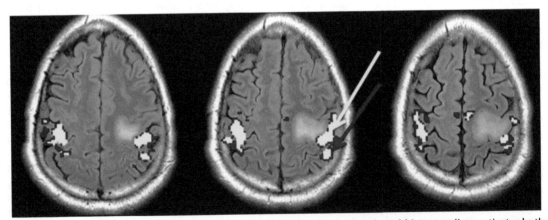

Fig. 7. Sensory fMRI paradigms often activate the motor gyrus. Bilateral hand-scrubbing paradigm activates both primary motor (*yellow arrow*) and sensory motor (*red arrow*).

EFFECT OF TUMOR ON FUNCTIONAL MR IMAGING

Presence of a tumor can affect the BOLD fMRI signal. The BOLD signal depends on a predictable vascular response, which can be affected by a tumor's abnormal neovasculature. The BOLD contrast is a measure of the proportional changes in the amount of oxygenated blood that replaces deoxygenated blood during a task. Tissue that is negative in and around a tumor on fMRI can become active after surgery when mass effect associated with tumor is removed and normal perfusion is restored.[40] This false-negative phenomenon is referred to as tumor-induced neurovascular uncoupling, and was first described by Holodny and colleagues.[41] These investigators showed that the fMRI activation volume on the tumor side of the brain was diminished in relation to the healthy contralateral side. This effect is hypothesized to be caused by a loss of autoregulation in the tumor vasculature. **Fig. 9** shows an example of this commonly seen phenomenon during a finger-tapping fMRI paradigm. The study by Krings and colleagues[42] in 2002 supported the decoupling theory. The patients in this study, suffering from moderate paresis, had tumors affecting the motor cortex and reduced signal magnitude within the primary motor cortex. In cases where patients were completely paretic, the fMRI signal was even further diminished. However, in these patients the signal from the supplementary motor cortex and the contralateral hemisphere increased. This effect is most likely explained by compensation. In Ludemann and colleagues'[43] work the BOLD signal of patients with larger highly vascularized tumors tended to be smaller than the signals of patients with smaller less vascularized gliomas. Lastly, it has been suggested that bilateral motor paradigms be used in fMR preoperative mapping so that the contralateral

hemisphere BOLD activation acts as a control reference.[44] In this way it is easier to make determinations about displaced anatomy and reduced BOLD magnitudes.

The effects of BOLD decoupling on the interpretation of fMRI maps vary. In motor mapping, where the main goal is often localization of a single gyrus, a diminished fMR signal is irrelevant as long as it correctly identifies the gyrus in question. For example, Holodny and colleagues[45] found that there was a significant difference in the volume of activation in the primary motor cortex on the tumor side of the brain versus the nontumor side. This effect was most seen in glioblastoma multiforme. Despite decoupling effects on the BOLD fMRI signal, the motor cortex was still correctly identified. However, caution should still be exercised in the case where tumor and other factors associated with the tumor completely eliminate the fMRI signal, as these maps are at risk of errors in interpretation. Holodny and colleagues[41] have shown that BOLD fMRI activation can be not only diminished but also eliminated.

COMBINATION OF METHODS

A variety of other mapping techniques can be complementary to fMRI for presurgical planning. These techniques vary in aspects such as resolution (both spatial and temporal), or their ability to preferentially localize or lateralize function. The methods also vary in invasiveness. Common methods used in place of or in addition to fMRI are magnetoencephalography (MEG), electroencephalography (EEG), PET, and diffusion tractography (DTI).

Magnetoencephalography

In the 2006 study by Korvenoja and colleagues,[46] both MEG and fMRI were used to locate the primary sensorimotor cortex. Their study showed

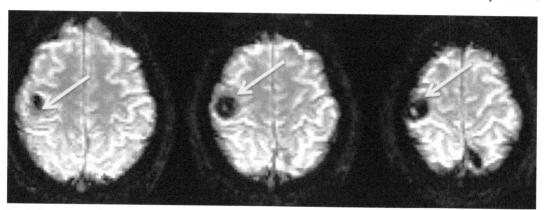

Fig. 8. Dropout artifact. T2* signal loss can cause false-negative determinations of function in fMRI (*arrow*). In this case the artifact was caused by hemorrhage.

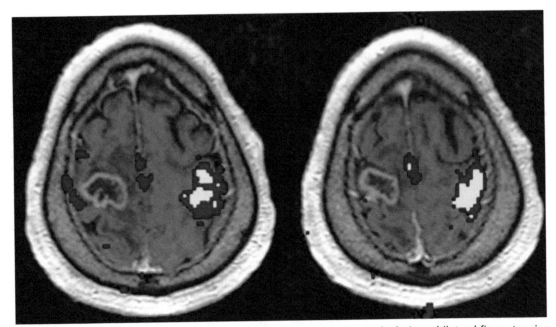

Fig. 9. Diminished BOLD response adjacent to a tumor. fMRI signal magnitude during a bilateral finger-tapping task is diminished adjacent to a glioblastoma multiforme. The exact mechanism that accounts for this phenomenon is unknown, and caution in interpretation should be exercised in and around lesions.

that MEG predicated a more accurate and specific location of the gyrus of interest in comparison with fMRI. In all 15 patients, the localization of the central sulcus with MEG was correct. Because fMRI activation activates the entire network of structures required for a motor task (both essential and secondary areas) it can be difficult to interpret the localization of the motor gyrus where the premotor, primary motor, and sensory gyri may activate on fMRI simultaneously, compromising specificity. This aspect is not an issue with MEG. The spatial resolution for these 2 methods also varies; MEG can achieve 5 mm whereas fMRI can be as low as 1 mm.

Other studies, such as one performed by Kober and colleagues[47] in 2001, indicated comparable identification of the primary motor gyrus using either MEG or fMRI, and thus showed a strong degree of clinical usefulness for identifying the sensory/motor region of the brain. Both of these techniques allow for much more precise preoperative planning for surgery than traditional anatomic MR markers. However, of the two, MR imaging scanners are much more readily available than MEG scanners, and are thus more popular.

Electroencephalography

A method similar to MEG is EEG, which directly measures the cortical electrical activity of the brain through potentials. Both of these techniques have superb temporal resolution. Using somatosensory

evoked potentials (SSEPs) as measured by EEG and fMRI together, the central sulcus is often identified, particularly in the operating room just preceding direct cortical stimulation.[33] However, EEG is a much more invasive methodology than fMRI. Furthermore, owing to their electrical sensitivity SSEPs often fail to identify the rolandic region, making fMRI integration into the neurosurgical navigation system helpful in these cases.[48]

Positron Emission Tomography

PET, a neuroimaging technique described elsewhere in this issue, is a brain-mapping technique that preceded fMRI historically and is based on blood glucose metabolism. When performing a paradigm, the cerebral metabolism is measured and statistical operations similar to those used for fMRI are used to create a map of function.[23] In a 1999 study, Bittar and colleagues[28] showed that there was good concordance between PET and fMRI in regard to locating the primary motor and somatosensory cortex. In their work the distance of peak PET and fMRI activation centroids averaged 7.9 mm (range 1–18 mm; $P > .05$) Unlike PET, fMRI has the added benefit of not requiring an invasive radioactive tracer.

Diffusion Tractography

DTI, an MR method that measures water diffusivity in the brain, is used to map the white matter tracts. This topic also is considered more thoroughly in an article elsewhere in this issue. Combining DTI with gray matter fMRI localizations provides a more complete picture of the functional anatomy around a tumor. Once the precentral gyrus is localized, further consideration is given to the descending white matter tracts.[38,39,49–52] If violated, the corticospinal tract, the major tract leading from the primary motor cortex to the spinal cord, can lead to irreversible paresis.[53] Furthermore, with regard to brain tumors, this combination of fMRI and DTI allows for the presurgical evaluation of the effects of rolandic brain tumors on the pyramidal (corticospinal) tract.[50] fMRI has also been used

to enhance the ability to identify tracts of interest within a brain where deformed anatomy is present by providing a seed point for DTI postprocessing.[53]

INTRAOPERATIVE MAPPING

fMRI is often integrated into the intraoperative mapping environment. **Fig. 10** shows a motor map integrated into the Brainlab Neuronavigation System (Feldkirchen, Germany). Intraoperative direct cortical stimulation is considered the gold standard for functional localization in the operating room. It entails stimulating the exposed cortex with electrical current to localize the motor

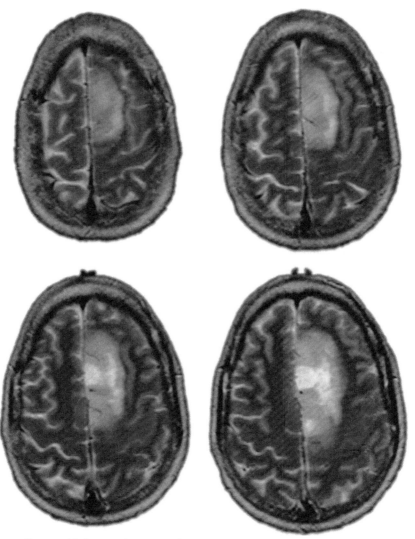

Fig. 10. Intraoperative graphic integrating motor fMRI. A bilateral finger-tapping fMRI paradigm can easily be integrated into a neurosurgical navigation system, and may decrease the time required for invasive mapping procedures. (*Courtesy of* Brainlab, Feldkirchen, Germany; with permission.)

gyrus.[54] It is this gold standard that fMRI and any other functional technique is compared against. BOLD fMRI commonly guides intraoperative mapping. When the motor gyrus is localized using fMRI preoperatively, these maps can guide direct cortical stimulation and save time in assaying the rolandic anatomy in some cases. Furthermore, direct cortical stimulation can only measure the gyral surfaces and does not always elicit a motor response. Therefore, fMRI has been proved valuable and can act as a significant addition to the neuronavigational toolbox.[2,3,55]

Coregistered fMR images can be formatted to a surgical microscope, and functional areas can be projected directly onto the surface of the exposed brain. Krishnan and colleagues[56] used neuronavigation around the motor strip during surgery, superimposing motor localizations for foot, hand, and tongue. Visualizing fiber tracks and connections within the navigational system also helps minimize the risk of iatrogenic injury by acting as a functional reference point during surgery. Intraoperative mapping using direct cortical stimulation has the advantage of assaying cortex essential for a function while fMRI shows all areas, both essential and supportive, for a task.[56]

There are small subsets of centers performing intraoperative BOLD fMRI in surgical units that include an MR scanner. Feigl and colleagues[57] concluded that intraoperative fMR mapping safely guided the neurosurgeons in avoiding damage to functional areas during surgery. Real-time data from a 3-T MR imaging scanner can be used efficiently, especially because no off-line postprocessing is needed. Work done by Nabavi and colleagues[58] yielded similar results. Their study looked at patients undergoing awake craniotomies with cortical stimulation in an MR imaging–assisted operating room. Intraoperative imaging added about 20 to 60 minutes to the procedure, but 94% of the patients in the study stated they would undergo the procedure again if needed.

Real-Time Functional MR Imaging

Real-time fMRI allows live evaluation of brain activation. Trials that are contaminated with head motion can be detected and corrected during the scanning session rather than rendering a study not usable in postprocessing after the scan. More widespread implementation of real-time imaging may shorten procedures and yield a higher proportion of usable fMRI data.[1,59]

SUMMARY AND FUTURE DIRECTIONS

Over the past decade, fMRI has become a common tool for presurgical sensory motor mapping.

fMRI is a significant preoperative asset for tumors located within the central region.[33] Using various motor paradigms, fMRI has significantly improved the neurosurgeon's confidence in functional localization during resection and also has changed surgical options for many patients. This noninvasive tool allows for easy display and integration with other neuroimaging techniques. Although fMRI is a useful preoperative tool, it is not perfect. Tumors that affect the normal vascular coupling of neuronal activity will affect fMRI measurement.

fMRI continues to be developed in novel fields, such as digit mapping, a more specified mapping of the hand motor area. Sanchez-Panchuelo and colleagues[60] used a 7-T scanner to make high-resolution maps of digit representation. Thus, high-field scanners are providing increasing detail of motor representations. Robust maps have been made using high-field magnets showing the thumb (digit 1) as the most inferior and lateral while digits 2 to 5 are represented as increasingly superior. The higher spatial resolution and high-field mapping provides a promising tool for increased precision of the functional organization and specificity of different areas within the central region.

Visual inspection of a patient performing a bilateral finger-tapping paradigm, common in the clinical mapping environment, does not allow for an accurate correlation between a precise task and the BOLD fMRI response, a particular issue when analyzing the effects of tumor on the motor gyrus. fMRI maps can be difficult to interpret in the context of increased or decreased magnitude and the pattern of activation. Some groups have tried to enhance interpretative power in these cases by developing MR-compatible devices that measure finger kinematics. For example, Schaechter and colleagues[61] developed a system to measure angular velocity from each of the 10 digits while performing a motor task. In this way, more inferences can be drawn about the differences between tumor-infiltrated motor gyri and normal patterns of hand motor activation.

fMRI continues to make strides in preoperative neurosurgical planning.

REFERENCES

1. Decharms RC. Applications of real-time fMRI. Nat Rev Neurosci 2008;9(9):720–9.
2. Wilkinson ID, Romanowski CA, Jellinek DA, et al. Motor functional MRI for pre-operative and intraoperative neurosurgical guidance. Br J Radiol 2003;76(902):98–103.
3. Paleologos TS, Wadley JP, Kitchen ND, et al. Clinical utility and cost-effectiveness of interactive image-guided craniotomy: clinical comparison between

conventional and image-guided meningioma surgery. Neurosurgery 2000;47(1):40–7 [discussion: 47–8].

4. Kasahara M, Menon DK, Salmond CH, et al. Altered functional connectivity in the motor network after traumatic brain injury. Neurology 2010;75(2): 168–76.

5. Tieleman A, Deblaere K, Van Roost D, et al. Preoperative fMRI in tumour surgery. Eur Radiol 2009; 19(10):2523–34.

6. Stippich C, Blatow M. Clinical functional MRI: presurgical functional neuroimaging. Berlin; New York: Springer; 2007.

7. Zentner J, Hufnagel A, Pechstein U, et al. Functional results after resective procedures involving the supplementary motor area. J Neurosurg 1996; 85(4):542–9.

8. Fontaine D, Capelle L, Duffau H. Somatotopy of the supplementary motor area: evidence from correlation of the extent of surgical resection with the clinical patterns of deficit. Neurosurgery 2002;50(2): 297–303 [discussion: 303–5].

9. Krainik A, Lehericy S, Duffau H, et al. Postoperative speech disorder after medial frontal surgery: role of the supplementary motor area. Neurology 2003; 60(4):587–94.

10. Bannur U, Rajshekhar V. Post operative supplementary motor area syndrome: clinical features and outcome. Br J Neurosurg 2000;14(3):204–10.

11. Brennan NP. Preparing the patient for the fMRI study and optimization of paradigm selection and delivery. In: Holodny AI, editor. Functional neuroimaging. New York: Informia Healthcare; 2008. p. 13–21.

12. Dassonville P, Zhu XH, Ugurbil K, et al. Functional activation in motor cortex reflects the direction and the degree of handedness. Proc Natl Acad Sci U S A 1997;94:14015–8 [Erratum appears in Proc Natl Acad Sci U S A 1998;95(19): 11499].

13. Matsuzaka Y, Aizawa H, Tanji J. A motor area rostral to the supplementary motor area (presupplementary motor area) in the monkey: neuronal activity during a learned motor task. J Neurophysiol 1992;68(3):653–62.

14. Luppino GM, Matelli M, Camarda RM, et al. Multiple representations of body movements in mesial area 6 and the adjacent cingulate cortex: an intracortical microstimulation study in the macaque monkey. J Comp Neurol 1991;311(4):463–82.

15. Fried I, Katz A, McCarthy G, et al. Functional organization of human supplementary motor cortex studied by electrical stimulation. J Neurosci 1991; 11(11):3656–66.

16. Mitz AR, Wise SP. The somatotopic organization of the supplementary motor area: intracortical microstimulation mapping. J Neurosci 1987;7(4): 1010–21.

17. Arienzo D, Babiloni C, Ferretti A, et al. Somatotopy of anterior cingulate cortex (ACC) and supplementary motor area (SMA) for electric stimulation of the median and tibial nerves: an fMRI study. Neuroimage 2006;33(2):700–5.

18. Chainay H, Krainik A, Tanguy ML, et al. Foot, face and hand representation in the human supplementary motor area. Neuroreport 2004;15(5):765–9.

19. Rijntjes M, Dettmers C, Buchel C, et al. A blueprint for movement: functional and anatomical representations in the human motor system. J Neurosci 1999;19(18):8043–8.

20. Nachev P, Kennard C, Husain M. Functional role of the supplementary and pre-supplementary motor areas. Nat Rev Neurosci 2008;9(11):856–69.

21. Tanji J, Kurata K. Comparison of movement-related activity in 2 cortical motor areas of primates. J Neurophysiol 1982;48(3):633–53.

22. Brinkman C, Porter R. Supplementary motor area in the monkey - activity of neurons during performance of a learned motor task. J Neurophysiol 1979;42(3):681–709.

23. Tharin S, Golby A. Functional brain mapping and its applications to neurosurgery. Neurosurgery 2007;60(4):185–201.

24. VanOostende S, VanHecke P, Sunaert S, et al. FMRI studies of the supplementary motor area and the premotor cortex. Neuroimage 1997;6(3): 181–90.

25. Peck KK, Bradbury M, Hou BL, et al. The role of the supplementary motor area (SMA) in the execution of primary motor activities in brain tumor patients: functional MRI detection of time-resolved differences in the hemodynamic response. Med Sci Monit 2009;15(4):Mt55–62.

26. Tanji J. The supplementary motor area in the cerebral-cortex. Neurosci Res 1994;19(3):251–68.

27. Peck KK, Bradbury M, Psaty EL, et al. Joint activation of the supplementary motor area and presupplementary motor area during simultaneous motor and language functional MRI. Neuroreport 2009;20(5):487–91.

28. Bittar RG, Olivier A, Sadikot AF, et al. Presurgical motor and somatosensory cortex mapping with functional magnetic resonance imaging and positron emission tomography. J Neurosurg 1999; 91(6):915–21.

29. Pujol J, Deus J, Acebes JJ, et al. Identification of the sensorimotor cortex with functional MRI: frequency and actual contribution in a neurosurgical context. J Neuroimaging 2008;18(1):28–33.

30. Petrella JR, Shah LM, Harris KM, et al. Preoperative functional MR imaging localization of language and motor areas: effect on therapeutic decision making in patients with potentially resectable brain tumors. Radiology 2006;240(3): 793–802.

31. Kim PE, Singh M. Functional magnetic resonance imaging for brain mapping in neurosurgery. Neurosurg Focus 2003;15(1):E1.

32. Birn RM, Cox RW, Bandettini PA. Detection versus estimation in event-related fMRI: choosing the optimal stimulus timing. Neuroimage 2002;15(1): 252–64.

33. Rombouts SA, Barkhof F, Scheltens P. Clinical applications of functional brain MRI. Oxford (United Kingdom): Oxford University Press; 2007.

34. Zarahn E, Aguirre G, Desposito M. A trial-based experimental design for fMRI. Neuroimage 1997; 6(2):122–38.

35. Aguirre G, D'Esposito M. Experimental design for brain fMRI. In: Moonen CT, Bandettini PA, editors. Functional MRI. Berlin: Springer; 2000. p. 369–80.

36. Liu TT, Frank LR, Wong EC, et al. Detection power, estimation efficiency, and predictability in event-related fMRI. Neuroimage 2001;13(4):759–73.

37. Marquart M, Birn R, Haughton V. Single- and multiple-event paradigms for identification of motor cortex activation. AJNR Am J Neuroradiol 2000; 21(1):94–8.

38. Stippich C. Presurgical functional magnetic resonance imaging (fMRI). Clin Neuroradiol 2007;2: 69–87.

39. Krings T, Reinges MH, Erberich S, et al. Functional MRI for presurgical planning: problems, artefacts, and solution strategies. J Neurol Neurosurg Psychiatry 2001;70(6):749–60.

40. Roux FE, Boulanouar K, Ibarrola D, et al. Functional MRI and intraoperative brain mapping to evaluate brain plasticity in patients with brain tumours and hemiparesis. J Neurol Neurosurg Psychiatry 2000; 69(4):453–63.

41. Holodny AI, Schulder M, Liu WC, et al. Decreased BOLD functional MR activation of the motor and sensory cortices adjacent to a glioblastoma multiforme: implications for image-guided neurosurgery. AJNR Am J Neuroradiol 1999;20(4):609–12.

42. Krings T, Topper R, Willmes K, et al. Activation in primary and secondary motor areas in patients with CNS neoplasms and weakness. Neurology 2002;58(3):381–90.

43. Lüdemann L, Förschler A, Grieger W, et al. BOLD signal in the motor cortex shows a correlation with the blood volume of brain tumors. J Magn Reson Imaging 2006;23(4):435–43.

44. Schreiber A, Hubbe U, Ziyeh S, et al. The influence of gliomas and nonglial space-occupying lesions on blood-oxygen-level-dependent contrast enhancement. AJNR Am J Neuroradiol 2000;21: 1055–63.

45. Holodny AI, Schulder M, Liu WC, et al. The effect of brain tumors on BOLD functional MR imaging activation in the adjacent motor cortex: implications for

image-guided neurosurgery. AJNR Am J Neuroradiol 2000;21(8):1415–22.

46. Korvenoja A, Kirveskari E, Aronen HJ, et al. Sensorimotor cortex localization: comparison of magnetoencephalography, functional MR imaging, and intraoperative cortical mapping. Radiology 2006; 241(1):213–22.

47. Kober H, Nimsky C, Moller M, et al. Correlation of sensorimotor activation with functional magnetic resonance imaging and magnetoencephalography in presurgical functional imaging: a spatial analysis. Neuroimage 2001;14(5):1214–28.

48. Petrovich N, Holodny AI, Tabar V, et al. Discordance between functional magnetic resonance imaging during silent speech tasks and intraoperative speech arrest. J Neurosurg 2005;103(2):267–74.

49. Parmar H, Sitoh YY, Yeo TT. Combined magnetic resonance tractography and functional magnetic resonance imaging in evaluation of brain tumors involving the motor system. J Comput Assist Tomogr 2004;28(4):551–6.

50. Stippich C, Kress B, Ochmann H, et al. Preoperative functional magnetic resonance tomography (FMRI) in patients with rolandic brain tumors: indication, investigation strategy, possibilities and limitations of clinical application. Rofo 2003; 175(8):1042–50 [in German].

51. Ulmer JL, Salvan CV, Mueller WM, et al. The role of diffusion tensor imaging in establishing the proximity of tumor borders to functional brain systems: implications for preoperative risk assessments and postoperative outcomes. Technol Cancer Res Treat 2004;3(6):567–76.

52. Holodny AI, Schwartz TH, Ollenschleger M, et al. Tumor involvement of the corticospinal tract: diffusion magnetic resonance tractography with intraoperative correlation - case illustration. J Neurosurg 2001;95(6):1082.

53. Schonberg T, Pianka P, Hendler T, et al. Characterization of displaced white matter by brain tumors using combined DTI and fMRI. Neuroimage 2006; 30(4):1100–11.

54. Xie J, Chen XZ, Jiang T, et al. Preoperative blood oxygen level-dependent functional magnetic resonance imaging in patients with gliomas involving the motor cortical areas. Chin Med J (Engl) 2008; 121(7):631–5.

55. Gasser T, Ganslandt O, Sandalcioglu E, et al. Intraoperative functional MRI: implementation and preliminary experience. Neuroimage 2005;26(3):685–93.

56. Krishnan R, Raabe A, Hattingen E, et al. Functional magnetic resonance imaging integrated neuronavigation: correlation between lesion-to-motor cortex distance and outcome. Neurosurgery 2004;55(4): 904–14.

57. Feigl GC, Safavi-Abbasi S, Gharabaghi A, et al. Real-time 3 T fMRI data of brain tumour

patients for intra-operative localization of primary motor areas. Eur J Surg Oncol 2008; 34(6):708–15.

58. Nabavi A, Dörner L, Stark AM, et al. Intraoperative MRI with 1.5 Tesla in neurosurgery. Neurosurg Clin N Am 2009;20(2):163–71.

59. Schwindack C, Siminotto E, Meyer M, et al. Real-time functional magnetic resonance imaging (rt-fMRI) in patients with brain tumours: preliminary findings using motor and language paradigms. Br J Neurosurg 2005;19(1):25–32.

60. Sanchez-Panchuelo RM, Francis S, Bowtell R, et al. Mapping human somatosensory cortex in individual subjects with 7T functional MRI. J Neurophysiol 2010;103(5):2544–56.

61. Schaechter JD, Stokes C, Connell BD, et al. Finger motion sensors for fMRI motor studies. Neuro-image 2006;31(4):1549–59.

Visual Mapping Using Blood Oxygen Level Dependent Functional Magnetic Resonance Imaging

Edgar A. DeYoe, PhD[a],*, Ryan V. Raut[b]

KEYWORDS

- Human • Functional MR imaging • Brain mapping • Visual cortex • Cancer
- Arteriovenous malformation • Epilepsy

KEY POINTS

- Functional MR (fMR) can be used to map the visual cortex and identify healthy brain tissue near a site of operable brain abnormality.
- fMR mapping using an advanced stimulus/task paradigm permits identification of brain subregions supporting central vision that is critical for reading and other visual functions.
- Novel functional field map (FFMap) displays permit instant appreciation of the behavioral relevance of visual cortex activation, especially with respect to existing and treatment-induced visual field deficits.
- Neurovascular uncoupling (NVU) can complicate the interpretation of fMRI data, but this can be ameliorated by use of new methods to detect and map NVU.
- Resting-state fMRI can be used to map the visual cortex in patients who are behaviorally compromised.

INTRODUCTION

Being the most essential of our senses, the intricacy and brilliance of vision are perhaps most appreciated when compromised by damage or disease. Although a comprehensive account of the processes by which quanta of light falling on the retinae are translated into subjective visual experience is lacking, recent advances, particularly from functional neuroimaging, have allowed researchers to sketch out the functional organization of the human visual system, and thus provide a framework for understanding the sensory and perceptual effects of central vision pathology. For instance, it is now known that vision-related cortex, once thought to reside primarily in the calcarine fissure of the occipital lobe, extends throughout the entire lobe and into adjoining portions of the temporal and parietal lobes (Fig. 1) and even to remote locations in the frontal lobes.[1–4] Though highly interconnected, this extensive network can be subdivided into more than a dozen functionally distinct visual areas which, if selectively damaged, can result in deficits ranging from simple scotomata (localized regions of blindness) to complex agnosias and higher-order perceptual deficiencies.[5–12] For the clinician, staying abreast of all these developments can be daunting and of questionable therapeutic value given their limited ability to "cure" central nervous system damage. However, there are clinical applications, such as the guidance of neurosurgery and the documentation of disease progression, for which detailed assessment of visual system involvement may be warranted to avoid potentially

---

[a] Department of Radiology, Medical College of Wisconsin, 8701 Watertown Plank Road, Milwaukee, WI 53226, USA; [b] Department of Radiology, University of Wisconsin-Madison, Madison, WI 53792, USA
* Corresponding author.
E-mail address: deyoe@mcw.edu

Neuroimag Clin N Am 24 (2014) 573–584
http://dx.doi.org/10.1016/j.nic.2014.08.001
1052-5149/14/$ – see front matter © 2014 Elsevier Inc. All rights reserved

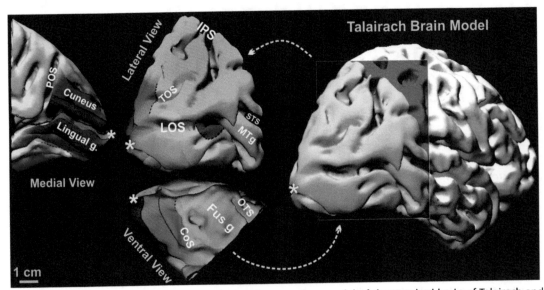

Fig. 1. Subdivisions of human visual cortex displayed on a surface model of the standard brain of Talairach and Tournoux.[59] Whole brain at right shows plane used to create a separate occipital lobe model. Yellow asterisks mark the tip of the occipital pole. Colored patches on occipital models mark the approximate locations of functionally distinct visual areas. (*Medial view*) Pink with yellow asterisk: primary visual cortex, V1, which is flanked above and below by purple V2. Magenta (cuneus): dorsal division of V3. (*Ventral view*) Blue-gray: ventral division of V3. Dark blue: V4. Light blue: ventral occipital complex.[3] Dark green: fusiform face area.[60] (*Lateral view*) Red in LOS-TOS complex.[3] Yellow: lateral occipital complex.[61,62] CoS, collateral sulcus; Fus g, fusiform gyrus; IPS, intraparietal sulcus; LOS, lateral occipital sulcus; MTg, middle temporal gyrus; OTS, occipitotemporal sulcus; POS, parietal occipital sulcus; STS, superior temporal sulcus; TOS, transverse occipital sulcus.

debilitating vision deficits. Accordingly, this article outlines some of the more clinically relevant tools developed in the last decade for mapping the human visual system, and highlights key interpretational issues and future trends.

From a clinical applications perspective, it is noteworthy that some of the earliest accounts of vision loss attributable to brain damage noted the relationship between the anatomic site of damage and the location and severity of a visual scotoma within the patient's field of view.[13–19] This perspective is reiterated today in the use of functional magnetic resonance imaging (fMRI) to provide retinotopic maps of the visual cortex potentially at risk from invasive surgical and radiation treatment of nearby brain tumors, arteriovenous malformations, or epileptic foci. fMRI is used to map eloquent neural responses evoked by sensory, motor, or cognitive tasks by measuring localized changes in the oxygenation of blood hemoglobin that are triggered by focal changes in neural activity. Although fMRI is, therefore, an indirect measure of neuronal function, it is noninvasive, well tolerated by patients, rapidly acquired in as little as 20 minutes, and can provide extensive maps of eloquent brain tissue that, if damaged, could result in a posttreatment visual deficit.

VISUAL MAPPING PARADIGM AND ANALYSIS

Early approaches to mapping human visual cortex were as simple as turning the lights on and off, or flashing a large checkerboard. Although such stimuli can evoke activation of the visual cortex, the resulting fMRI maps do not reveal even the most rudimentary features of functional organization such as the distinction between the cortical representations of peripheral versus central vision, the latter being particularly critical for many day-to-day visual tasks such as reading. Today, more comprehensive and informative approaches are available. (For detailed reviews of methodology and the functional organization of the visual cortex, see Gill and colleagues[20] and DeYoe and colleagues[21]). Mapping of visual field eccentricity and angular position using fMRI scans of approximately 4 minutes each can yield more informative cortical maps that delineate multiple, functionally distinct, visual areas and differentiate subregions supporting central versus peripheral vision. This mapping can be done efficiently through sequential display of a slowly expanding checkered annulus and a slowly rotating checkered wedge, respectively (**Fig. 2**). The checkerboard patterns are composed of high-contrast, black and white checks that counterphase flicker at 8 Hz, resulting

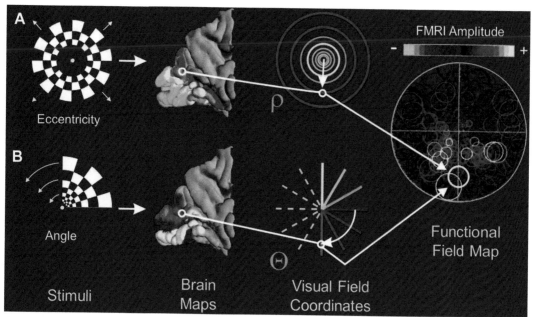

Fig. 2. Stimuli for visual field mapping and construction of Functional Field Maps (FFMaps). Retinotopic mapping stimuli consist of an expanding, black and white, checkered annulus (*A*) or a rotating wedge (*B*) counterphase flickered at 8 Hz presented in a temporal phase-mapping paradigm. A single expansion/rotation sequence takes 32 seconds and is repeated 5 times within a 168-second scan run. (The initial 8 seconds of the scan containing the equilibration transient are discarded.) Outer radius of visual display extends to 20° eccentricity. Expanding annuli are not scaled linearly in size and eccentricity, but rather are scaled nonlinearly so as to activate roughly equal areas of V1 as estimated using the retinocortical mapping function of Balasubramanian and colleagues.[63] The subject's task during each mapping sequence is to fixate a small dot at the center of the display and press a button when the dot blinks off for 0.125 second varied randomly every 4 to 8 seconds. This task helps ensure that the patient attends to the mapping stimulus and maintains the gaze at the center of the display. Postprocessing of the resulting fMRI data yield an estimate of the visual field coordinates (eccentricity [*rho*], angle [*theta*]), at which the mapping stimuli activate each voxel most strongly. Using these coordinates, a circle symbol can be placed at the corresponding location on a diagram of the patient's view of the stimulus display (*right*). The symbol is colored to show the amplitude of the fMRI response according to the pseudocolor scale above. The size of the symbol represents the error in estimating the preferred stimulus location for that voxel (approximately 70% confidence interval). Symbols for all visually responsive voxels are placed on the diagram to yield an FFMap that allows the physician to determine instantly if the patient's visual cortex is responding to all locations within his or her field of view.

in strong neural activation and, subsequently, relatively large increases in the blood oxygen level dependent (BOLD) fMRI signal in visually responsive brain areas. The stimuli are presented in a temporal phase mapping sequence, meaning that locations in the visual field differing in eccentricity (distance from center of gaze) or angular (clock) position are stimulated at different times (temporal phases). Consequently, this approach uses the timing of the fMRI response to identify the location in the patient's visual field that most strongly activates each responsive brain voxel when stimulated. Although this stimulus sequence can be viewed passively with good results, the patient can be asked to watch a small marker at the center of the video display and press a button whenever the marker briefly disappears at random intervals.

The button task is advantageous in that it provides independent verification that the patient is viewing the display throughout the fMRI scan, and documents that the patient is paying attention to the stimulus. Moreover, actively attending to the visual stimulus can significantly enhance the brain response in both primary and later stage (extrastriate) visual areas. Complementary information garnered by using both the annulus and wedge stimuli yields detailed retinotopic maps of the visual cortex in addition to any focal defects resulting from abnormality.

Together, the eccentricity and angular mapping data can be used to generate a novel Functional Field Map (FFMap), which displays the brain activation in the form of a map of the patient's visual field (see **Fig. 2**). Each circle symbol in the FFMap corresponds to a visually responsive voxel in the cortex, its position determined by the eccentricity and angle of the ring and wedge stimuli to which the voxel has responded most strongly. The color of each circle indicates the strength of the fMRI response while the size represents an estimate of the error in measuring the preferred stimulus position. For a healthy individual, the FFMap will contain circle symbols distributed throughout the visual field. However, if the visual cortex is focally damaged, symbols will be missing or less numerous within the retinotopic zone of the visual field affected by the disorder, as illustrated in **Fig. 3**, which shows the FFMap from a patient with an upper left quadrant scotoma (indicated by the black area in the underlying Humphrey visual perimetry map). In sum, the FFMap provides a unique display that can instantly reveal the relationship between a cortical pattern of focal pathologic disorder and its effects on the patient's vision.

CLINICAL APPLICATION

In general, the primary clinical application of fMRI vision mapping has been for presurgical planning in patients with pathologic abnormality or potential surgical involvement of the visual pathways. When resection is necessary, neurosurgeons are able to use knowledge gained from the fMRI maps to help plan an optimal approach and extent of resection that maximizes therapeutic value, yet avoids damage to neighboring eloquent cortex that may be critical for daily visual functions. Although aggressive resection of a tumor can significantly improve long-term outcome, potentially debilitating postoperative deficits can arise if neighboring eloquent cortex is damaged.[22–24] Identification of eloquent brain tissue using intraoperative cortical stimulation (ICS) has traditionally been the method of choice for neurosurgeons. Consequently, several studies have compared task-based fMR (tbfMR) imaging activation with ICS maps to help establish the validity of fMRI for presurgical planning. (For reviews see Sunaert,[24] Dimou and colleagues,[25] and Giussani and colleagues[26]). fMRI maps of sensorimotor areas are generally in good agreement with ICS, although results have been more variable in language areas, possibly because of higher variation in the behavioral task activation and the more diffuse anatomy of language networks. Nevertheless, fMRI has been widely implemented for presurgical mapping of both sensorimotor and language areas. Studies comparing fMRI and ICS maps in the visual cortex have also reported good correspondence.[27,28] However, for a variety of reasons fMRI vision

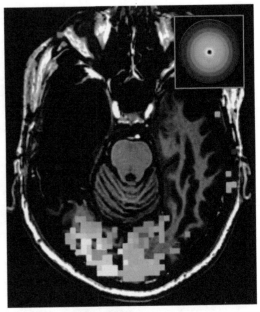

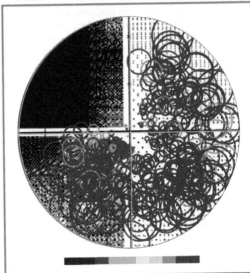

Fig. 3. fMRI mapping of visual field eccentricity in an epileptic patient whose right anterior temporal lobe (*left side of upper panel*) was previously resected to remove epileptogenic tissue in that region. (*Upper*) Axial view. fMRI activation (*small squares*) is colored according to the eccentricity of the stimulus (cf **Fig. 2**) that maximally activated each voxel. Color code is shown by inset at upper right. (*Lower*) FFMap showing robust fMRI activation (*red-orange circles*) associated with portions of the visual field having normal visual sensitivity as indicated by light stippling in the Humphrey perimetry chart shown in the background. Note the lack of fMRI response in the blind upper left quadrant extending into peripheral lower left quadrant. FFMap color scale shows relative amplitude of fMRI activation.

mapping has not been used as widely in the clinic despite its potential utility (see DeYoe and colleagues[21]).

As the clinical use of fMRI grows, reliance on visual mapping paradigms optimized for clinical rather than research applications will also become increasingly important. Such optimization includes use of visual stimuli extending out to visual field eccentricities of 10° to 20° or more to obtain reasonably complete retinotopic maps. Use of time-efficient paradigms such as temporal phase mapping can reduce scanning time, which promotes patient compliance and permits acquisition of additional scan paradigms such as diffusion tensor imaging to map white matter tracts, and breath-hold cerebrovascular reactivity to detect hemodynamic abnormality (see the section on NVU). As already mentioned, use of a button-press task is highly recommended because it helps the physician to distinguish fMRI signals that are compromised by brain abnormality from signals compromised by poor patient compliance, sedation, or other nonspecific effects. Even so, fMR vision mapping under passive viewing conditions can successfully reveal fMRI activation when other task paradigms fail. Finally, fMR visual field mapping and the FFMap display technology have been shown to yield diagnostic information that can help to differentiate an apparent sensory deficit from higher-order perceptual problems such as hemispatial neglect.[21]

RESTING-STATE FUNCTIONAL MR IMAGING OF THE VISUAL CORTEX

Despite the widespread availability of fMRI, behavioral task requirements can limit the number of patients for whom it can be used successfully. Patients who are behaviorally or cognitively impaired and young children who may struggle with performing a specific task or adhering to instructions can be excluded.[29] To circumvent this limitation, resting-state fMR (rsfMR) imaging provides a potential alternative to tbfMR imaging for clinical brain mapping. rsfMR imaging can reveal functional organization through the analysis of intrinsic BOLD signals that are temporally correlated within, but not between, functional subsystems.[30-32] The technique has been used in a wide variety of studies since 1995, when Biswal and colleagues[30] reported its usefulness for mapping "functional connectivity" in subjects who simply rest quietly with eyes open or closed during an otherwise conventional fMRI scan. Moreover, several studies have shown that the visual cortex can be selectively mapped using rsfMR imaging.[33-35]

At the time of writing, the validity of rsfMR imaging for clinical presurgical mapping, and mapping of the visual cortex in particular, has yet to be fully established. A handful of preliminary studies have compared rsfMR imaging maps in tumor patients with tbfMR imaging and sometimes with ICS.[36-41] The results of these studies have suggested that rsfMR imaging maps can indeed provide useful information for presurgical planning. So far, however, validity assessments of rsfMR imaging for clinical brain mapping have focused almost exclusively on the sensorimotor cortex. As mentioned earlier, tbfMR imaging vision mapping and ICS mapping of the visual cortex show good concordance, suggesting that this is also likely to be true for rsfMR imaging mapping. In this context, it is noteworthy that the visual cortex may provide an ideal "test bed" for such validity assessments. Like sensorimotor cortex, the visual cortex is functionally and anatomically well defined. However, the visual cortex can be mapped with tbfMR imaging using a passive viewing task, which may minimize behavioral sources of variation and thus maximize the likelihood of obtaining concordance with rsfMR imaging maps.

In a preliminary comparison of rsfMR and tbfMR imaging in the visual cortex of both tumor patients and healthy individuals, the authors found the that the 2 paradigms generate similar activation maps (**Fig. 4**B, C). Indeed a subsequent analysis showed that the pattern of rsfMR imaging activation can be used as a predictor of the presence of tbfMR imaging activation on a voxel-by-voxel basis. **Fig. 4**D shows the color-coded comparison for each voxel within an occipital region of interest (see **Fig. 4**A). Exact matches are indicated by green colors (true-positive and true-negative predictions), whereas mismatches are shown in contrasting orange and red colors (false-positive and false-negative predictions). The results suggest that rsfMR imaging may provide more complete maps that include voxels representing portions of the visual field at eccentricities beyond the outer limits of the video stimulus display, or hidden by the fixation marker at the center of the display (orange colors in **Fig. 4**D). Overall, this type of analysis indicates that, as an indicator of BOLD activation, rsfMR imaging is at least as valid or better than tbfMR imaging for 80% of voxels.

Although these results are encouraging, it is likely premature to treat rsfMR imaging as a replacement for tbfMR imaging in presurgical planning. More likely, rsfMR imaging can be used as an adjunct to tbfMR imaging under select conditions in which a task-based paradigm is impractical. One example of this potential is illustrated in

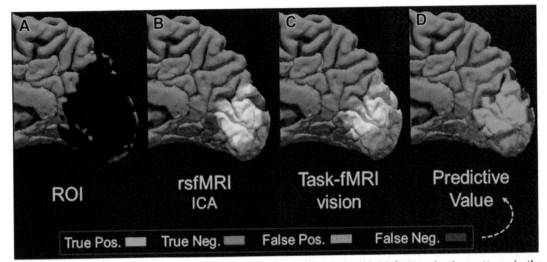

Fig. 4. Quantitative comparison of resting-state (rs) (*B*) and task-based (tb) (*C*) fMRI activation patterns in the medial occipital cortex. (*A*) Region of interest in which the presence/absence of statistically significant fMRI activation was compared on a voxel-by-voxel basis. For each voxel, the status of rsfMR imaging was taken as a predictor of the status of tbfMR imaging activation. Matched activation status is colored light green (true positive) or dark green (true negative) in (*D*). Mismatched activation status is colored orange (false positive) or red (false negative). Note the presence of a significant zone of orange, indicating that resting-state activation may engage portions of the visual cortex that are not stimulated by the limited extent of the task-based visual stimuli (see text).

Fig. 5. rsfMR imaging was used to map the visual cortex in a patient who had recently been rendered blind by a midbrain tumor causing increased intracranial cerebrospinal fluid pressure and subsequent dysfunction of visual afferent pathways (eg, optic radiations: note distended ventricles in left 2 columns of **Fig. 5**). Although tbfMR vision mapping was obviously impossible for this patient, the authors were able to use rsfMR imaging to demonstrate that cortical components of the visual system were still functionally connected in an apparently normal manner, consistent with the pattern observed in a healthy volunteer (center 2 columns) using identical methods and with atlas components from the 100 Connectomes database[42] (right 2 columns).

At present, widespread acceptance of rsfMR imaging as a clinical tool is hampered by a lack of consensus regarding the preferred method of data analysis. In particular, both seed-based and independent component analysis (ICA)[43] have been widely used for rsfMR imaging data, although both have limitations for clinical use. ICA yields multiple networks that are not necessarily mutually exclusive or wholly consistent across patients and that can split conventional networks, such as the visual system, into multiple subcomponents (cf **Fig. 5**). The resulting ICA components must be either manually identified based on expert knowledge (a prohibitively time-consuming process) or autoclassified by computational comparison with

an atlas such as the 1000 Connectomes,[42] Human Connectome,[44] or other published data.[45] Seed-based analyses can suffer from many of the same weaknesses, but offer the advantage that the functional connectivity of individual voxels or zones bordering a planned resection can be selectively visualized. However, the resulting connectivity pattern may or may not correspond to a network whose brain function, and hence its clinical importance, is easily identified. Additional analytical tools based on graph theory hold promise for identifying critical brain sites that, if damaged, may produce debilitating functional deficits because of their widespread connectivity.[46,47] At present, however, the reliability and validity of such analyses across patients having variable brain abnormality has yet to be established. Even seemingly rudimentary issues such as the most appropriate setting of the statistical threshold for differentiating valid rsfMR imaging signals from noise have yet to be fully explored in a clinical context (though this is also true for tbfMR imaging). This issue is particularly problematic for the analysis of data from single subjects or patients.[40,48–51] Despite these issues, rsfMR imaging offers potentially overriding advantages for clinical use, including the simplicity and brevity of data acquisition combined with comprehensive coverage of key functional networks for virtually any patient capable of resting quietly in an MR imaging scanner.

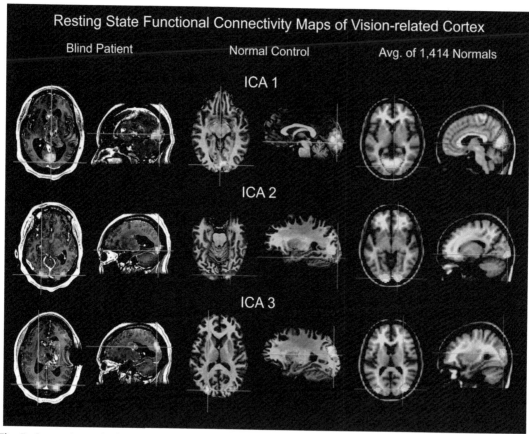

Fig. 5. Comparison of rsfMR imaging brain maps for a recently blind patient (*left 2 columns*), a single healthy control (*middle 2 columns*), and the average of more than 1400 subjects taken from the 1000 Connectomes database.[42] This example demonstrates the viability of using rsfMR imaging as an alternative to tbfMR imaging with patients for whom a task (eg, viewing a visual stimulus) may be impractical or impossible. (*Data from* Biswal BB, Mennes M, Zuo XN, et al. Toward discovery science of human brain function. Proc Natl Acad Sci U S A 2010;107:4734–9.)

NEUROVASCULAR UNCOUPLING IN THE VISUAL CORTEX

An important consideration for the clinical interpretation of both tbfMR and rsfMR imaging data is that they both are indirect measures of neural activity/connectivity. As outlined in **Fig. 6** excerpted from Attwell and colleagues,[52] the BOLD fMRI signal arises from a cascade of cellular and chemical events that link neural activity to local changes in cerebral blood flow, volume, and oxygenation,[52–54] which together alter the relative volume of oxygenated to deoxygenated hemoglobin contained in each imaging voxel. Typically, as neural activity within a voxel increases the proportion of oxygenated hemoglobin also rises, thereby reducing local magnetic field distortion which, in turn, allows water protons to emit a stronger, more coherent magnetic resonance signal. However, focal brain disorder can directly disrupt this hemodynamic cascade without grossly affecting the underlying neural activity. This process can then reduce or eliminate the BOLD fMRI response in voxels that are nevertheless neuronally responsive, a phenomenon known as neurovascular uncoupling (NVU). NVU can arise from dysfunction at any point along the aforementioned cascade, and from defects in the underlying vasculature.[55] NVU poses a significant challenge for the use of functional neuroimaging in clinical applications because it compromises the validity of the BOLD signal as a biomarker of neural activity.

If fMRI is used to identify eloquent brain tissue near a planned resection site, failure to consider NVU could result in inadvertent resection of healthy tissue. The danger of NVU in this context lies primarily in the generation of false-negative indicators of brain activity. If a brain region is, in fact, neurally active but is not indicated as such in the fMRI brain map, the surgeon may falsely assume

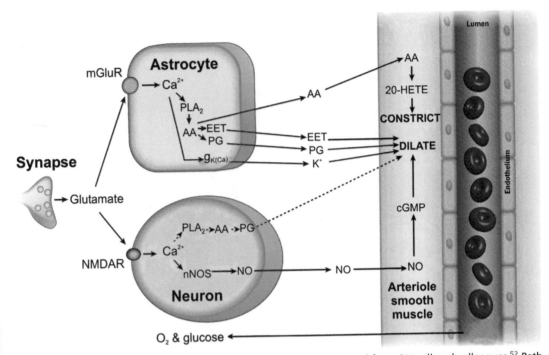

Fig. 6. Diagram illustrating the neurovascular coupling cascade, excerpted from Attwell and colleagues.[52] Pathways from astrocytes and neurons (*left*) regulate blood flow by sending messengers (*arrows*) to influence the smooth muscles around the arterioles that supply oxygen and glucose to the cells (*right*, shown as the vessel lumen surrounded by endothelial cells and smooth muscle). In neurons, synaptically released glutamate acts on *N*-methyl-D-aspartate receptors (NMDAR) to raise $[Ca^{2+}]_i$, causing neuronal nitric oxide synthase (nNOS) to release nitric oxide (NO), which activates smooth muscle guanylate cyclase; this generates cyclic guanosine monophosphate (cGMP) to dilate vessels. Raised $[Ca^{2+}]_i$ may also (*dashed line*) generate arachidonic acid (AA) from phospholipase A_2 (PLA_2), which is converted by cyclooxygenase (COX)-2 to prostaglandins (PG) that dilate vessels. Glutamate raises $[Ca^{2+}]_i$ in astrocytes by activating metabotropic glutamate receptors (mGluR), generating AA and, thus, 3 types of metabolite: prostaglandins (by COX-1/3, and COX-2 in pathologic situations), epoxyeicosatrienoic acids (EETs) (by P450 epoxygenase) in astrocytes, which dilate vessels, and 20-hydroxyeicosatetraenoic (20-HETE) (by ω-hydroxylase) in smooth muscle, which constricts vessels. An increase in $[Ca^{2+}]_i$ in astrocyte endfeet may activate Ca^{2+}-gated K^+ channels ($g_{K(Ca)}$), releasing K^+, which also dilates vessels. Note that pathologic disruption of this cascade could occur at many stages, both early and late, to cause neurovascular uncoupling. (*From* Attwell D, Buchan AM, Charpak S, et al. Glial and neuronal control of brain blood flow. Nature 2010;468:234; with permission.)

that the region can be resected without causing postoperative impairment. Consequently, testing for NVU in prospective neurosurgical patients is highly recommended. This approach can be especially important for patients suspected of having existing cerebrovascular abnormality such as local ischemia, arteriovenous malformations, highly vascularized tumors, or cerebral infarcts.

Fortunately, testing for NVU is now becoming a standard component of the patient workup for presurgical planning,[55] although the most appropriate method to assess NVU is still under consideration. Cerebrovascular reactivity (CVR) mapping using a simple breath-hold task or administration of inhaled CO_2 can provide brain-wide maps of vascular responsiveness, a necessary, though not sufficient, condition for BOLD activation.

These techniques induce a transient state of hypercapnia, which normally produces observable changes in the BOLD signal throughout the brain.[55–58] A reduced or absent CO_2 response can mark zones of potential NVU. Though helpful, such tests only probe the ability of the vascular smooth muscles to respond to changes in blood CO_2, leaving open the potential for disruption of the neurovascular cascade at any stage preceding the smooth muscle response (cf **Fig. 6**). Whether NVU can actually be caused by factors acting at different stages of the neurovascular cascade remains unclear at the time of writing. Therefore, while it is true that the absence of a CVR response indicates the likely presence of NVU, the inverse is not necessarily true; the presence of a CVR response does not definitively indicate that NVU

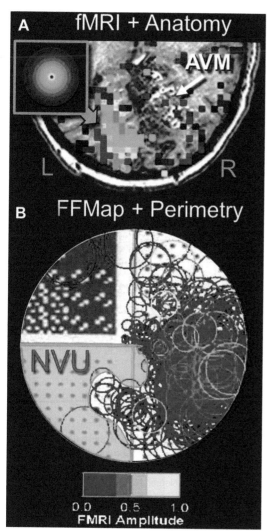

Fig. 7. fMRI (fMRI)-based mapping of the visual cortex in a patient with an arteriovenous malformation (AVM) in the right occipitoparietal cortex. (*A*) fMRI activation is color coded to indicate the visual field eccentricity of the ring stimulus that most strongly activated each voxel (inset shows color code). (*B*) FFMap showing robust fMRI activation (*orange circles*) limited mainly to the right visual field. However, the patient's Humphrey perimetry chart shown in the background indicates that vision was normal (*sparse stipple*) in the lower left quadrant, thus marking a zone of neurovascular uncoupling (*blue shading*). NVU, neurovascular uncoupling.

is absent. For example, it is conceivable that, in some cases, NVU might be caused by a selective pathologic effect on glial cells that link neuronal activation to the vascular smooth muscles (cf Fig. 6). In such a case a CVR test may appear normal, yet the fMR BOLD response could be absent. To distinguish between these potentially distinct causes of NVU, the authors refer to a CO_2 challenge as a test for late-stage NVU. Making such a distinction is potentially important because other methods are capable of detecting both early-stage and late-stage NVU. For example, **Fig. 7**A illustrates the case of a patient with a right occipital arteriovenous malformation showing minimal fMRI activation. In apparent agreement, the patient's FFMap shows little fMRI activation in the contralesional, left visual field, suggestive of a nearly complete hemianopia. (Note the paucity of orange circles in the left visual field of **Fig. 7**B). However, the patient's Humphrey perimetry chart shown in the background of **Fig. 7**B indicates normal vision in the lower left quadrant (light stipple with blue shading). Normal visual sensitivity in this quadrant verifies that the corresponding neural function is viable, yet fails to trigger a BOLD hemodynamic response: de facto NVU. Though definitive for detecting both early-stage and late-stage NVU, such a behavioral test is mainly of use for patients with visual system abnormality. Identification of a practical test that is definitive for both early-stage and late-stage NVU and that is anatomically comprehensive awaits future development.

SUMMARY

tbfMR imaging has proved to be a valuable technology for elucidating the functional anatomy of the visual cortex in patients with operable brain diseases. Clinically it can provide key information for planning and guiding brain surgery or other invasive treatments in patients with pathologic conditions affecting the visual cortex of the occipital, temporal, and parietal lobes. Vision mapping paradigms can provide detailed maps of the retinotopic organization of the visual cortex, thereby permitting identification of brain sites supporting critical central vision in individual patients. FFMaps provide a novel display of brain activation that can be used to quickly assess the behavioral relevance of fMRI patterns potentially compromised by pathologic disorder or a specific surgical approach. FFMaps can also be used to detect regions of NVU, making them additionally valuable for presurgical planning. Taskless, rsfMR imaging has received increasing attention from clinicians, owing to its ease of application and potential use with a wider range of patients. However, along with these exciting technological developments has come an increased awareness of potential limitations and interpretational issues. Researchers should remain cognizant that fMRI is an indirect indicator of neuronal activity, and NVU should always be taken into consideration, especially in clinical populations. Ongoing research is likely to identify improved methods for detecting NVU and to develop more clinically practical methods for the analysis of rsfMR imaging data. Despite its limitations, fMRI, in conjunction with diffusion tensor imaging and other methodologies, now provides physicians with an unprecedented array of information that can be used to inform and refine the diagnosis and treatment of operable brain abnormalities involving the human visual system.

REFERENCES

1. Wandell BA, Dumoulin SO, Brewer AA. Visual field maps in human cortex. Neuron 2007;56:366–83.
2. Silver MA, Kastner S. Topographic maps in human frontal and parietal cortex. Trends Cogn Sci 2009; 13:488–95.
3. Wandell BA, Winawer J. Imaging retinotopic maps in the human brain. Vision Res 2011;51(7):718–37.
4. Szczepanski SM, Pinsk MA, Douglas MM, et al. Functional and structural architecture of the human dorsal frontoparietal attention network. Proc Natl Acad Sci U S A 2013;110:15806–11. http://dx.doi.org/10.1073/pnas. 1313903110.
5. Vaina LM, Cowey A. Impairment of the perception of second order motion but not first order motion in a patient with unilateral focal brain damage. Proc R Soc Lond B Biol Sci 1996;263:1225–32.
6. Barton JJ. Higher cortical visual function. Curr Opin Ophthalmol 1998;9:40–5.
7. Clarke S, Walsh V, Schoppig A, et al. Colour constancy impairments in patients with lesions of the prestriate cortex. Exp Brain Res 1998;123:154–8.
8. Beauchamp MS, Haxby JV, Rosen AC, et al. A functional MRI case study of acquired cerebral dyschromatopsia. Neuropsychologia 2000;38: 1170–9.
9. Girkin CA, Miller NR. Central disorders of vision in humans. Surv Ophthalmol 2001;45:379–405.
10. Goodwin J. Disorders of higher cortical visual function. Curr Neurol Neurosci Rep 2002;2:418–22.
11. Trick GL. Beyond visual acuity: new and complementary tests of visual function. Neurol Clin 2003; 21:363–86.
12. Das A, Huxlin KR. New approaches to visual rehabilitation for cortical blindness: outcomes and putative mechanisms. Neuroscientist 2010;16:374–87. http://dx.doi.org/10.1177/1073858409356112.
13. Inouye T. Die Sehstorungen bei Schussverletzungen der kortikalen Sehsphare. Leipzig: W Engelmann; 1909.
14. Marie P, Chatelin C. Les troubles visuels dus aux lésions des voies optiques intracérébrales et de la sphère visuelle corticale dans les blessures du crane par coup de feu. Rev Neurol (Paris) 1914–15;28:882–925.
15. Holmes G, Lister WT. Disturbances of vision from cerebral lesions, with special reference to the cortical representation of the macula. Brain 1916; 39:34–73.
16. Holmes G. Disturbances of vision by cerebral lesions. Br J Ophthalmol 1918;2:353–84.
17. Holmes G. A contribution to the cortical representation of vision. Brain 1931;56:470–9.
18. Holmes G. Representation of mesial sectors of retinae in the calcarine cortex. Jahrbücher für Psychiatrie und Neurologie 1934;51:39–48.
19. Holmes G. The organization of the visual cortex in man (Ferrier lecture). Proceedings of the Royal Society B: Biological Sciences 1945;132:348–61.
20. Gill S, Ulmer J, DeYoe EA. Vision and higher cortical function. In: Holodny AI, editor. Functional neuroimaging: a clinical approach. New York: Informa Healthcare; 2008. p. 67–80.
21. DeYoe EA, Ulmer J, Mueller WM, et al. FMRI of Human Visual Pathways. In: Faro S, Mohamed FB, editors. Functional neuroradiology: principles and clinical applications. New York: Springer; 2011. p. 485–511.
22. Schulder M, Maldjian JA, Liu WC, et al. Functional image-guided surgery of intracranial tumors located in or near the sensorimotor cortex. J Neurosurg 1998;89:412–8. http://dx.doi.org/10.3171/jns.1998.89.3.0412.
23. Roessler K, Donat M, Lanzenberger R, et al. Evaluation of preoperative high magnetic field motor functional MRI (3 Tesla) in glioma patients by navigated electrocortical stimulation and postoperative outcome. J Neurol Neurosurg Psychiatr 2005;76: 1152–7. http://dx.doi.org/10.1136/jnnp.2004.050286.
24. Sunaert S. Presurgical planning for tumor resectioning. J Magn Reson Imaging 2006;23:887–905.
25. Dimou S, Battisti RA, Hermens DF, et al. A systematic review of functional magnetic resonance imaging and diffusion tensor imaging modalities used in presurgical planning of brain tumour resection. Neurosurg Rev 2013;36: 205–14. http://dx.doi.org/10.1007/s10143-012-0436-8 [discussion: 214].
26. Giussani C, Roux FE, Ojemann J, et al. Is preoperative functional magnetic resonance imaging reliable for language areas mapping in brain tumor surgery? Review of language functional magnetic resonance imaging and direct cortical stimulation correlation studies. Neurosurgery 2010;66:113–20. http://dx.doi.org/10.1227/01.NEU.0000360392.15450.C9.
27. Hirsch J, Ruge MI, Kim KH, et al. An integrated functional magnetic resonance imaging procedure for preoperative mapping of cortical areas associated with tactile, motor, language, and visual functions. Neurosurgery 2000;47:711–21 [discussion: 721–2].

28. Kapsalakis IZ, Kapsalaki EZ, Gotsis ED, et al. Preoperative evaluation with FMRI of patients with intracranial gliomas. Radiol Res Pract 2012; 2012:727810. http://dx.doi.org/10.1155/2012/727810.

29. Pujol J, Conesa G, Deus J, et al. Clinical application of functional magnetic resonance imaging in presurgical identification of the central sulcus. J Neurosurg 1998;88:863–9. http://dx.doi.org/10.3171/jns.1998.88.5.0863.

30. Biswal B, Yetkin FZ, Haughton VM, et al. Functional connectivity in the motor cortex of resting human brain using echo-planar MRI. Magn Reson Med 1995;34:537–41.

31. Fox MD, Snyder AZ, Vincent JL, et al. The human brain is intrinsically organized into dynamic, anti-correlated functional networks. Proc Natl Acad Sci U S A 2005;102:9673–8.

32. Fox MD, Raichle ME. Spontaneous fluctuations in brain activity observed with functional magnetic resonance imaging. Nat Rev Neurosci 2007;8:700–11.

33. Lowe MJ, Mock BJ, Sorenson JA. Functional connectivity in single and multislice echoplanar imaging using resting-state fluctuations. Neuroimage 1998;7:119–32.

34. Cordes D, Haughton V, Arfanakis K, et al. Mapping functionally related regions of brain with functional connectivity MR imaging. AJNR Am J Neuroradiol 2000;21:1636–44.

35. van de Ven VG, Formisano E, Prvulovic D, et al. Functional connectivity as revealed by spatial independent component analysis of fMRI measurements during rest. Hum Brain Mapp 2004;22:165–78.

36. Liu H, Buckner RL, Talukdar T, et al. Task-free presurgical mapping using functional magnetic resonance imaging intrinsic activity. J Neurosurg 2009;111:746–54.

37. Kokkonen SM, Nikkinen J, Remes J, et al. Preoperative localization of the sensorimotor area using independent component analysis of resting-state fMRI. Magn Reson Imaging 2009;27:733–40. http://dx.doi.org/10.1016/j.mri.2008.11.002.

38. Zhang D, Johnston JM, Fox MD, et al. Preoperative sensorimotor mapping in brain tumor patients using spontaneous fluctuations in neuronal activity imaged with functional magnetic resonance imaging: initial experience. Neurosurgery 2009;65:226–36.

39. Manglore S, Bharath RD, Panda R, et al. Utility of resting fMRI and connectivity in patients with brain tumor. Neurol India 2013;61:144–51. http://dx.doi.org/10.4103/0028-3886.111120.

40. Rosazza C, Aquino D, D'Incerti L, et al. Preoperative mapping of the sensorimotor cortex: comparative assessment of task-based and resting-state FMRI. PLoS One 2014;9:e98860. http://dx.doi.org/10.1371/journal.pone.0098860.

41. Tie Y. Defining language networks from resting-state fMRI for surgical planning–a feasibility study. Hum Brain Mapp 2014;35:1018–30. http://dx.doi.org/10.1002/hbm.22231.

42. Biswal BB, Mennes M, Zuo XN, et al. Towards discovery science of human brain function. Proc Natl Acad Sci U S A 2010;107(10):4734–9.

43. Beckmann CF, DeLuca M, Devlin JT, et al. Investigations into resting-state connectivity using independent component analysis. Philos Trans R Soc Lond B Biol Sci 2005;360:1001–13.

44. Van Essen DC, Ugurbil K, Auerbach E, et al. The Human Connectome Project: a data acquisition perspective. Neuroimage 2012;62(4):2222–31.

45. Allen EA, Erhardt EB, Damaraju E, et al. A baseline for the multivariate comparison of resting-state networks. Front Syst Neurosci 2011;5:2. http://dx.doi.org/10.3389/fnsys.2011.00002.

46. Bullmore E, Sporns O. Complex brain networks: graph theoretical analysis of structural and functional systems. Nat Rev Neurosci 2009;10:186–98.

47. Rubinov M, Sporns O. Complex network measures of brain connectivity: uses and interpretations. Neuroimage 2009;52(3):1059–69.

48. Anderson JS, Ferguson MA, Lopez-Larson M, et al. Reproducibility of single-subject functional connectivity measurements. AJNR Am J Neuroradiol 2011;32:548–55. http://dx.doi.org/10.3174/ajnr.A2330.

49. Gorgolewski KJ, Storkey AJ, Bastin ME, et al. Adaptive thresholding for reliable topological inference in single subject fMRI analysis. Front Hum Neurosci 2012;6:245. http://dx.doi.org/10.3389/fnhum.2012.00245.

50. Ragnehed M, Engstrom M, Knutsson H, et al. Restricted canonical correlation analysis in functional MRI-validation and a novel thresholding technique. J Magn Reson Imaging 2009;29:146–54. http://dx.doi.org/10.1002/jmri.21494.

51. Genovese CR, Lazar NA, Nichols T. Thresholding of statistical maps in functional neuroimaging using the false discovery rate. Neuroimage 2002;15:870–8. http://dx.doi.org/10.1006/nimg.2001.1037.

52. Attwell D, Buchan AM, Charpak S, et al. Glial and neuronal control of brain blood flow. Nature 2010;468:232–43.

53. Logothetis NK. The underpinnings of the BOLD functional magnetic resonance imaging signal. J Neurosci 2003;23:3963–71.

54. Hillman EM. Coupling mechanism and significance of the BOLD signal: a status report. Annu Rev Neurosci 2014;37:161–81. http://dx.doi.org/10.1146/annurev-neuro-071013-014111.

55. Pillai JJ, Mikulis DJ. Cerebrovascular reactivity mapping: an evolving standard for clinical

functional imaging. AJNR Am J Neuroradiol 2014. http://dx.doi.org/10.3174/ajnr.A3941.

56. Pillai JJ, Zaca D. Clinical utility of cerebrovascular reactivity mapping in patients with low grade gliomas. World J Clin Oncol 2011;2:397–403.

57. Zaca D, Hua J, Pillai JJ. Cerebrovascular reactivity mapping for brain tumor presurgical planning. World J Clin Oncol 2011;2:289–98.

58. Pillai JJ, Zaca D. Comparison of BOLD cerebrovascular reactivity mapping and DSC MR perfusion imaging for prediction of neurovascular uncoupling potential in brain tumors. Technol Cancer Res Treat 2012;11(4):361–74.

59. Talairach J, Tournoux P. Co-planar stereotaxic atlas of the human brain. New York: Thieme Medical Publishers; 1988.

60. Kanwisher N, McDermott J, Chun MM. The fusiform face area: a module in human extrastriate cortex specialized for face perception. J Neurosci 1997; 17:4302–11.

61. Malach R, Reppas JB, Benson RR, et al. Object-related activity revealed by functional magnetic resonance imaging in human occipital cortex. Proc Natl Acad Sci U S A 1995;92:8135–9.

62. Grill-Spector K, Kushnir T, Hendler T, et al. A sequence of object-processing stages revealed by fMRI in the human occipital lobe. Hum Brain Mapp 1998;6:316–28.

63. Balasubramanian M, Polimeni J, Schwartz EL. The V1-V2-V3 complex: quasiconformal dipole maps in primate striate and extra-striate cortex. Neural Netw 2002;15:1157–63.

Memory Assessment in the Clinical Context Using Functional Magnetic Resonance Imaging
A Critical Look at the State of the Field

Mary Pat McAndrews, PhD[a,b,]*

KEYWORDS

- Episodic memory • Functional MR imaging • Epilepsy • Medial temporal lobe • Activation
- Connectivity

KEY POINTS

- Encoding and retrieval tasks that emphasize relational processes show greatest activation of medial temporal lobe (MTL) structures.
- Reduced task-related MTL activation in epilepsy and mild cognitive impairment or Alzheimer disease can indicate functional integrity of that region for supporting memory.
- Resting-state functional connectivity of the MTL regions may provide a more reliable metric of clinical memory capacity.
- The diagnostic and predictive value of functional magnetic resonance imaging (fMRI), relative to structural MR imaging and baseline memory performance, remains to be elucidated.

TRANSITIONS IN TRANSLATIONAL IMAGING

There has been a huge increase in functional magnetic resonance imaging (fMRI) studies over the past 3 decades devoted to characterizing the neural architecture of memory processes, including encoding and retrieval of different types of material, identifying patterns that correlate with intraindividual and between-group variance in memory success, and parsing different types of memory operations such as retrieval of item versus relational information. The field is so rich in data and the taxonomy of memory terminology sufficiently well-defined that semiautomated meta-analyses of relevant data have been undertaken using techniques such as activation likelihood estimation.[1,2]

Furthermore, fMRI studies are now affording key insights about the merits of different memory theories in ways that were unimaginable just a decade ago. Given the abundance of cognitive neuroscience data and techniques available to identify different associations and dissociations among brain regions and memory operations, it is reasonable to assume that the clinical application would also be well advanced. Certainly the rapid movement from the laboratory to the clinic for functional mapping of sensorimotor and language systems, where these data are used to inform neurosurgical decisions in a growing number of centers, might imply that memory would not be far behind. However, this is not yet the case; clinical applications of memory fMRI remain in the realm of research

The author has no conflicts to disclose.
[a] Krembil Neuroscience Centre, Toronto Western Research Institute, University Health Network, 4F-409, 399 Bathurst Street, Toronto, Onatrio M5T 2S8, Canada; [b] Department of Psychology, University of Toronto, 100 St George Street, 4th Floor, Sidney Smith Hall, Toronto, Onatrio M5S 3G3, Canada
* Neuropsychology Clinic, Toronto Western Hospital, 4F-409, 399 Bathurst Street, Toronto, Ontario M5T 2S8, Canada.
E-mail address: Mary.McAndrews@uhn.ca

neuroimaging.theclinics.com

rather than being standard of care at present. Nonetheless, there are some successes to celebrate, some important lessons learned in trying to establish a strong evidentiary basis for the translation to clinical utility, and some exciting new paths forward that are discussed in this review. Throughout, examples are drawn mainly from the context of temporal lobe epilepsy (TLE), as it is in this context that many important advances have been made (see recent reviews[3–5]). However, data from other conditions including mild cognitive impairment (MCI), Alzheimer disease, and transient global amnesia are also helpful, as they illustrate key points with respect to interpretation of the fMRI blood oxygenation level dependent (BOLD) signal in memory processes.

THE GOALS OF CLINICAL FUNCTIONAL MR IMAGING FOR MEMORY

It is important to start by considering the goals of memory fMRI memory in clinical contexts. In patients with recurrent seizures arising from one temporal lobe, the concern is whether its removal in an effort to eliminate seizures will come at a significant cost in the form of postsurgical memory decline. It is well established that the functional adequacy of epileptogenic tissue in the medial temporal lobe (MTL) is a risk factor for postoperative change, in that better preoperative performance is associated with greater decline.[6,7] Neuropsychological testing reveals that generally the left MTL is most involved in verbal memory functions whereas the right mediates visuospatial memory,[8–10] and that information is used to inform both diagnosis (ie, does the memory impairment align with structural magnetic resonance [MR] imaging and electroencephalographic evidence) and prediction (ie, how much of a loss might be expected in a particular memory domain). Nonetheless, there are some weaknesses in the material specificity alignment, which undermine strong inferences about functional adequacy of MTL to be resected; these may be attributed to variation in processing strategies, test sensitivity, or possible reorganization of memory systems in epilepsy.[11] In principle, fMRI is uniquely suited to investigate the functional anatomy of memory, and is thus poised to contribute a more direct metric of functional adequacy of the epileptogenic tissue. With a robust metric relating functional activation to clinical memory performance, one might predict more confidently whether an individual patient is likely to suffer a clinically significant decline. Leaving aside the issue of how best to characterize such a decline (eg, a statistically significant drop in memory test scores, subjective concerns,

evidence of impairments in everyday functioning), the aim of identifying fMRI metrics of functional integrity has generated considerable research in epilepsy surgery centers.

In addition to epilepsy surgery, there are other clinical contexts in which determining the functional integrity of memory-relevant regions is important. The hippocampus and entorhinal cortex have long been recognized as structures showing early damage in the pathologic progression to Alzheimer disease,[12,13] and measurement of hippocampal volume and entorhinal cortex thickness are now foundational elements of protocols for diagnosis and staging progression in MCI and Alzheimer disease.[14,15] As described later, recent fMR imaging studies of memory in that population have begun to reveal interesting patterns of activation in these MTL structures that may well provide another useful biomarker of disease progression and may even illuminate the fundamental biological mechanisms of that progression. Furthermore, although there are relatively few studies at present, the use of memory activation tasks to assess the impact of rehabilitation strategies (whether cognitive, pharmacologic, or behavioral) on regional functioning and as an index of plasticity offers enormous promise.

THE PRAGMATICS OF CLINICAL FUNCTIONAL MRI FOR MEMORY

The procedures for imaging in clinical contexts involve several choices. As outlined in **Box 1**, there are many decision points throughout the investigation and there are no simple plug-and-play solutions for imaging memory. The choices begin with selecting an activation task that is likely to be sufficiently reliable, sensitive, and readily implemented in a clinical context. Although there are elegant examples of activation tasks that demonstrate robust MTL activity in healthy young adults, they often require many repetitions (to accumulate sufficient data to achieve adequate signal-to-noise ratio), leading to unacceptably long imaging times (eg, 30 minutes or longer) for ease of clinical implementation. In addition, it is important to consider whether a task has proved to be sensitive to individual differences and to correlate with clinical features of memory, because deriving meaningful cutoffs for what will be interpreted as adequate, as opposed to defective activation, will necessitate proving its relationship to outcome data. This aspect is exemplified herein with the studies on TLE.

In identifying focal activation, there is nothing in the "raw" BOLD signal that is informative, so analysis typically requires contrasts between conditions, such as memory versus baseline or items subsequently recalled versus items subsequently forgotten. Having then determined the statistical threshold to use (too stringent and nothing shows as activated, too liberal and most of the brain might appear engaged), the next decision is the metric to be used to characterize functional integrity. In epilepsy, one could look at asymmetry of activation between MTL regions in each hemisphere, which is best if it can be expected that the normative patterns for both hemispheres show the same magnitude and/or extent of activation under the probe task. If there is no expectation of symmetry, comparison against some other standard is required, which may rely on a considerable amount of normative data on the same task over many individuals who are matched for important features (including age) with the

epilepsy group, to ascertain whether the degree of activation in the affected MTL appears to be outside of the normal range. As discussed later, both strategies have been used in epilepsy. Validation of the clinical utility of any measure requires comparing it with appropriate neuropsychological measures of current memory performance and/or with scores that reflect presurgical to postsurgical changes on those measures. However, the field is not yet sufficiently mature that clinical cutoffs have been derived, and very few studies have looked at sensitivity and specificity of the fMRI indicator. The general rubric of poor activation signaling a defective neural substrate and, thus, less overall risk is one that has general consensus but, as discussed later, bigger is not invariably better in the sense of greater functional integrity.

MEMORY IN TEMPORAL LOBE EPILEPSY: ACTIVATION TASKS AND CORRESPONDENCE WITH CLINICAL MEMORY DATA

A survey of the cognitive neuroscience literature indicates that tasks that reliably activate the MTL in healthy individuals share a few characteristics. Those that rely on encoding of complex novel visual information, such as scenes, in comparison with baseline repeated images are strong activators of MTL, including posterior regions such as the parahippocampal gyrus.[16–18] Tasks that involve relational processing (eg, pairs of elements such as word-word or word-face; item-context associations) typically engage this region to a greater extent than those focusing on single elements, at both encoding and retrieval.[19–24] Finally, very robust activation of the MTL bilaterally is typically observed when individuals retrieve memories of events from their own personal past (ie, details of autobiographical memories) in comparison with other forms of semantic retrieval (typically word meaning but also facts about one's life).[25–27] Of importance, the latter 2 distinctions (relational and autobiographical) also have strong behavioral evidence for the necessity of hippocampal involvement, as such processes are impaired in patients with medial TLE (mTLE) or following unilateral excision of a temporal lobe.[28–33]

This review concentrates on studies in which fMRI results were correlated with or used to predict performance on neuropsychological memory tests in patients with mTLE. Scene encoding was one of the earlier paradigms used, likely because of the robust bilateral MTL activation generated by the contrast of complex novel scenes against a baseline (either "scrambled" picture or the same scene presented multiple times), the simple instructions ("try to remember the new scenes"), and the statistical power of a block-design presentation (alternating 20–30-second blocks of novel and baseline conditions), thus lending itself to relatively short scanning times (approximately 5 minutes) (**Fig. 1**). In the earliest study of patients with unilateral mTLE, Detre and colleagues[34] showed that asymmetry of activation in a region of interest (ROI) including posterior hippocampus, parahippocampal gyrus, and fusiform gyrus corresponded to memory results of the sodium amobarbital inactivation procedure, such that the spatial extent of activation was smaller on the side with worse memory performance. Subsequent studies using the same paradigm extended these results, indicating that both asymmetry ratios and absolute activation within the epileptogenic hippocampus were correlated with postoperative memory outcomes.[35–39] A similar result regarding asymmetric activation and its

relation to memory performance has been shown for a task involving mental navigation in a familiar environment, namely, imagining walking through your home town.[40,41] These studies indicate that the left or right MTL found to be compromised on clinical memory tests generates a weaker BOLD response during a memory challenge.

Another strategy has been to use material-specific memory probes for fMR imaging that are more likely to preferentially activate one or the other mesial temporal region (eg, words for the left hemisphere, abstract designs for the right hemisphere). In this case one can investigate the functional adequacy of the epileptogenic MTL as described earlier, but also the possibility that the contralateral MTL has augmented processing for nonpreferred material, and thus whether there is evidence of neural plasticity attributable to recurrent seizures. A caveat is that this material specificity does not always map onto hemispheric

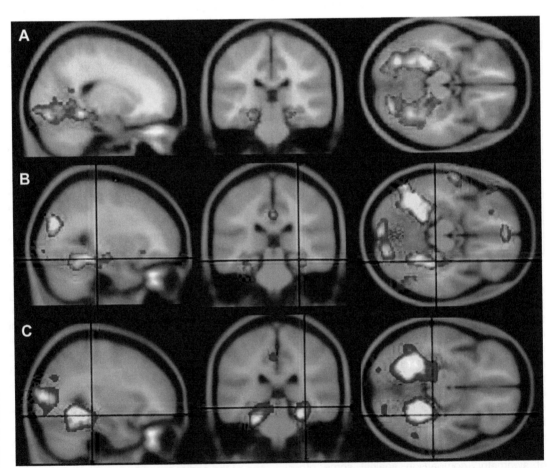

Fig. 1. Scene-encoding fMR imaging. Regions in color reflect areas of greater activation for novel scenes versus a repeated scene. (A) Average of 10 healthy controls, threshold P<.001 (corrected for multiple comparisons by False Discovery Rate). (B, C) Individual patients with right medial temporal lobe epilepsy (mTLE), at a similar threshold. Note that it is difficult to discern differences between patients and normative control data, with respect to spatial extent or magnitude of activation, based on visual inspection.

asymmetry in fMRI signals, even in healthy individuals.[42] A word-recollection paradigm was found in several studies to demonstrate that the degree of activation in the left MTL in left mTLE patients predicted the magnitude of postoperative verbal memory decline.[43,44] However, another group using a different verbal memory task demonstrated instead a somewhat complex pattern of activation changes in multiple brain regions relative to controls that seems to undermine the simple functional adequacy approach.[45,46] Some studies have examined multiple tasks expected to be more selective to left (words) or right (pictures, faces) MTL engagement, in an attempt to see whether correlation with material-specific declines in memory performance can be enhanced by this strategy. Several of these have demonstrated greater activation in the nonaffected relative to the epileptogenic MTL, in addition to material-specific differences between controls and patients (eg, greater right hemisphere activation during word encoding in left mTLE patients).[47,48] There was support for using either activation asymmetry or absolute magnitude of activation in the epileptogenic MTL as an index of functional adequacy, in that BOLD magnitude therein correlated positively with material-specific memory preoperatively and also with the magnitude of postoperative decline.[48,49] One study suggests that this pattern is characteristic of signals from the anterior MTL, with posterior MTL activation showing the converse pattern of a positive correlation between preoperative activation and postoperative performance.[50]

The preoperative imaging data in these studies typically show greater activation in the contralateral MTL during memory tasks, but it is not clear as to whether this is a marker of adaptive plasticity or attempted compensation. Most of these studies are underpowered (eg, comprising 7–15 participants per group) to adequately address factors related to plasticity such as age of onset and duration of seizures. Furthermore, greater atypical contralateral (eg, right MTL for verbal material) activation in several studies has been shown to be associated with poorer memory for that type of material,[39,48,50] suggesting that it is not truly adaptive or compensatory. In addition, one study reported that increased activation in the posterior MTL following anterior temporal lobe resection in patients with left mTLE was actually correlated with worse postoperative verbal memory performance.[51] The question of whether "more is better" in terms of activation magnitude is discussed again later.

Although much of the energy in this clinical memory imaging has been devoted to identifying optimal memory tasks for activating the MTL and, thus, serving as a biomarker for functional integrity, several investigators have shown that the degree of left hemisphere activation during language comprehension or production tasks can be a powerful predictor of verbal memory decline following left anterior temporal lobe resection.[52,53] Indeed, a direct comparison of a language lateralization measure and hippocampal asymmetry on a scene-encoding task showed that the former was a better predictor of verbal memory decline following dominant resections.[54] There are several possible explanations for this result. It may be critical to look at activation in regions beyond the MTL to enhance prediction, as memory is undoubtedly supported by wider brain networks. In addition, the full capacity of the MTL and extended memory architecture may not be characterized best by activation tasks whereby there is likely to be considerable variability in performance adequacy or effort. Both of these themes are now explored in greater depth.

CHALLENGES TO THE LINK BETWEEN ACTIVATION MAGNITUDE AND FUNCTIONAL INTEGRITY

Much of the foregoing interpretations are predicated on the expectation that a greater magnitude of activation signifies a more functionally intact anatomic substrate. It is a reasonable assumption, but one that may be incomplete or incorrect, particularly when activation is taking place in damaged regions of brain, as in the hippocampus of a patient with mesial temporal sclerosis (MTS). Furthermore, even in the healthy brain, the degree of MTL activation may reflect a combination of objective encoding and retrieval of details, and a subjective experience of recollection that may be divorced from reality under certain conditions.[55–57] The author's own experience with a memory task that produces very robust activation in the MTL, autobiographical recall, is a good object lesson regarding the complex relationship between memory-induced functional activation and clinical indicators. Retrieval of episodes from the personal past is well established as generating reliable activation in mesial temporal regions (Fig. 2)[25,27,58] and patients with TLE demonstrate marked deficits in recalling details of autobiographical experiences.[29,31,59] Furthermore, mesial temporal damage in these patients results in a markedly reduced activation in the affected region and in the whole network of regions typically engaged during autobiographical recall.[9,60] Nonetheless, the author's group has found relatively poor correspondence between the magnitude or extent of

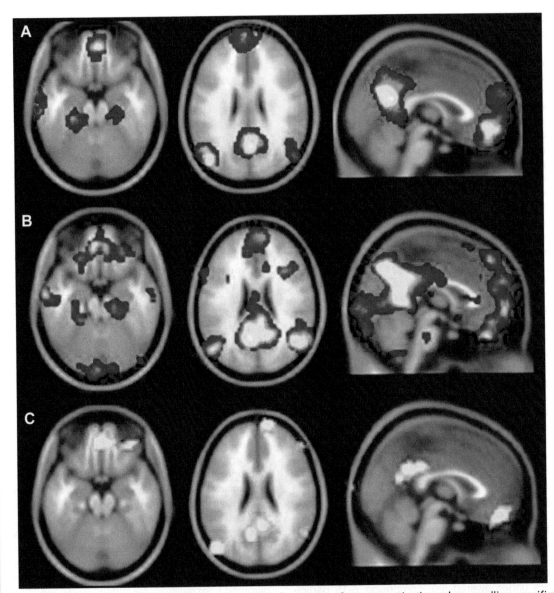

Fig. 2. Autobiographical memory. Regions in color reflect areas of greater activation when recalling specific events from one's own life experience versus sentence completion. (*A*) Average of 12 healthy controls, threshold *P*<.001 (corrected for multiple comparisons by False Discovery Rate). (*B*) Single healthy control, threshold *P*<.005 (uncorrected). (*C*) Patient with left mTLE, threshold *P*<.01 (uncorrected). Note that despite a more liberal statistical threshold, activation is much weaker and more restricted in the patient and is absent in both MTL regions despite a focal left epileptogenic abnormality.

hippocampal activation and performance on clinical memory tests, and even some negative correlations in certain tasks (McAndrews, unpublished data). Thus, one can have a task that clearly engages the MTL during scanning and is dependent on the MTL for execution, and yet not be able to identify a clear fMRI biomarker of integrity (see also Ref.[54]).

One possibility is that there is a nonmonotonic function relating activation levels to clinical

impairment in TLE. In comparison with controls, mTLE patients with good postscanning recognition showed increased bilateral MTL activation during an encoding task, whereas those with poor subsequent memory showed reduced activation.[61] This same pattern has been observed in another disorder involving MTL damage, MCI. Sperling and colleagues[62] observed that, compared with controls, patients with very mild memory deficits show hyperactivation in the

MTL, whereas patients with more significant deficits show hypoactivation.[63] This pattern could suggest an attempt at compensation early in the course of neurodegeneration, which then fails following a critical level of neuronal damage. However, there are also data suggesting that this hyperactivation in MCI may actually reflect a pathologic process, as individuals with greater activation at baseline show more pronounced cognitive decline several years later,[64] and reducing hippocampal excitability pharmacologically has been shown to reduce activity and improve memory in MCI patients on a memory task sensitive to hippocampal integrity.[65] Finally, the author's group had the opportunity to scan scene encoding and recognition with an individual during and after an episode of transient global amnesia (TGA).[66] This female patient failed to show MTL activation for the standard contrasts (novel scenes > fixation at encoding; old scenes > new scenes at recognition). However, she showed substantial bilateral hippocampal activation when all scenes were contrasted (old and new) against the fixation stimulus (a blurred repeating scene) during the recognition run; this was not seen in any controls or in the patient when she returned for scanning 3 months later when her memory had returned to normal. Although this result confirmed that the hippocampal tissue was viable in the sense that it was capable of generating a BOLD signal, it was clearly not an indicator of good memory during the TGA episode. These findings illustrate a critical point, namely that variations in engagement or strategies during an fMRI memory task may add a great deal of noise to the simple calculation that activation magnitude equals memory competence.

RESTING-STATE fMRI AND MEMORY

The MTL, specifically hippocampus and parahippocampal gyrus, are components of the default-mode network (DMN), a set of midline and lateral brain regions characterized by strong anatomic connectivity and significant functional connectivity during rest or introspective thought.[67–69] Of interest, the DMN shows considerable overlap with the constellation of brain regions commonly engaged during episodic recollection (**Fig. 3**),[58,70] and several studies have demonstrated abnormal connectivity between the MTL and other DMN regions in patients with mTLE.[71–74] The consequence of disrupted connectivity to memory performance is a novel area of investigation. The author's group investigated connectivity between the hub of the DMN, the posterior cingulate cortex (PCC), and both ipsilateral and contralateral hippocampi in patients with unilateral mTLE.[75] Compared with controls, PCC-hippocampal connectivity was reduced in the epileptogenic

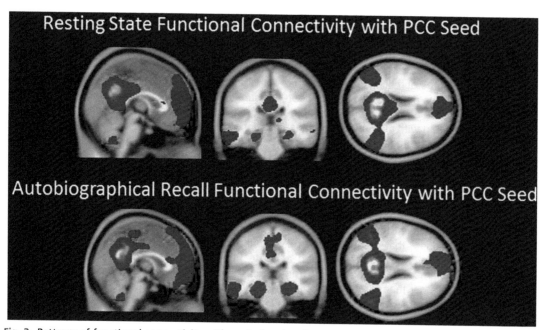

Fig. 3. Patterns of functional connectivity with posterior cingulate cortex (PCC). Seed connectivity from the PCC reveals strikingly similar patterns during resting state/mind wandering (*top panel*) and when participants are instructed to retrieve specific personal episodic memories according to verbal cues (*bottom panel*). These images demonstrate that resting-state fMR imaging appears to engage memory-relevant brain networks.

hemisphere and increased in the contralateral hemisphere, and stronger connectivity on the epileptogenic side was associated with better presurgical memory and greater decline in postsurgical memory. Connectivity on the contralateral side was protective with respect to memory decline and, based on postoperative scanning of a small cohort of patients, the author's group reported an increase in contralateral connectivity after removal of the epileptogenic side, suggestive of plasticity.

Although there is considerable overlap between regions in the DMN and those activated by an autobiographical retrieval task, preliminary data in a sample of 10 patients with left mLTE suggest that this connectivity measure collected during rest was a better predictor of verbal memory performance on a standard clinical measure than was the same connectivity during autobiographical retrieval in the same patient cohort (correlation values of 0.78 vs 0.55, unpublished data). Although this needs to be established in a larger sample and with postoperative memory change as an outcome, it is possible that resting-state functional connectivity (rsFC) measures are superior to task-based ones, as they eliminate variance or noise associated with alternative strategies and/or alternative networks being utilized during the activation task by patients in whom some degree of functional reorganization may have already taken place. Of interest, similar findings regarding rsFC in the MTL in other memory-impaired populations provide converging evidence for these conclusions. Amnesic patients with bilateral MTL damage show decreased connectivity between PCC and MTL components of the DMN.[76] The degree of resting connectivity between these regions is predictive of memory performance in older adults,[77] and disrupted connectivity correlated with memory performance separates patients with amnestic MCI from non-amnestic MCI.[78] Finally, other rsFC patterns, both involving the hippocampus and extratemporal regions, have been shown to relate to the degree of memory impairment in mTLE and MCI/Alzheimer disease.[79–82]

Even with rsFC, however, there are likely to be important complexities that need to be addressed. For example, a few studies looked at connectivity and memory capacity seeded from the hippocampus (rather than PCC as the author had done) to explore more widespread connectivity throughout the brain. One found a similar pattern, in that hippocampus-PCC connectivity was among the few indices to show a positive correlation with episodic memory,[83] whereas another demonstrated a negative correlation

between memory performance and connectivity involving an atrophic epileptogenic hippocampus and the ipsilateral posterior cingulate.[80] The source of these discrepancies requires considerable further empirical work. Fortunately, the barrier to conducting resting-state studies is considerably lower than with activation memory tasks in terms of amount of data required, the complexity of task influences, and the possibility of pooling data from multiple centers.

THE ADDED VALUE OF fMRI IN DIAGNOSIS AND PREDICTION

MTS is readily identified on structural MR imaging, characterized by volume loss and high signal on T2-weighted scans. This is the most frequently seen pathologic feature in mTLE, and has been shown to contribute to prediction of postoperative memory decline in that patients with greater MTS show smaller losses following removal of the affected hippocampus.[84–86] Thus, it is important to understand how structural integrity may affect the capacity for activation, and to ascertain the added value of fMR imaging data in clinical contexts. To date there is scant empirical evidence on either point. In several studies of mTLE, investigators have reported minimal activation in the sclerotic hippocampus but more in adjacent MTL and extratemporal regions.[87,88] Results are mixed regarding the correlation between functional and structural measures of hippocampal integrity, with some investigators reporting a moderate to strong relationship[39] and others no correlation.[50] The relative merits of each putative biomarker in explaining variation in memory performance in mTLE is not yet clear, although there is some suggestion that functional activation or connectivity measures may make a stronger contribution.[50,75,89] Clearly these are important issues, as specialized expertise is required to include fMRI in preoperative epilepsy evaluations, and the clinical utility it affords beyond other conventional metrics must be demonstrated before it will be widely adopted (**Box 2**).

Although establishing group differences and correlations with clinical measures is a crucial step in advancing clinical fMRI for memory, for it to be useful at the individual patient level it is imperative to establish sensitivity, specificity, and positive predictive value (PPV) for fMR imaging measures. Using the probability of clinically meaningful postoperative decline in mTLE as an example, would 3 activated voxels present no risk whereas 15 would signify a strong risk? Although few studies have attempted to quantify this, Bonelli and colleagues[51] reported that

Box 2

Using fMR imaging to assess functional adequacy in medial temporal lobe (MTL) epilepsy

Putative Indices

- Asymmetry of activation in MTL regions
- Absolute magnitude of activation in epileptogenic MTL
- Connectivity (during task or resting state) between epileptogenic MTL and other brain regions

Expectations for Memory Outcomes

- Greater engagement of epileptogenic MTL correlated with better preoperative memory performance on clinically relevant tests
- Greater engagement of epileptogenic MTL correlated with greater material-specific memory loss following anterior temporal lobectomy surgery
- Greater/increased contralateral engagement associated with less risk of postoperative decline

activation of the MTL alone showed poor PPV (20%–30%, depending on hemisphere), but also that it did significantly contribute to strong prediction when language lateralization and preoperative test performance were included in the models (PPV 70% for left mTLE/verbal memory change and 100% for right mTLE and visual memory change). Overall, the field is not sufficiently mature to have highly reliable activation tasks or rsFC metrics with appropriate cutoffs for clinical decision making, but this issue is likely years rather than decades away from being resolved.

FINAL CONCEPTUAL AND METHODOLOGICAL CAVEATS IN IMAGING MEMORY

This review has concentrated throughout on the medial temporal regions, specifically the hippocampus and parahippocampal cortices, as key to the clinical utility of memory fMR imaging. This bias is not meant to imply that other brain regions do not participate in memory operations in both health and disease, nor that they may be very relevant to clinical questions such as diagnosis, disease progression, or treatment-induced plasticity. However, MTL regions have been identified as crucial in certain clinical conditions in which fMRI might play an important role. It is acknowledged that fMRI in this region is subject to some challenges because of increased susceptibility-related signal dropout and distortion. There is a considerable body of literature devoted to optimization of acquisition parameters or postscanning estimation processes for this region.[90–93] Furthermore, Beisteiner and colleagues[94] have raised concerns that conventional postprocessing techniques, such as normalization through the use of standard template-based ROI definitions, can change the clinical interpretation of results for individual patient data. These investigators advocate for analysis based on nontransformed functional data and also point to the importance of using multiple metrics to quantify activation. As already discussed, the choice of task-activation methods (particular probe task, the more sensitive block design versus the more specific event-related design) or models for assessing functional connectivity are also important considerations.

For a measure to be valid, its reliability must be demonstrated. Concerns have been raised about test-retest reliability in memory task activations, particularly in complex tasks that may be likely to induce different strategies. Even in simple novelty encoding paradigms, poor intrasubject reliability has been shown in healthy controls despite group-level consistency in activation patterns across test sessions.[95] There is some evidence that rsFC may show greater reliability,[96,97] although variables such as participant age, scan length, and other acquisition parameters can have modest influences.[98,99] The validity of interpretation regarding between-subject differences in activation metrics and their relationship to functional memory status will be influenced by many factors, including structural integrity of the substrate, etiology and duration of disease, cerebral reserve, and task engagement and competence. In addition, the extent to which the microscopic pathology in mTLE or MCI/Alzheimer disease and the use of medications in these conditions may influence (either globally or locally) the neurovascular coupling that is crucial for observing the BOLD effect is not yet known.[100–102] Many of these influences will be difficult to estimate in small-scale studies, let alone the individual case. Finally, the essentially correlational methods involved in fMR imaging studies require convergent validation with other causal manipulations (eg, stimulation or inactivation, lesion) to increase confidence that activated regions are indeed essential to memory performance.

REFERENCES

1. Spaniol J, Davidson PS, Kim AS, et al. Event-related fMRI studies of episodic encoding and

retrieval: meta-analyses using activation likelihood estimation. Neuropsychologia 2009;47 (8–9):1765–79.

2. Kim H. Differential neural activity in the recognition of old versus new events: an activation likelihood estimation meta-analysis. Hum Brain Mapp 2013; 34(4):814–36.

3. Duncan J. The current status of neuroimaging for epilepsy. Curr Opin Neurol 2009;22(2):179–84.

4. Richardson M. Current themes in neuroimaging of epilepsy: brain networks, dynamic phenomena, and clinical relevance. Clin Neurophysiol 2010;121(8):1153–75.

5. Binder JR. Preoperative prediction of verbal episodic memory outcome using FMRI. Neurosurg Clin N Am 2011;22(2):219–32, ix.

6. Chelune GJ. Hippocampal adequacy versus functional reserve: predicting memory functions following temporal lobectomy. Arch Clin Neuropsychol 1995; 10(5):413–32.

7. Harvey DJ, Naugle RI, Magleby J, et al. Relationship between presurgical memory performance on the Wechsler Memory Scale-III and memory change following temporal resection for treatment of intractable epilepsy. Epilepsy Behav 2008; 13(2):372–5.

8. Milner B. Memory and the medial temporal regions of the brain. In: Pribram KH, Broadbent DE, editors. Biology of memory. NewYork: Academic Press; 1970. p. 29–50.

9. McAndrews MP, Cohn M. Neuropsychology in temporal lobe epilepsy: influences from cognitive neuroscience and functional neuroimaging. Epilepsy Res Treat 2012;2012:925238.

10. Jones-Gotman M, Smith ML, Risse GL, et al. The contribution of neuropsychology to diagnostic assessment in epilepsy. Epilepsy Behav 2010; 18(1–2):3–12.

11. Saling MM. Verbal memory in mesial temporal lobe epilepsy: beyond material specificity. Brain 2009; 132(Pt 3):570–82.

12. Braak H, Braak E. Evolution of the neuropathology of Alzheimer's disease. Acta Neurol Scand Suppl 1996;165:3–12.

13. Whitwell JL, Przybelski SA, Weigand SD, et al. 3D maps from multiple MRI illustrate changing atrophy patterns as subjects progress from mild cognitive impairment to Alzheimer's disease. Brain 2007; 130(Pt 7):1777–86.

14. Jack CR Jr, Petersen RC, Xu Y, et al. Rates of hippocampal atrophy correlate with change in clinical status in aging and AD. Neurology 2000;55(4):484–9.

15. Risacher SL, Saykin AJ, West JD, et al. Baseline MRI predictors of conversion from MCI to probable AD in the ADNI cohort. Curr Alzheimer Res 2009; 6(4):347–61.

16. Binder JR, Bellgowan PS, Hammeke TA, et al. A comparison of two FMRI protocols for eliciting hippocampal activation. Epilepsia 2005;46(7): 1061–70.

17. Stern CE, Corkin S, Gonzalez RG, et al. The hippocampal formation participates in novel picture encoding: evidence from functional magnetic resonance imaging. Proc Natl Acad Sci U S A 1996;93(16):8660–5.

18. Harrington GS, Tomaszewski FS, Buonocore MH, et al. The intersubject and intrasubject reproducibility of FMRI activation during three encoding tasks: implications for clinical applications. Neuroradiology 2006;48(7):495–505.

19. Davachi L, Wagner AD. Hippocampal contributions to episodic encoding: insights from relational and item-based learning. J Neurophysiol 2002;88(2): 982–90.

20. Kirwan CB, Stark CE. Medial temporal lobe activation during encoding and retrieval of novel face-name pairs. Hippocampus 2004;14(7):919–30.

21. Giovanello KS, Schnyer DM, Verfaellie M. A critical role for the anterior hippocampus in relational memory: evidence from an fMRI study comparing associative and item recognition. Hippocampus 2004;14(1):5–8.

22. Cohn M, Moscovitch M, Lahat A, et al. Recollection versus strength as the primary determinant of hippocampal engagement at retrieval. Proc Natl Acad Sci U S A 2009;106(52):22451–5.

23. Rugg MD, Vilberg KL, Mattson JT, et al. Item memory, context memory and the hippocampus: fMRI evidence. Neuropsychologia 2012;50(13):3070–9.

24. Ranganath C, Yonelinas AP, Cohen MX, et al. Dissociable correlates of recollection and familiarity within the medial temporal lobes. Neuropsychologia 2004;42(1):2–13.

25. Maguire EA. Neuroimaging studies of autobiographical event memory. Philos Trans R Soc Lond B Biol Sci 2001;356(1413):1441–51.

26. Addis DR, Moscovitch M, Crawley AP, et al. Recollective qualities modulate hippocampal activation during autobiographical memory retrieval. Hippocampus 2004;14(6):752–62.

27. Svoboda E, McKinnon MC, Levine B. The functional neuroanatomy of autobiographical memory: a meta-analysis. Neuropsychologia 2006;44(12): 2189–208.

28. Cohn M, McAndrews MP, Moscovitch M. Associative reinstatement: a novel approach to assessing associative memory in patients with unilateral temporal lobe excisions. Neuropsychologia 2009; 47(13):2989–94.

29. St-Laurent M, Moscovitch M, Levine B, et al. Determinants of autobiographical memory in patients with unilateral temporal lobe epilepsy or excisions. Neuropsychologia 2009;47(11):2211–21.

30. Thaiss L, Petrides M. Source versus content memory in patients with a unilateral frontal cortex or a

temporal lobe excision. Brain 2003;126(Pt 5): 1112–26.

31. Viskontas IV, McAndrews MP, Moscovitch M. Remote episodic memory deficits in patients with unilateral temporal lobe epilepsy and excisions. J Neurosci 2000;20(15):5853–7.

32. Moran M, Seidenberg M, Sabsevitz D, et al. The acquisition of face and person identity information following anterior temporal lobectomy. J Int Neuropsychol Soc 2005;11(3):237–48.

33. Smith ML, Bigel M, Miller LA. Visual paired-associate learning: in search of material-specific effects in adult patients who have undergone temporal lobectomy. Epilepsy Behav 2011;20(2): 326–30.

34. Detre JA, Maccotta L, King D, et al. Functional MRI lateralization of memory in temporal lobe epilepsy. Neurology 1998;50(4):926–32.

35. Rabin ML, Narayan VM, Kimberg DY, et al. Functional MRI predicts post-surgical memory following temporal lobectomy. Brain 2004;127 (Pt 10):2286–98.

36. Szaflarski JP, Holland SK, Schmithorst VJ, et al. High-resolution functional MRI at 3T in healthy and epilepsy subjects: hippocampal activation with picture encoding task. Epilepsy Behav 2004; 5(2):244–52.

37. Vannest J, Szaflarski JP, Privitera MD, et al. Medial temporal fMRI activation reflects memory lateralization and memory performance in patients with epilepsy. Epilepsy Behav 2008;12(3):410–8.

38. Mechanic-Hamilton D, Korczykowski M, Yushkevich PA, et al. Hippocampal volumetry and functional MRI of memory in temporal lobe epilepsy. Epilepsy Behav 2009;16(1):128–38.

39. Bigras C, Shear PK, Vannest J, et al. The effects of temporal lobe epilepsy on scene encoding. Epilepsy Behav 2013;26(1):11–21.

40. Jokeit H, Okujava M, Woermann FG. Memory fMRI lateralizes temporal lobe epilepsy. Neurology 2001; 57(10):1786–93.

41. Janszky J, Jokeit H, Kontopoulou K, et al. Functional MRI predicts memory performance after right mesiotemporal epilepsy surgery. Epilepsia 2005; 46(2):244–50.

42. Kennepohl S, Sziklas V, Garver KE, et al. Memory and the medial temporal lobe: hemispheric specialization reconsidered. Neuroimage 2007; 36(3):969–78.

43. Richardson MP, Strange BA, Thompson PJ, et al. Pre-operative verbal memory fMRI predicts postoperative memory decline after left temporal lobe resection. Brain 2004;127(Pt 11):2419–26.

44. Richardson MP, Strange BA, Duncan JS, et al. Memory fMRI in left hippocampal sclerosis: optimizing the approach to predicting postsurgical memory. Neurology 2006;66(5):699–705.

45. Dupont S, Van de Moortele PF, Samson S, et al. Episodic memory in left temporal lobe epilepsy: a functional MRI study. Brain 2000;123(Pt 8): 1722–32.

46. Dupont S, Samson Y, Van de Moortele PF, et al. Delayed verbal memory retrieval: a functional MRI study in epileptic patients with structural lesions of the left medial temporal lobe. Neuroimage 2001;14(5):995–1003.

47. Golby AJ, Poldrack RA, Illes J, et al. Memory lateralization in medial temporal lobe epilepsy assessed by functional MRI. Epilepsia 2002;43(8): 855–63.

48. Powell HW, Richardson MP, Symms MR, et al. Reorganization of verbal and nonverbal memory in temporal lobe epilepsy due to unilateral hippocampal sclerosis. Epilepsia 2007;48(8):1512–25.

49. Powell HW, Richardson MP, Symms MR, et al. Preoperative fMRI predicts memory decline following anterior temporal lobe resection. J Neurol Neurosurg Psychiatr 2008;79(6):686–93.

50. Bonelli SB, Powell RH, Yogarajah M, et al. Imaging memory in temporal lobe epilepsy: predicting the effects of temporal lobe resection. Brain 2010; 133(Pt 4):1186–99.

51. Bonelli SB, Thompson PJ, Yogarajah M, et al. Memory reorganization following anterior temporal lobe resection: a longitudinal functional MRI study. Brain 2013;136(Pt 6):1889–900.

52. Binder JR, Sabsevitz DS, Swanson SJ, et al. Use of preoperative functional MRI to predict verbal memory decline after temporal lobe epilepsy surgery. Epilepsia 2008;49(8):1377–94.

53. Labudda K, Mertens M, Aengenendt J, et al. Presurgical language fMRI activation correlates with postsurgical verbal memory decline in left-sided temporal lobe epilepsy. Epilepsy Res 2010; 92(2–3):258–61.

54. Binder JR, Swanson SJ, Sabsevitz DS, et al. A comparison of two fMRI methods for predicting verbal memory decline after left temporal lobectomy: language lateralization versus hippocampal activation asymmetry. Epilepsia 2010;51(4): 618–26.

55. Pustina D, Gizewski E, Forsting M, et al. Human memory manipulated: dissociating factors contributing to MTL activity, an fMRI study. Behav Brain Res 2012;229(1):57–67.

56. Qin S, van Marle HJ, Hermans EJ, et al. Subjective sense of memory strength and the objective amount of information accurately remembered are related to distinct neural correlates at encoding. J Neurosci 2011;31(24):8920–7.

57. Dennis NA, Bowman CR, Vandekar SN. True and phantom recollection: an fMRI investigation of similar and distinct neural correlates and connectivity. Neuroimage 2012;59(3):2982–93.

58. McDermott KB, Szpunar KK, Christ SE. Laboratory-based and autobiographical retrieval tasks differ substantially in their neural substrates. Neuropsychologia 2009;47(11):2290–8.

59. St-Laurent M, Moscovitch M, Jadd R, et al. The perceptual richness of complex memory episodes is compromised by medial temporal lobe damage. Hippocampus 2014;24(5):560–76.

60. Addis DR, Moscovitch M, McAndrews MP. Consequences of hippocampal damage across the autobiographical memory network in left temporal lobe epilepsy. Brain 2007;130(Pt 9):2327–42.

61. Guedj E, Bettus G, Barbeau EJ, et al. Hyperactivation of parahippocampal region and fusiform gyrus associated with successful encoding in medial temporal lobe epilepsy. Epilepsia 2011;52(6):1100–9.

62. Sperling RA, Dickerson BC, Pihlajamaki M, et al. Functional alterations in memory networks in early Alzheimer's disease. Neuromolecular Med 2010;12(1):27–43.

63. Miller SL, Fenstermacher E, Bates J, et al. Hippocampal activation in adults with mild cognitive impairment predicts subsequent cognitive decline. J Neurol Neurosurg Psychiatr 2008;79(6):630–5.

64. Dickerson BC, Salat DH, Greve DN, et al. Increased hippocampal activation in mild cognitive impairment compared to normal aging and AD. Neurology 2005;65(3):404–11.

65. Bakker A, Krauss GL, Albert MS, et al. Reduction of hippocampal hyperactivity improves cognition in amnestic mild cognitive impairment. Neuron 2012;74(3):467–74.

66. Westmacott R, Silver FL, McAndrews MP. Understanding medial temporal activation in memory tasks: evidence from fMRI of encoding and recognition in a case of transient global amnesia. Hippocampus 2008;18(3):317–25.

67. Raichle ME, Krauss GL, Albert MS, et al. A default mode of brain function. Proc Natl Acad Sci U S A 2001;98(2):676–82.

68. Honey CJ, Sporns O, Cammoun L, et al. Predicting human resting-state functional connectivity from structural connectivity. Proc Natl Acad Sci U S A 2009;106(6):2035–40.

69. Buckner RL, Andrews-Hanna JR, Schacter DL. The brain's default network: anatomy, function, and relevance to disease. Ann N Y Acad Sci 2008;1124:1–38.

70. Rugg MD, Vilberg KL. Brain networks underlying episodic memory retrieval. Curr Opin Neurobiol 2013;23(2):255–60.

71. Voets NL, Adcock JE, Stacey R, et al. Functional and structural changes in the memory network associated with left temporal lobe epilepsy. Hum Brain Mapp 2009;30(12):4070–81.

72. Zhang Z, Lu G, Zhong Y, et al. Altered spontaneous neuronal activity of the default-mode network in mesial temporal lobe epilepsy. Brain Res 2010;1323:152–60.

73. Liao W, Zhang Z, Pan Z, et al. Default mode network abnormalities in mesial temporal lobe epilepsy: a study combining fMRI and DTI. Hum Brain Mapp 2011;32(6):883–95.

74. James GA, Tripathi SP, Ojemann JG, et al. Diminished default mode network recruitment of the hippocampus and parahippocampus in temporal lobe epilepsy. J Neurosurg 2013;119(2):288–300.

75. McCormick C, Quraan M, Cohn M, et al. Default mode network connectivity indicates episodic memory capacity in mesial temporal lobe epilepsy. Epilepsia 2013;54(5):809–18.

76. Hayes SM, Salat DH, Verfaellie M. Default network connectivity in medial temporal lobe amnesia. J Neurosci 2012;32(42):14622–9.

77. Wang L, Laviolette P, O'Keefe K, et al. Intrinsic connectivity between the hippocampus and posteromedial cortex predicts memory performance in cognitively intact older individuals. Neuroimage 2010;51(2):910–7.

78. Dunn CJ, Laviolette P, O'Keefe K, et al. Deficits in episodic memory retrieval reveal impaired default mode network connectivity in amnestic mild cognitive impairment. Neuroimage Clin 2014;4:473–80.

79. Wagner K, Frings L, Halsband U, et al. Hippocampal functional connectivity reflects verbal episodic memory network integrity. Neuroreport 2007;18(16):1719–23.

80. Doucet G, Osipowicz K, Sharan A, et al. Extratemporal functional connectivity impairments at rest are related to memory performance in mesial temporal epilepsy. Hum Brain Mapp 2013;34(9):2202–16.

81. Han SD, Arfanakis K, Fleischman DA, et al. Functional connectivity variations in mild cognitive impairment: associations with cognitive function. J Int Neuropsychol Soc 2012;18(1):39–48.

82. Wang Z, Liang P, Jia X, et al. Baseline and longitudinal patterns of hippocampal connectivity in mild cognitive impairment: evidence from resting state fMRI. J Neurol Sci 2011;309(1–2):79–85.

83. Holmes M, Folley BS, Sonmezturk HH, et al. Resting state functional connectivity of the hippocampus associated with neurocognitive function in left temporal lobe epilepsy. Hum Brain Mapp 2014;35(3):735–44.

84. Baxendale SA, van Paesschen W, Thompson PJ, et al. The relationship between quantitative MRI and neuropsychological functioning in temporal lobe epilepsy. Epilepsia 1998;39(2):158–66.

85. Saling MM, Berkovic SF, O'Shea MF, et al. Lateralization of verbal memory and unilateral hippocampal sclerosis: evidence of task-specific effects. J Clin Exp Neuropsychol 1993;15(4):608–18.

86. Lineweaver TT, Morris HH, Naugle RI, et al. Evaluating the contributions of state-of-the-art assessment techniques to predicting memory outcome after unilateral anterior temporal lobectomy. Epilepsia 2006;47(11):1895–903.

87. Sidhu MK, Stretton J, Winston GP, et al. A functional magnetic resonance imaging study mapping the episodic memory encoding network in temporal lobe epilepsy. Brain 2013;136(Pt 6):1868–88.

88. Bonnici HM, Sidhu M, Chadwick MJ, et al. Assessing hippocampal functional reserve in temporal lobe epilepsy: a multi-voxel pattern analysis of fMRI data. Epilepsy Res 2013;105(1–2):140–9.

89. McCormick C, Protzner AB, Barnett AJ, et al. Linking DMN connectivity to episodic memory capacity: what can we learn from patients with medial temporal lobe damage? Neuroimage Clin 2014;5: 188–96.

90. Embleton KV, Haroon HA, Morris DM, et al. Distortion correction for diffusion-weighted MRI tractography and fMRI in the temporal lobes. Hum Brain Mapp 2010;31(10):1570–87.

91. Marshall H, Hajnal JV, Warren JE, et al. An efficient automated z-shim based method to correct through-slice signal loss in EPI at 3T. MAGMA 2009;22(3):187–200.

92. Halai AD, Welbourne SR, Embleton K, et al. A comparison of dual gradient-echo and spin-echo fMRI of the inferior temporal lobe. Hum Brain Mapp 2014;35(8):4118–28.

93. Takeda H, Kim B. Retrospective estimation of the susceptibility driven field map for distortion correction in echo planar imaging. Inf Process Med Imaging 2013;23:352–63.

94. Beisteiner R, Klinger N, Hollinger I, et al. How much are clinical fMRI reports influenced by standard postprocessing methods? An investigation of normalization and region of interest effects in the medial temporal lobe. Hum Brain Mapp 2010;31(12):1951–66.

95. Brandt DJ, Sommer J, Krach S, et al. Test-retest reliability of fMRI brain activity during memory encoding. Front Psychiatry 2013;4:163.

96. Shehzad Z, Kelly AM, Reiss PT, et al. The resting brain: unconstrained yet reliable. Cereb Cortex 2009;19(10):2209–29.

97. Zuo XN, Kelly C, Adelstein JS, et al. Reliable intrinsic connectivity networks: test-retest evaluation using ICA and dual regression approach. Neuroimage 2010;49(3):2163–77.

98. Song J, Desphande AS, Meier TB, et al. Age-related differences in test-retest reliability in resting-state brain functional connectivity. PLoS One 2012;7(12):e49847.

99. Birn RM, Molloy EK, Patriat R, et al. The effect of scan length on the reliability of resting-state fMRI connectivity estimates. Neuroimage 2013;83: 550–8.

100. Babiloni C, Vecchio F, Altavilla R, et al. Hypercapnia affects the functional coupling of resting state electroencephalographic rhythms and cerebral haemodynamics in healthy elderly subjects and in patients with amnestic mild cognitive impairment. Clin Neurophysiol 2014;125(4):685–93.

101. Gomez-Gonzalo M, Losi G, Brondi M, et al. Ictal but not interictal epileptic discharges activate astrocyte endfeet and elicit cerebral arteriole responses. Front Cell Neurosci 2011;5:8.

102. Rosengarten B, Paulsen S, Burr O, et al. Neurovascular coupling in Alzheimer patients: effect of acetylcholine-esterase inhibitors. Neurobiol Aging 2009;30(12):1918–23.

Preoperative Diffusion Tensor Imaging
Improving Neurosurgical Outcomes in Brain Tumor Patients

John L. Ulmer, MD[a],*, Andrew P. Klein, MD[a], Wade M. Mueller, MD[b],
Edgar A. DeYoe, PhD[a], Leighton P. Mark, MD[a]

KEYWORDS

• Neurosurgery • Outcome • Diffusion tensor imaging • Brain mapping

KEY POINTS

- Preoperative mapping has revolutionized the neurosurgical care of brain tumor patients.
- Maximizing resections more safely has improved diagnosis, optimized treatment algorithms, and significantly decreased potentially devastating postoperative deficits associated with injury to functional brain networks.
- Although this mapping process has multiple steps and complimentary localization sources, diffusion tensor imaging (DTI) stands out for its essential role in depicting individual white matter tracts.
- A thorough understanding of DTI technique, data visualization, and limitations with a mastery of functional and dysfunctional white matter anatomy is necessary to realize the potential of this technology.
- By establishing spatial relationships between specific lesion borders and functional networks preoperatively and perioperatively, DTI is cementing its role in high-risk neurosurgical resections and becoming the standard of care.

INTRODUCTION

Neurosurgical care of brain tumor patients is undergoing a major shift with the emergence of preoperative brain mapping using advanced imaging techniques. This shift involves improved diagnostic and prognostic measures as well as improved patient outcomes, including significantly decreased morbidity in an otherwise inherently high-risk arena. Although preoperative mapping in tumor patients is a multistep process, it is diffusion tensor imaging (DTI) that has made the most profound impact, taking an expedited translational route from research to clinical practice. As with any tool, it is only as powerful as the person using it. Understanding the DTI technique, data visualization methods, effect of pathologic processes, and technical limitations is essential in the application to preoperative brain mapping. Combining the DTI data with expertise in white matter anatomy and functional and dysfunctional brain networks enables the physician to create a patient-specific neurosurgical plan that defines the spatial relationships between the lesion and functional brain networks, thereby guiding intraoperative assessments. The following explores the emerging and powerful clinical application of preoperative DTI.

[a] Department of Radiology, Medical College of Wisconsin, 8701 Watertown Plank Road, Milwaukee, WI 53226, USA; [b] Department of Neurosurgery, Medical College of Wisconsin, 8701 Watertown Plank Road, Milwaukee, WI 53226, USA
* Corresponding author.
E-mail address: julmer@mcw.edu

Neuroimag Clin N Am 24 (2014) 599–617
http://dx.doi.org/10.1016/j.nic.2014.08.002
1052-5149/14/$ – see front matter © 2014 Elsevier Inc. All rights reserved

RATIONALE FOR BRAIN TUMOR SURGERY AND PREOPERATIVE DIFFUSION TENSOR IMAGING

The primary goals for neurosurgical resection of brain tumors are to establish a histologic diagnosis and achieve maximal cytoreduction. Because of the histologic heterogeneity in gliomas, gross total resections are preferable to subtotal resections or biopsies for accurate diagnosis, biomarker analysis, and optimization of treatment algorithms. Treatment algorithms usually include adjuvant radiotherapy, chemotherapy, or both. Maximal cytoreduction has been theorized to decrease cell populations that could convert to higher grade neoplasms[1,2] and improve the effectiveness of adjuvant therapies by altering cell kinetics and reducing cell populations resistant to chemoradiation. Point of fact, resection extent of high-grade and low-grade gliomas has been shown to correlate with improved survival.[1,3–6] Furthermore, up to 53% of glioma patients may show improved neurologic function after resection.[7] Operative excision of primary brain tumors can also decrease steroid dependence and seizure activity. For the foreseeable future, surgical resection of brain tumors will play a major role in brain tumor therapy.

Before the era of modern preoperative brain mapping, neurologic complication rates for brain tumor resections ranged from 7% to 26%.[7–15] However, preoperative mapping has the potential to decrease postoperative complications to well below these standards. DTI shows particular promise to improve surgical outcomes in guiding intraoperative functional resection boundaries. During initial internal translation of preoperative DTI at the Medical College of Wisconsin (MCW) in 2004, a pilot study compared postoperative outcomes after resections of left dominant high-risk posterior frontal lobe tumors in 18 patients before DTI implementation and 15 patients after DTI implementation.[16,17] The patient groups were matched by age, gender, histology, tumor size, and location, and with resections performed by the same neurosurgeon with identical technique. Postoperative edema and/or surgical injury resulted in speech and motor deficits in 44% and 47% of the patients in each group, respectively. However, 39% of patients without the advantage afforded by preoperative DTI had persistent speech and/or motor deficits at 1 month after surgery, resulting from surgical injury to eloquent networks. This compared with only 7% ($P<.05$) for those patients with preoperative DTI available to guide resection boundaries. Recovery of deficits was presumed to be owing to resolution of postoperative edema. Since then, with further refinements in the DTI application, postoperative neurologic complication rates have fallen to less than half of this benchmark.[17,18]

Other investigators utilized a prospective, randomized design to demonstrate the impact of DTI integrated tract data into neurosurgical navigational systems. In a prospective, randomized investigation, the effect of DTI on survival and postoperative neurologic outcomes was assessed. The results showed a significantly decreased incidence in postoperative motor deficits from 33% (120 patients) to 15% (118 patients) in brain tumor patients with motor tract involvement, by exporting preoperative DTI to the intraoperative navigational system.[19] Significantly higher 6-month Karnofsky performance scores were evident in the latter group. In addition, survival was positively impacted. For the high-grade tumor subgroup (81 patients), median survival increased significantly from 14 to 21 months with the intraoperative use of preoperative DTI data. Mounting experimental data and anecdotal experience are securing a place for preoperative DTI in treatment algorithms for brain tumor patients.

UNDERSTANDING WHITE MATTER ANATOMY

A thorough understanding of white matter anatomy as reflected by DTI is required for the technique to impact surgical decision making. This requires recognition that DTI is an imperfect indicator of white matter structure and function, and that the understanding of the same in the human animal is evolving. We are some distance from fully understanding the functionality of complex human white matter networks. To date, our understanding of white matter functional networks is derived from 2 main lines of evidence, namely experimental nonhuman animal tracings and human lesion deficit localization inferences. Inferences about white matter functionality based on anatomic connectivity studies are limited by our incomplete understanding of functional cortical networks. Inferences about white matter deficits associated with surgical injury based on lesion-localization studies are limited by several factors. Most reports of deficits associated with specific white matter injury provide no patient population denominator, and as such the deficit predictability of any one individual is unknown. This may be influenced by individual variability as well as redundancy inherent in the networks. Lesions involving adjacent functional cortex or functionally distinct white matter pathways in the same anatomic region complicate lesion localization analyses further.

More elementary functional networks, such as primary motor and vision, are fairly well understood and have been deliberately avoided during neurosurgical procedures for many years. Preoperative DTI can be readily translated to complement surgical decision making in avoiding motor or vision deficits. Conversely, identifying critical white matter networks subserving higher cognitive functions is complicated by our evolving understanding of these functional networks, limitations of functional magnetic resonance imaging (fMRI), limitations of DTI, and patient variability. Autoradiographic tract tracing studies in nonhuman primates have revealed a tremendous amount of detail regarding white matter tract organization.[20] Much of this information is directly transferable to the human brain. In other cases, however, it is not. For example, the lack of complex speech and language capabilities in nonhuman primates remains a major obstacle in applying these data directly to the human language system on a patient-by-patient basis. Emerging theories of ventral and dorsal language organization[21–24] may aid in establishing which association tracts are necessary and thus to be avoided during surgery. Ultimately, our current understanding of cognitive white matter functional networks may only provide a frame of reference by which to impart preoperative risks to our neurosurgical colleagues. However, DTI as is can guide intraoperative mapping strategies. Reviews of white matter connectivity and deficits associated with lesions are available,[25,26] much of which is also reflected in Tables 1 and 2.

FUNCTIONAL LOCALIZATION SOURCES

Given the limitations of our understanding of white matter networks and the limitations of the DTI technique, complimentary preoperative and perioperative localization sources are necessary to establish functional network proximity risks. These sources include clinical presentation, functional anatomy at standard imaging, preoperative functional mapping techniques, intraoperative functional white matter testing, and intraoperative electrocortical mapping.[18,27–33] Each of these sources is an imperfect indicator of proximity risk alone, but together can provide critical functional information.

Clinical presentation is a localizing parameter in and of itself. A lesion-induced persistent deficit is an indicator of proximity and operative risk for that particular function. An understanding of localized lesion-induced deficits helps to determine the source of such deficits, and relevant reviews on the topic are available.[17,25,26,34] A presenting deficit that persists has a fairly high positive predictive value that the lesion has proximity to eloquent structures. However, a transient deficit associated with seizure activity lowers positive predictive value considerably, owing to the potential for propagation of epileptogenic activity. A high negative predictive value (NPV) should not be assumed because seizures and persistent deficits may be absent even though a lesion has proximity to eloquent structures. Handedness determines the likelihood of left hemisphere language dominance.[27] Right-handed individuals have a 98% chance of being left hemisphere dominant for language function. This means for every 100 mapping cases performed on right-handers, 2 of them will have significant language function in the right hemisphere. Left-handed individuals have a 67% chance of being left dominant. The remaining 33% of left handers are either right hemisphere dominant for language or have shared hemisphere function. Hemispheric dominance established by fMRI informs significance to potential language networks in the lesional hemisphere established at DTI.

Knowledge of *functional anatomy at standard imaging* is critical in the interpretation of preoperative DTI data. Alone, DTI can be limited in establishing functional network proximity because of pathophysiologic constraints. In clinical practice, the color-coded fractional anisotropy (CC-FA) maps are superimposed on anatomic imaging sequences to optimally characterize relationships of white matter structures to pathologic processes (Fig. 1). Anatomic distortion of perilesional white matter from edema and infiltrating tumor may obscure or reorient tracts, making them difficult to discern on CC DTI. With the use of standard imaging, expected relationships of tracts to each other and to gyral and sulcal landmarks can help to predict functional network proximity when tract directions are altered or FA is reduced.

Preoperative mapping techniques, including DTI and fMRI, are complementary in defining spatial relationships between lesion borders and functional brain networks. DTI evaluates white matter proximity, and fMRI evaluates eloquent cortex proximity. Investigators have found that the combined use of DTI and fMRI is superior to fMRI alone for preoperative functional system risk-proximity designations.[17,29] In fact, NPV for a postoperative functional deficit can approach 100% using these techniques.[17] Scenarios exist where deep brain lesions are remote from functional cortex, but may have proximity to multiple critical white matter networks (see Fig. 1). In general, the deeper the lesion is located within the brain, the more likely multiple functional white matter networks will be at risk. Preoperative DTI may provide critical information, even when fMRI is unnecessary. On the other hand, fMRI may inform the interpretation of DTI, helping to assign significance to adjacent white

Table 1
Association tract anatomy and proposed or observed deficits

Tract	Reciprocal Connections	Proposed Functions	Proposed or Observed Deficits
SLF I	Caudal aspect of the superior parietal lobule, and superior frontal gyrus (BA 6, 9, including SMA region).	Higher-order motor function. Initiation of planned motor movements and selection of competing conditional associative motor tasks, such as driving.	Compromised selection of competing conditional associative motor tasks.
SLF II	Caudal aspect of the inferior parietal lobule and lower bank of the intraparietal sulcus and frontal lobe (BA 6, 8, 9, 46).	Conveys visuospatial information to prefrontal cortex. Ventral component of the dorsal visual processing stream, involved in spatial attention and engagement in the environment.	Visuospatial and visual attention deficits.
SLF III	Rostral portion of the inferior parietal lobule and parietal operculum and frontal lobe (BA 6, 44, ventral 46).	Involved in goal-direction motor behavior. Involved in imitation, and gestural and possible linguistic communication. Likely involved in phonemic and articulatory aspects of language, as the dorsal language pathway of the dominant hemisphere.	Ideomotor apraxia (*left*). Phonemic and articulatory deficits (*left*).
SLF IV	Caudal aspect of the superior temporal lobe, including superior temporal gyrus and sulcus, and frontal lobe (dorsal BA 8, 46, 6).	Auditory spatial bundle. May not be directly linked to language areas as previously thought.	Deficits in auditory discrimination.
SFOF	Medial preoccipital area, lateral-dorsal preoccipital area, medial parietal area, caudal cingulate gyrus, caudal inferior parietal lobule, and dorsolateral prefrontal cortex. Ventrally rests on the SCF.	Dorsal component of the dorsal visual processing stream. Involved in action tracking and reaching, visual guidance of movements, maintenance of vigilance and spatial aspects of attention through connections to supplementary eye fields.	Deficits in visuospatial processing. Optic ataxia.
IFOF	Presence is disputed, but believed by advocates to connect occipital and posterior temporal lobes, and dorsal/ventral prefrontal cortex. Posterior terminations include posterior MTG and ITG, fusiform/lingual gyri.	Conveys information between visual association areas and frontal lobes. Implicated in ventral (semantic) language network functions, based on intraoperative stimulation studies.	Semantic paraphasias with intraoperative stimulation. Possible visuospatial and visual recognition deficits.

ILF	Ventral occipital lobe, parietal lobe including intraparietal sulcus, and temporal lobe including parahippocampal gyrus.	Component of ventral processing stream that is involved in object/place/face/word (left) recognition. Involved in visual associative memory, analysis of visual motion, visual spatial analysis and attention. Plays subsidiary role in the ventral language stream.	Visual agnosias (objects, words, faces, places). Visual memory deficits. Visual hypo-emotionality.
UF	Anterior and medial temporal lobe (rostral STG and ITG, parahippocampal gyrus, amygdala), and orbitofrontal/medial prefrontal/ventrolateral prefrontal cortex. Also amygdala to anterior and inferior temporal cortex.	Connects areas of sound recognition, memory recognition, and is involved in processing of emotion, inhibition and self-regulation. Important in the interactions between auditory stimuli, cognition and emotion. *Right:* Engaging visual or multimodal imagery necessary for retrieval of autobiographical or event memories. *Left:* Storage and access to remote semantic and lexical memories.	*Right:* Disturbances in retrieval of episodic, context-dependent memory (memory of personal experiences). *Left:* Semantic, context-free memory (learned concepts and facts).
CG	Limbic pathway connecting septal area to the uncus, coursing within the cingulate and parahippocampal gyri. *Anterior CG:* Connects frontal lobe, parietal lobe, amygdala, hippocampus, medial dorsal thalamus, basal ganglia, brainstem motor nuclei, and hypothalamus. *Posterior CG:* Connects temporal association, medial temporal, parietal, orbitofrontal, and dorsolateral prefrontal cortex.	*Anterior CG:* Attention, volitional control of cognition and motor functions. *Anterior CG (rostral):* Involved in emotion and visceral functions. *Anterior CG (caudal):* Involved in cognition and higher-order motor control. *Posterior CG:* Monitoring sensory events and behavior in the service of memory and spatial orientation. Visuospatial processing and verbal memory. Processing of phasic pain and transforming aversive input into movements. Possible role in stimulus-driven, smooth pursuit, and reflexive eye movements.	*Anterior CG:* Pain unconsciousness. Akinetic mutism (*left*). Deficits of saccades and internally driven eye movements. *Posterior CG:* Retrosplenial amnesia. Visuospatial, visual memory and verbal memory deficits.

"Left" assumes left dominant and "right" assumes nondominant.

Abbreviations: BA, Brodmann areas; CG, cingulum; IFOF, inferior fronto-occipital fasciculus; ILF, inferior longitudinal fasciculus; ITG, inferior temporal gyrus; MTG, middle temporal gyrus; SCF, subcallosal fasciculus; SFOF, superior fronto-occipital fasciculus; SLF, superior longitudinal fasciculus; SMA, supplementary motor area; STG, superior temporal gyrus; UF, uncinate fasciculus.

Table 2
Projection tract and corpus callosum anatomy and observed deficits

Tract	Projections and Connections	Observed Deficits
SCF	Corticosubcortical connections from anterior cingulate gyrus and pre-SMA/SMA region to the corpus striatum.	*Left:* Akinetic mutism. Disorders of preparation and initiation of speech. Transcortical motor aphasia, anomia, and delayed initiation of speech with preserved articulation observed with intraoperative stimulation.
ALIC	Corticofugal motor and thalamocortical sensory projection fibers form compact WM bundles in the corona radiata and internal capsule. The ALIC contains anterior thalamic sensory and FPT motor fibers.	Impairment of inhibitory reflexive eye saccades with injury to the FPT connecting the dorsolateral PFC to superior colliculi. Ipsilesional conjugate eye deviation with injury to the FPT connected to the superior colliculus or paramedian pontine reticular formation.
GIC	Corticofugal motor and thalamocortical sensory projection fibers make up compact WM bundles in the corona radiata and internal capsule. The GIC contains anterior and inferior thalamic fibers and the corticobulbar tract.	*GIC:* Contralateral faciolingual weakness. Subcortical dementia and executive memory disorder with injuries to thalamofrontal/ thalamolimbic fibers. Contralesional intermittent failure to maintain sustained muscle contraction. *GIC and ALIC:* Impaired motor control circuit with injury to vestibulocerebellar and cerebello-rubro-thalamic pathways and fibers from SMA and prefrontal region projecting to the thalamus. *GIC–PLIC junction:* Contralesional motor and sensory deficits of fingers, face, and tongue. Verbal memory deterioration (left dominant). Dizziness/vertigo with injury to the vestibulothalamic pathway (right or left).
PLIC	Corticofugal motor and thalamocortical sensory projection fibers make up compact WM bundles in the corona radiata and internal capsule. The PLIC contains superior, posterior, and inferolateral thalamic fibers, the corticospinal tract, and the TPOPT. The retrolenticuar portion of the PLIC contains components of the optic and acoustic radiations.	Apathy and impaired consciousness. Contralesional hemiparesis/ hemiplegia. Contralesional hemianesthesia with injury to the thalamocortical sensory pathway. Contralesional hemiataxia with injury to cerebellar dentato-rubro-thalamocortical and corticopontocerebellar pathways. Verbal memory loss (*left*). Ipsilesional conjugate eye deviation with injury to the TPOPT connected to the superior colliculus or paramedian pontine reticular formation. Impairment in the reflexive eye saccades owing to the injury to the parietotectal fibers.

FX	Limbic structure connecting the hippocampus with the hypothalamus and basal forebrain nuclei.	Memory deficits, learning dysfunction, antegrade amnesia, temporally graded retrograde amnesia. Visual memory deficits (*right*). Verbal memory deficits (*left*).
OR	Project from the lateral geniculate nucleus to the primary visual cortex. Superior fibers course backward toward the occipital lobe, and inferior fibers course anteroinferiorly around the temporal horn before coursing posteriorly to the primary visual cortex and form Meyer's loop.	Contralesional visual field deficits. Lower visual field deficit from injury to superior fibers. Superior visual field deficit from injury to inferior fibers. Visual field deficits may occur from injury to the optic radiation located in the retrolenticular portion of the PLIC.
AR	Project from medial geniculate nucleus to the primary auditory cortex. AR fibers course through the retrolenticular portion of the PLIC.	Auditory agnosia. Word deafness (bilateral or left). Amusia (right > left). Environmental sound agnosia (bilateral or right).
CC	Connects homologous neocortical areas across hemispheres.	*Genu and anterior body:* Nondominant limb apraxia, frontocallosal alien hand syndrome, cognitive dysfunction. *Posterior body and splenium:* Left ideomotor apraxia, left hand tactile anomia, left visual field color anomia, associative visual agnosia, left visual field dyslexia, left hand agraphia, right hand constructural apraxia, left hemispatial neglect, left motor neglect, callosal alien hand syndrome, visuomotor delay, optic ataxia, and auditory disconnection.

"Left" assumes left dominant and "right" assumes nondominant.

Abbreviations: ALIC, anterior limb internal capsule; AR, acoustic radiation; CC, corpus callosum; FPT, frontopontine tract; FX, fornix; GIC, genu internal capsule; OR, optic radiation; PFC, prefrontal cortex; PLIC, posterior limb internal capsule; SCF, subcallosal fasciculus; SMA, supplementary motor area; TPOPT, temporo-parieto-occipital pontine tract.

A

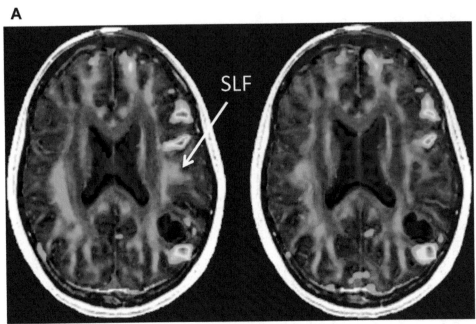

Fig. 1. A 34-year-old, right-handed woman with a posterior parasylvian low-grade glioma, presenting with seizure-induced transient aphasia and agraphia. SPGR gadolinium-enhanced underlays with 50% faded color-coded fractional anisotropy (CC-FA) diffusion tensor imaging (DTI) map overlays optimize viewing of eloquent white matter relationships. Functional activation at functional magnetic resonance imaging (fMRI) is associated with reading comprehension. Note focal activation within the posterior aspect of the left middle temporal gyrus and the angular gyrus, areas thought to play a key role in semantic storage and retrieval, immediately adjacent to the lesion. Left dominant language activation at fMRI, a clinical presentation with language deficits, and right-handedness provide concordant evidence of left hemispheric language dominance, thereby informing the significance of regional white matter networks. (A) Axial CC-FA DTI maps show the horizontal aspect of the superior longitudinal fasciculus (SLF) anterior to the lesion. SLF III is positioned most laterally within the horizontal bundle, but is not distinguishable at CC-FA from SLF II and IV running more medially. (B) Coronal DTI shows the relationships of the lesion to the fiber bundle (*yellow arrows*) containing optic radiations (OR), inferior longitudinal fasciculus (ILF), and inferior fronto-occipital fasciculus (IFOF), although specific functional networks cannot be distinguished from one another with CC-FA maps. The lesion has no immediate proximity to visual cortex, but visual function is nevertheless at surgical risk. (C) Sagittal DTI shows the relationship of the lesion to the horizontal bundle of the SLF (*yellow arrow*), the vertical portion of the SLF (SLF IV; *blue arrow*), and the fiber bundle containing the ILF, IFOF, and OR (*white arrow*). The relationship to the lesion of terminal innervation of surrounding eloquent language cortex is unknown, owing to limitations of DTI and fMRI in defining juxtacortical white matter and critical cortical nodes, respectively. The preoperative mapping results indicate key lesion borders for intraoperative functional white matter testing, as well as the need for electrocortical mapping of language functions.

matter. This is especially true in matters of hemispheric dominance.

Intraoperative localization techniques, including functional white matter testing and electrocortical stimulation, are critical in border risk assessments and in defining functional resection boundaries. When used in conjunction with lesion border risk designations derived from preoperative mapping, these techniques can be utilized most powerfully (**Fig. 2**). Electrocortical stimulation is a direct means of identifying eloquent cortex and is complimentary to preoperative fMRI. To establish functional white matter resection boundaries, preoperative DTI seeks to designate borders

specifically by functional risks and guide intraoperative testing. Intraoperative electrical white matter stimulation is 1 method used for functional white matter testing.[30,31] At MCW, intraoperative functional dissection testing is performed by the *Mueller* method.[17,18] In conjunction with border risk designations derived from preoperative DTI, an ultrasonic aspirator is used that not only provides tissue fragmentation, irrigation, aspiration, and coagulation, but has a close-distance, nonlethal, and transient effect on neuronal tissue. Thus, the technique affords a particularly efficient means of establishing functional resection boundaries intraoperatively. The approach has been

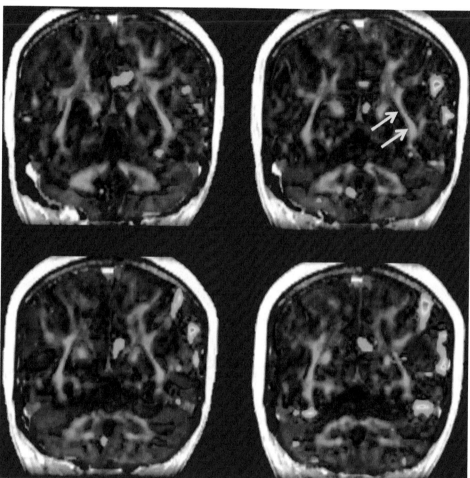

Fig. 1.

utilized and refined in more than 800 preoperative mapping cases at our institution. Periodic retrospective review of our neurosurgical outcomes at MCW reveals a benchmark of less than 3% postoperative neurologic complications using this approach. In current practice, nearly all postoperative neurologic complications at our institution arise from small vessel injury and stroke. The importance of a high NPV for preoperative lesion border risk assessments cannot be overstated. A false-negative border risk designation at DTI could lead to failure to test functions along a dissection border and consequent injury to critical white matter structures.

DIFFUSION TENSOR IMAGING ACQUISITION AND VISUALIZATION
Color-Coded Fractional Anisotropy Maps

For CC-FA maps, a dual-refocused spin echo technique is used to minimize distortions and maximize signal-to-noise ratio (SNR). At least 6 orthogonal gradient encoding directions are required to construct a diffusion ellipsoid, but 12 or more are preferred to minimize directional undersampling at fiber crossings and at acute angulations. Higher read out times and diffusion weighting can be chosen to achieve higher DTI resolution, but at the expense of lower SNR and increased scan duration. For 1.5 T at MCW, CC-FA maps are acquired as 3 modular datasets with 3-mm slice thickness, 13 gradient encoding directions, b value of 900, number of excitations of 2, echo time (TE) of 70 ms, and minimum repetition time (TR) of 11 s are used to acquire a total of 40 contiguous slices. Typically, 128 × 128 matrix and a field of view of 20 to 24 cm will be acquired, with in-plane resolution generally at 1.8 × 1.8 mm. Acquisition time is 5.5 minutes for each dataset, with a total time of 16.5 minutes for all 3 datasets. Three averaged datasets at 1.5 T provide an SNR equivalent to a single run with a number of

C

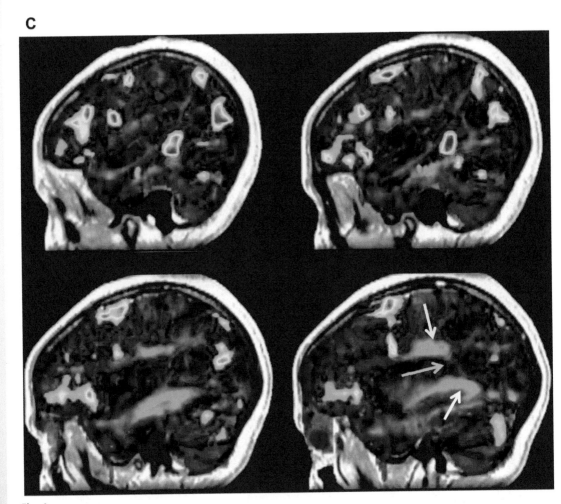

Fig. 1.

excitations of 6, with SNR to spare. If a patient can only withstand 1-, or 2-, 5.5-min acquisitions, the data are aesthetically compromised, but still diagnostic. For 2.5- and 2-mm slice thicknesses, however, 4 and 6 averaged 5.5-min datasets, respectively, are required to achieve diagnostic SNR. Movement between data acquisitions can be corrected in post processing. The DTI data are suitable, although not optimal, for fiber tracking if needed (see Fiber Tracking).

At 3 T, MRI sequence parameters are similar, although slice thickness is typically reduced. Higher TR may be needed, a b value of 1000 or greater, and up to 50 slices are acquired. We generally acquire data at 2-mm slice thickness requiring 3 acquisitions to achieve nearly isotropic voxels of 1.87 × 1.87 × 2 mm with sufficient signal. DTI data at 1.5 or 3 T are acquired in the axial plane and reconstructed in coronal and sagittal planes and superimposed onto desired underlay images for all cases. Because DTI is

acquired with other mapping data, including fMRI, patients with prior surgeries or biopsies are scanned at 1.5 T to reduce susceptibility. Sequence parameters are customized to optimize patient compliance and minimize motion effects, depending the length of time required to acquire DTI and other mapping data. Generally, however, 3 runs at 3-mm (1.5 T) or 2-mm (3 T) slice thicknesses suffice. The ellipsoid, or diffusion tensor, is the basis by which relative directional information of white matter can be displayed on a voxel-by-voxel basis. Information from the 3 components of the diffusion tensor vector are displayed in CC-FA maps.[35] These maps enable one to visualize the anatomic organization of white matter tracts with the added value of directionality. At any 1 voxel on the image, 1 of 3 colors is assigned according to the eigenvector with the greatest eigenvalue. By convention, green represents the anteroposterior (or posteroanterior) direction, red the transverse (right to left or left

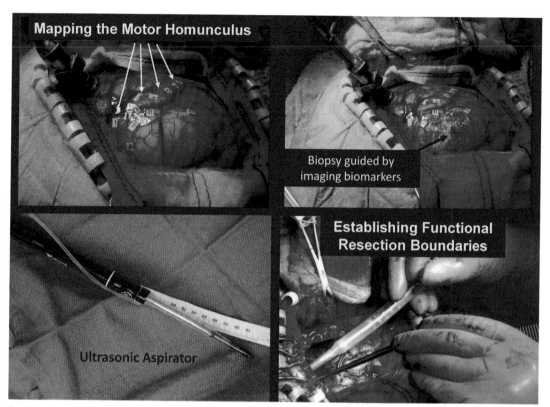

Fig. 2. Intraoperative functional localization techniques. (*Upper left*) Electrocortical stimulation mapping (ECS) of eloquent cortex provides for safe surgical trajectory in approaching a brain tumor. Letter tags identify lesion borders defined by intraoperative ultrasonography, and number tags identify the motor homunculus defined by ECS. (*Upper right*) Biopsy samples targeting highly cellular or metabolically active tumor tissues are chosen to avoid eloquent cortex. (*Lower left*) The ultrasonic aspirator, a surgical tool used to dissect tissues, has a close-distance, stunning effect on neural tissue causing transient intraoperative neurologic deficits. (*Lower right*) Intraoperative testing of white matter function along specific borders defined by preoperative diffusion tensor imaging (DTI) provides functional resection boundaries, avoiding permanent neurologic deficits.

to right) direction, and blue the craniocaudad (or caudocranial) direction; color intensities reflect the magnitude of the FA value.

A benefit of CC-FA maps is the ability to visualize global white matter architecture by the same method conventional MR images is displayed, in the axial, coronal, and sagittal planes. For optimal visualization, CC-FA maps are faded to 50% and superimposed on anatomic fluid-attenuated inversion recovery images and post contrast spoiled gradient recalled (SPGR) images (if the lesion enhances). With a thorough understanding of white matter anatomy, a tremendous amount of valuable information can be garnered before surgery. DTI atlases are available for a detailed illustration of white matter anatomy,[36] and tracts of greatest interest to neurosurgeons are included in **Fig. 3**. At our institution, the CC-FA map is the primary method by which DTI data are utilized in the preoperative mapping process.

Preoperative DTI has several important limitations. Because tract orientation information for a single voxel is based on the major eigenvector, the DTI model fails to accommodate complex intravoxel heterogeneity resulting from multiple fiber populations within each voxel. For example, the compact horizontal portion of the superior longitudinal fasciculus hinders identification of corticobulbar fibers as they originate from the lower precentral gyrus, traverse the superior longitudinal fasciculus, and emerge as part of the corona radiata. Likewise, functionally distinct tracts running in parallel within the same fiber bundle cannot be distinguished. An understanding of white matter anatomic relationships is thus critical in the interpretation of DTI, mitigating limitations of tract visualization, and improving estimations of tract locations.

Pathophysiologic factors, including tumor and edema, can reduce anisotropy and hinder depiction of white matter tracts altogether, whereas mass effect from either of these can cause regional changes

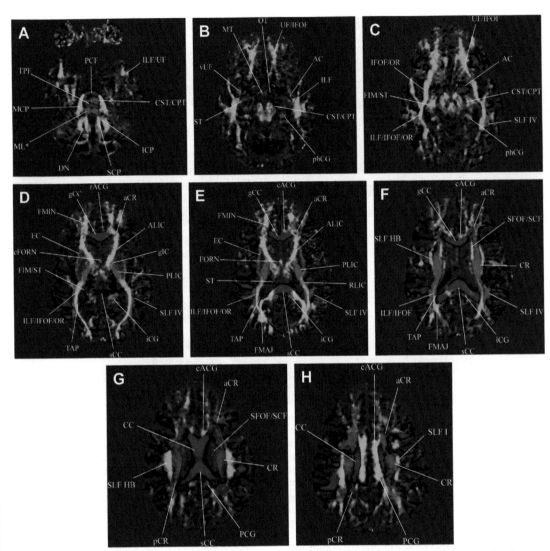

Fig. 3. White matter anatomy at color-coded fractional anisotropy (CC-FA) diffusion tensor imaging (DTI), represented in axial (*A–H*; inferior to superior), coronal (*I–L*; anterior to posterior), and sagittal (*M–P*; lateral to medial) planes. AC, anterior commissure; aCR, anterior corona radiata; ALIC, anterior limb of the internal capsule; cACG, caudal anterior cingulum; cFORN, column of the fornix; CN V, cranial nerve V; CPT, corticopontine tract; CR, corona radiata; CST, corticospinal tract; DN, dentate nucleus; DSCP, decussation of the superior cerebellar peduncles; EC, external capsule; FIM, fimbria; FMAJ, forceps major; FMIN, forceps minor; FORN, fornix; gCC, genu of the corpus callosum; gIC, genu of the internal capsule; iCG, isthmus of the cingulum; ICP, inferior cerebellar peduncle; IFOF, inferior fronto-occipital fasciculus; ILF, inferior longitudinal fasciculus; MCP, middle cerebellar peduncle; ML*, medial lemniscus (and smaller adjacent tracts including lateral lemniscus, anterior and lateral spinothalamic tract, and central tegmental tract); MT, mamillothalamic tract; OR, optic radiation; OT, optic tract; PCF, pontocerebellar fibers; phCG, parahippocampal cingulum; PLIC, posterior limb of the internal capsule; rACG, rostrum of the anterior cingulum; RLIC, retrolenticular internal capsule; sCC, splenium of the corpus callosum; SCF, subcallosal fasciculus; SCP, superior cerebellar peduncle; SFOF, superior fronto-occipital fasciculus; SLF HB, horizontal bundle of the superior longitudinal fasciculus (SLF II-IV); SLF IV, superior longitudinal fasciculus (IV); ST, stria terminalis; TAP, tapetum; TPF, transverse pontine fibers; UF, uncinate fasciculus; vUF, vertical bundle of the uncinate fasciculus.

in tract orientation.[37,38] DTI with echoplanar imaging is sensitive to regional field distortions at bone–tissue or air–tissue interfaces. This has important implications in preoperative brain mapping when assessing the proximity of eloquent white matter to brain tumors. Superimposing DTI data onto anatomic MR images is critical in evaluating the magnitude of geometric distortions. Although higher-order shimming may help to minimize these distortions, overlay nudge functions may be used

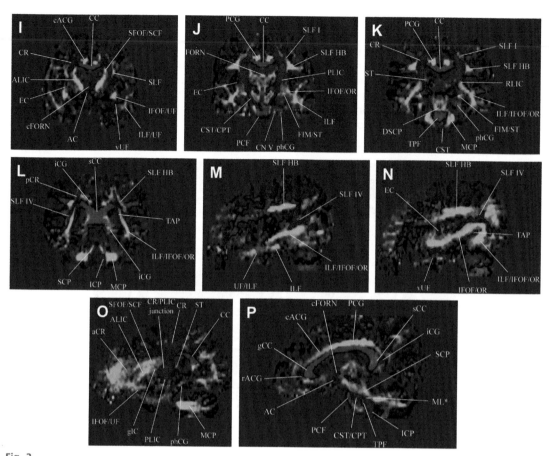

Fig. 3.

to realign DTI data to their corresponding white matter structures on MRI when these distortions exist in the vicinity of a lesion. Optimized re-registration of the 2 datasets should be centered at the surgical target to minimize DTI distortions. New acquisition and post-processing techniques addressing the issue of DTI geometric distortions have been proposed.[39,40]

Fiber Tracking

Fiber tracking, or tractography, is an additional means of displaying DTI data.[37,41–47] A 3-dimensional (3-D) representation of a white matter tract is constructed based on the directionality information derived from FA values. Using mathematical algorithms, fiber tract trajectories are estimated based on the major eigenvector at sampled locations, propagating from "seed points," or in whole brain analysis. Numerous different DTI tractography algorithms have been proposed in the literature, either deterministic or probabilistic.[41–45] The former method only uses the best estimate of the major eigenvector to propagate the fiber trajectories,

whereas the latter includes a method for estimating and displaying the uncertainty in propagation between 2 points. Most commercially available fiber tracking software packages use a deterministic mathematical algorithm. A unique characteristic of fiber tracking is the potential of distinguishing specific functional white matter tracts running in the same bundle.[37,46,47] The goal here is to increase specificity of DTI data in establishing critical spatial relationships.[48] In clinical settings, fiber tracking has been shown to distinguish specific white matter tracts adjacent to brain tumors.[49–51]

Anatomic constraints and limitations inherent in the technique may limit the applications of fiber tracking in clinical practice. It is important to remember that the 3-D depictions of fiber trajectories at tractography do not correspond with individual axons. They are merely indirect visual representations of the major eigenvector within voxels propagated along the course of the white matter tract. Owing to limitations in spatial resolution at MR imaging, 3-D tract components are much larger than the actual size of the axons. Crossing fiber tracts within individual voxels present a challenge for available DTI fiber tracking algorithms. Acute fiber angulations at the interface between cortex and white matter pose a challenge for current techniques as well. This limits the ability to determine exact fiber origins and terminations, a critical component of fiber tracking. Image noise, crossing fiber populations, diverging/converging trajectories all can alter the orientation of the major

eigenvector and cause falsely premature termination of a fiber tract.[52,53] Newer diffusion imaging techniques such as high angular diffusion imaging, diffusion spectrum imaging, and diffusion kurtosis imaging show promise in better resolving crossing tracts and could be on the horizon for clinical translation.[54–59] However, until these approaches become more widely available beyond a few

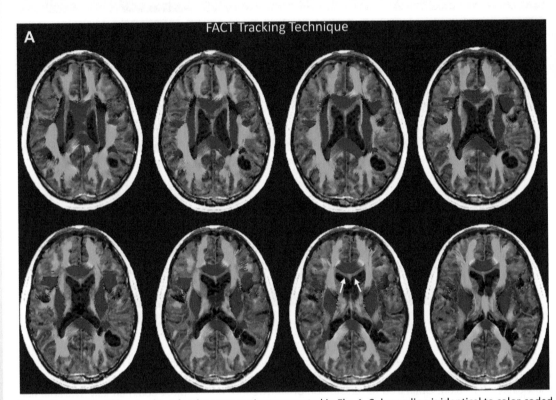

Fig. 4. Color-coded fiber tracking for the same patient presented in **Fig. 1**. Color coding is identical to color-coded fractional anisotropy (CC-FA) data, allowing for comparison between the datasets. Fiber tracking data can be suitable for 3-D visualization. However, overlying fiber tracking data onto faded CC-FA maps is critical to provide a case-by-case quality assurance. (*A*) Color-coded fiber tracking, using a commercially available fiber assignment by continuous tracking (FACT) algorithm, overlaid onto faded CC-FA maps, overlaid onto gadolinium-enhanced SPGR images. Only the large, central, white matter bundles are tracked. Note the geometric distortion evident by anterior displacement of anterior commissural fibers compared with the anatomic genu of the corpus callosum (*small white arrows*). (*B*) Commercially available FACT-based streamline tracking technique using the identical diffusion tensor imaging (DTI) data reveals smaller, more peripheral fiber tracks compared with A. Fibers are now seen wrapping around the peripheral borders of the lesion (*large yellow arrows*). Small fiber bundles that are indistinguishable in A are distinguishable in B (*large white arrow*). The bundle of fibers adjacent to the inferomedial border of the tumor containing the ILF, IFOF, and optic radiation can now be clearly distinguished from SLF IV and the tapetum. Geometric distortion of DTI data (*small white arrows*). (*C*) Although fiber tracking detail is improved using the streamline technique in *B*, 3-dimensional visualization of the tumor (*yellow outlined, yellow arrows*) in relation to major fiber bundles is hindered by smaller peripheral fiber bundles. (*D*) The standard FACT algorithm in A provides better visualization of tumor border (*red arrows, red tumor outline*) relationships to major white matter bundles, although recognition of missing peripheral tracks is critical to the interpretation. (*E*) Track-ball filtering of whole brain fiber tracking DTI data reveals better detail of spatial relationships between the tumor and SLF HB, SLF IV, IFOF, ILF, and OR. Recognition on the axial images in A that the normally green ILF/IFOF/OR is represented as a blue–purple bundle owing to blending of colors with the tapetum and SLF IV, provides for proper interpretation of the same on the 3-dimensional fiber tracking data. IFOF, inferior fronto-occipital fasciculus; ILF, inferior longitudinal fasciculus; OR, optic radiation; SLF HB, superior longitudinal fasciculus horizontal bundle; SLF IV, superior longitudinal fasciculus IV; UF, uncinate fasciculus.

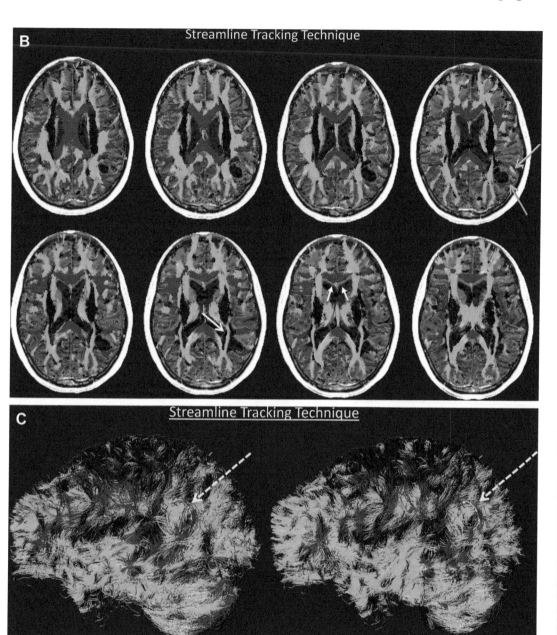

Fig. 4.

academic institutions, they remain largely irrelevant to patient care.

As is the case for CC-FA maps, pathophysiologic constraints also may limit the clinical application of fiber tracking for preoperative assessments. For example, peritumoral edema or tumor infiltration of white matter may reduce the anisotropy below the designated threshold for the tractography algorithm. This leads to erroneous termination of fibers at tractography when in fact the fibers may still exist. Lowering the anisotropy threshold to enable propagation of the tract through low anisotropy regions does not optimally solve this problem, because it results in reduced accuracy of the major eigenvector.[43] Relying disproportionately on fiber tracking results can lead to false-negative judgments about lesion border risk assessments. In a study of 10 patients with low-grade gliomas or malformations near language tracts, 17 of 21 intraoperative subcortical stimulations (81%) were concordant with preoperative fiber tracking results.[60] Negative fiber tracking does not rule out the presence of a fiber tract, especially when invaded by tumor. This

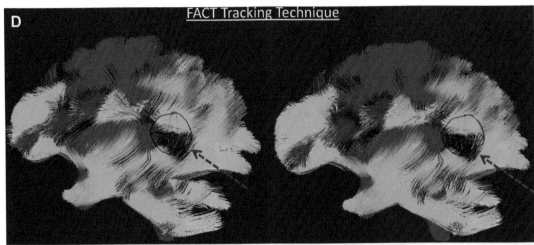

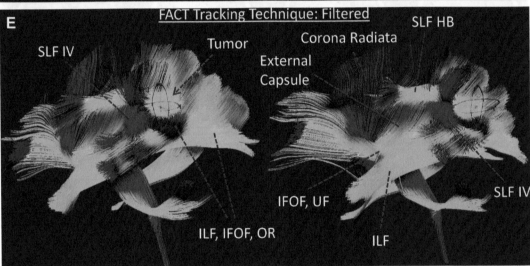

Fig. 4.

underscores a crucial advantage of CC-FA maps over fiber tracking. With the former, there is no loss of data, minimizing the chance for a false-negative prediction. In effect, the routine use of fiber tracking has been limited by insufficient NPV, lack of standardization, processor personnel-dependent results, and significant workflow limitations. Global white matter anatomic visualization with CC-FA maps remains a mainstay of preoperative brain mapping.

Recently, we have begun to use fiber tracking routinely for preoperative 3-D visualization of spatial relationships. Diagnostic analysis of spatial relationships is still based in CC-FA maps. Whole brain CC fiber tracking data (CC-FT) is presented with identical color coding as the FA maps, and later filtered for optimal visualization of the surgical target (Fig. 4). This processing strategy can be achieved in a matter of minutes, standardized, and exported to PACS. The fundamental concept

that empowers fiber tracking with this approach is that the interpreter's brain distinguishes functional white matter based on known regional anatomic relationships and color coding, just as is the case with FA-CC maps. In other words, there is no reliance on the software or post-processing personnel to distinguish functional white matter relationships. However, CC-FT should also be presented on axial images to reveal those tracts not detected by fiber tracking (see Fig. 4).

DIFFUSION TENSOR IMAGING INTERPRETATION

Neurosurgeons are interested in identifying sensorimotor, premotor, vision, and language functional networks and their relationships to the resectable lesion. Attempts have been made to estimate "safe" distances between a lesion border and functional cortex or white matter on fMRI and

DTI studies, respectively. However, there is no accepted "safe" distance, which may vary by surgical technique. Given the phenomenon of intraoperative brain shifting, it is risky to quantify preoperative distances and apply them to the intraoperative setting. DTI as well as fMRI are best used for qualitative assessment of spatial relationships. When interpreting DTI preoperatively, it is important to describe the relationships of white matter tracts to specific lesion borders. The term "immediate proximity" is used to describe a tract contacting or within a few millimeters to a lesion border. This relationship conveys to the neurosurgeon that there is significant risk of tract injury along this dissection border, and may trigger intraoperative functional white matter testing. Deficits are not expected to occur as a result of direct surgical injury if a tract location is "remote" (>1 cm) from a tumor border. "Relative proximity" is used to describe tract proximity somewhere between "immediate" and "remote."

FUTURE DIRECTIONS

One of the more recent advances with DTI and fMRI is the ability to import mapping data into neuronavigation systems. This allows the neurosurgeon real-time and interactive access to spatial relationships between the lesion and functional systems. Some of the neuronavigation systems incorporate their own basic DTI and fMRI processing software. However, lack of compatibility between other commercially available DTI/fMRI software and the select few neuronavigation platforms has proven to be an obstacle for the widespread use of this powerful technology. Forging ahead is likely, given that intraoperative use of preoperative mapping data has already displayed its strengths. Not only is there is a high correlation (but not perfect) between results of preoperative DTI data used intraoperatively with intraoperative subcortical mapping,[61] but use of preoperative DTI in neuronavigation has been shown to significantly improve postoperative outcome and survival in glioma patients.[19] Further, subcentimeter spatial agreement (8.7 ± 3.1 mm) between neuronavigational DTI and subcortical white matter stimulation has been demonstrated, although it will be compromised by brain shift at craniotomy and throughout the resection.[62] It is clear that, going forward, neuronavigation represents an important element in the evolution of clinical functional imaging.[63]

SUMMARY

Preoperative mapping has revolutionized the neurosurgical care of brain tumor patients. Maximizing resections more safely has improved diagnosis, optimized treatment algorithms, and, most important, has significantly decreased potentially devastating postoperative deficits associated with injury to functional brain networks. Although this mapping process has multiple steps and complimentary localization sources, it is DTI that stands out for its essential role in depicting individual white matter tracts. A thorough understanding of the DTI technique, data visualization methods, and limitations with a mastery of functional and dysfunctional white matter anatomy is necessary to realize the full potential of this powerful technology in clinical practice. By helping to establish spatial relationships between specific lesion borders and functional networks before and during surgery, DTI is cementing its role in high-risk neurosurgical resections and becoming the standard of care.

REFERENCES

1. Smith JS, Chang EF, Lamborn KR, et al. Role of extent of resection in the long-term outcome of low-grade hemispheric gliomas. J Clin Oncol 2008;26:1338–45.
2. Bernstein M, Berger M. Neurooncology – the essentials. 2nd edition. New York: Thieme; 2008.
3. Lacroix M, Abi-Said D, Fourney DR, et al. A multivariate analysis of 416 patients with glioblastoma multiforme: prognosis, extent of resection, and survival. J Neurosurg 2001;95:190–8.
4. Stummer W, Pichlmeier U, Meinel T, et al, ALA-Glioma Study Group. Fluorescence-guided surgery with 5-aminolevulinic acid for resection of malignant glioma: a randomized controlled multicentre phase III trial. Lancet Oncol 2006;7:392–401.
5. Ryken TC, Frankel B, Julien T, et al. Surgical management of newly diagnosed glioblastoma in adults: role of cytoreductive surgery. J Neurooncol 2008;89:271–86.
6. Claus EB, Horlacher A, Hsu L, et al. Survival rates in patients with low-grade glioma after intraoperative magnetic resonance image guidance. Cancer 2005;103:1227–33.
7. Chang S, Parney IF, McDermott M, et al. Perioperative complications and neurological outcome of first versus second craniotomy among patients enrolled in the glioma outcomes project. J Neurosurg 2003;98:1175–81.
8. Ciric I, Ammirati M, Vick N, et al. Supratentorial gliomas: surgical considerations and immediate postoperative results. gross total resection versus partial resection. Neurosurgery 1987;21:21–6.
9. Fadul C, Wood J, Thaler H, et al. Morbidity and mortality for excision of supratentorial gliomas. Neurology 1988;38:1374–9.

10. Sawaya R, Hammoud M, Schoppa D, et al. Neurosurgical outcomes in a modern series of 400 craniotomies for treatment parenchymal tumors. Neurosurgery 1998;42:1044–55.

11. Brell M, Ibanez J, Caral L, et al. Factors influencing surgical complications of intra-axial brain tumors. Acta Neurochir (Wien) 2000;142:739–50.

12. Deveaux BC, O'Fallon JR, Kelly PR. Resection, biopsy, and survival in malignant glial neoplasms: a retrospective study of clinical parameters, therapy, and outcome. J Neurosurg 1993;78(5):767–75.

13. Vorster SJ, Barnett GH. A proposed preoperative grading scheme to assess risk for surgical resection of primary and secondary intraaxial brain tumors. Neurosurg Focus 1998;4(6):e2.

14. Taylor MD, Berstein M. Awake craniotomy with brain mapping as the routine surgical approach to treating patients with supratentorial intraaxial tumors: a prospective trial of 200 cases. J Neurosurg 1999;90:35–41.

15. Bohinski RJ, Kokkino AK, Warnick RE, et al. Glioma resection in a shared resource operating room after optimal image-guided frameless stereotactic resection. Neurosurgery 2001;48:731–42.

16. Mueller W. DTI for neurosurgeons: cases and concepts. 2010 International Brain Mapping and Intraoperative Surgical Planning Society (IBMISPS) Brain, Spinal Cord Mapping and Image Guided Therapy Conference. Bethesda (MD), May 27, 2010.

17. Ulmer JL, Berman JI, Mueller WM, et al. Issues in translating imaging technology and presurgical diffusion tensor imaging. In: Faro SH, Mohamed FB, Law M, et al, editors. Functional neuroradiology: principles and clinical applications. 1st edition. New York: Springer; 2011.

18. Klein AP, Ulmer JL, Mueller WM, et al. DTI for presurgical mapping. In: Pillai JJ, editor. Functional brain tumor imaging. New York: Springer; 2014. p. 95–109.

19. Wu JS, Zhou LF, Tang WJ, et al. Clinical evaluation and follow-up outcome of diffusion tensor imaging-based functional neuronavigation: a prospective, controlled study in patients with gliomas involving pyramidal tracts. Neurosurgery 2007;61:935–48 [discussion: 948–9].

20. Schmahmann JD, Pandya DN. Fiber pathways of the brain. New York: Oxford University Press; 2006.

21. Makris N, Kennedy DN, McInerney S, et al. Segmentation of subcomponents within the superior longitudinal fascicle in humans: a quantitative, in vivo, DT-MRI Study. Cereb Cortex 2005;15(6):854–69.

22. Price CJ. The anatomy of language: contributions from functional neuroimaging. J Anat 2000;197(Pt 3):335–59.

23. Hickok G, Poeppel D. Dorsal and ventral streams: a framework for understanding aspects of the functional anatomy of language. Cognition 2004;92:67–99.

24. Duffau H. New insights into the anatomo-functional connectivity of the semantic system: a study using cortico-subcortical electrostimulations. Brain 2005;128:797–810.

25. Aralasmak A, Ulmer JL, Kocak M, et al. Association commissural, and projection pathways and their functional deficit reported in literature. J Comput Assist Tomogr 2006;30(5):695–716.

26. Maheshwari M, Klein AP, Ulmer JL. White matter: functional anatomy of key tracts. In: Faro SH, Mohamed FB, Law M, et al, editors. Functional neuroradiology: principles and clinical applications. 1st edition. New York: Springer; 2011.

27. Oldfield RC. The assessment and analysis of handedness: the Edinburgh inventory. Neuropsychologia 1971;9:97–113.

28. Ulmer JL, Hacein-Bey L, Mathews VP, et al. Lesion-induced Pseudo-dominance at fMRI: implications for pre-operative assessments. Neurosurgery 2004;55:569–81.

29. Ulmer JL, Salvan CV, Mueller WM, et al. The role of diffusion tensor imaging in establishing the proximity of tumor borders to functional brain systems: implications for preoperative risk assessments and postoperative outcomes. Technol Cancer Res Treat 2004;3:567–76.

30. Berger M. Minimalism through intraoperative functional mapping. Clin Neurosurg 1996;43:324–37.

31. Duffa H, Capelle L, Sichez N, et al. Intraoperative mapping of the subcortical language pathways using direct stimulations. Brain 2002;125(1):199–214.

32. Ulmer JL, Krouwer HG, Mueller WM, et al. Pseudo-reorganization of language cortical function at FMR imaging: a consequence of tumor-induced neurovascular uncoupling. AJNR Am J Neuroradiol 2003;24:213–7.

33. Sanai N, Mirzadeh Z, Berger MS. Functional outcome after language mapping for glioma resection. N Engl J Med 2008;358:18–27.

34. Brazos PW, Masdeu Jose C, Biller J. Localization in clinical neurology. 5th edition. Baltimore (MD): Lippincott Williams & Wilkins; 2007.

35. Pajevic S, Pierpaoli C. Color schemes to represent the orientation of anisotropic tissues from diffusion tensor data: application to white matter fiber tract mapping of the human brain. Magn Reson Med 1999;42:526–40.

36. Klein AP. Diffusion tensor imaging atlas of the brain. In: Faro SH, Mohamed FB, Law M, et al, editors. Functional neuroradiology: principles and clinical applications. 1st edition. New York: Springer; 2011.

37. Jellison BJ, Field AS, Medow JL, et al. Diffusion tensor imaging of cerebral white matter: a pictorial review of physics, fiber tract anatomy, and tumor

imaging patterns. AJNR Am J Neuroradiol 2004;25: 356–69.

38. Tropine A, Vucurevic G, Delani P, et al. Contribution of diffusion tensor imaging to delineation of gliomas and glioblastomas. J Magn Reson Imaging 2004;6: 905–12.

39. Wang FN, Huang TY, Lin FH, et al. PROPELLER EPI: an MRI technique suitable for diffusion tensor imaging at high field strength with reduced geometric distortions. Magn Reson Med 2005;54(5): 1232–40.

40. Gaggl W, Jesmanowicz A, Prost RW. Eddy current correction in diffusion tensor imaging using phase-correction in k-space. Annual meeting of the Organization for Human Brain Mapping. San Francisco, June 18–23, 2009.

41. Mori S, Crain BJ, Chacko VP, et al. Three dimensional tracking of axonal projections in the brain by magnetic resonance imaging. Ann Neurol 1999;45:265–9.

42. Conturo TE, Lori NF, Cull TS, et al. Tracking neuronal fiber pathways in the living human brain. Proc Natl Acad Sci U S A 1999;96:10422–7.

43. Basser P, Pajevic S, Pierpaoli C. In vivo fiber tractography using DT-MRI data. Magn Reson Med 2000;44:625–32.

44. Lazar M, Alexander A. Bootstrap white matter tractography (BOOT-TRAC). Neuroimage 2005;24: 524–32.

45. Parker G, Haroon H, Wheelr-Kingshott C. A framework for a streamline-based probabilistic index of connectivity (PICo) using a structural interpretation of MRI diffusion measurements. J Magn Reson Imaging 2003;18:242–54.

46. Mori S, Kaufmann WE, Davatzikos C, et al. Imaging cortical association tracts in the human brain using diffusion-tensor-based axonal tracking. Magn Reson Med 2002;47:215–23.

47. Catani M, Howard RJ, Pajevic S, et al. Virtual in vivo interactive dissection of white matter fasciculi in the human brain. Neuroimage 2002;17:77–94.

48. Han BS, Hong JH, Hong C, et al. Location of the corticospinal tract at the corona radiata in human brain. Brain Res 2010;1326:75–80.

49. Holodny A, Schwartz T, Ollenschleger M, et al. Tumor involvement of the corticospinal tract: diffusion magnetic resonance tractography with intraoperative correlation. J Neurosurg 2001;95:1082.

50. Clark C, Barrick T, Murphy M, et al. White matter fiber tracking in patients with space-occupying lesions of the brain: a new technique for neurosurgical planning? Neuroimage 2003;20:1601–8.

51. Berman J, Berger M, Mukherjee P, et al. Diffusion-tensor imaging-guided tracking of fibers of the pyramidal tract combined with intraoperative cortical stimulation mapping in patients with gliomas. J Neurosurg 2004;101:66–72.

52. Anderson A. Theoretical analysis of the effects of noise on diffusion tensor imaging. Magn Reson Med 2001;46:1174–88.

53. Lazar M, Alexander A. Divergence/convergence effects on the accuracy of white matter tractography algorithms. Toronto: International Society for Magnetic Resonance in Medicine; 2003. p. 2160.

54. Tuch D. Q-ball imaging. Magn Reson Med 2004;52: 1358–72.

55. Frank LR. Characterization of anisotropy in high angular resolution diffusion-weighted MRI. Magn Reson Med 2002;47:1083–99.

56. Tournier J, Calamante F, Gadian D, et al. Direct estimation of the fiber orientation density function from diffusion-weighted MRI data using spherical deconvolution. Neuroimage 2004;23: 1176–85.

57. Wedeen VJ, Hagmann P, Tseng W, et al. Mapping complex tissue architecture with diffusion spectrum magnetic resonance imaging. Magn Reson Med 2005;54:1377–86.

58. Jensen JH, Helpern JA, Ramani A, et al. Diffusional kurtosis imaging: the quantification of non-gaussian water diffusion by means of magnetic resonance imaging. Magn Reson Med 2005;53: 1432–40.

59. Wu EX, Cheung MM. MR diffusion kurtosis imaging for neural tissue characterization. NMR Biomed 2010;23:836–48.

60. Leclercq D, Duffau H, Delmaire C, et al. Comparison of diffusion tensor imaging tractography of language tracts and intraoperative subcortical stimulations. J Neurosurg 2010;112:503–11.

61. Coenen VA, Krings T, Axer H, et al. Intraoperative three-dimensional visualization of the pyramidal tract in a neuronavigation system (PTV) reliably predicts true position of principal motor pathways. Surg Neurol 2003;60:381–90.

62. Berman JI, Berger MS, Chung SW, et al. Accuracy of diffusion tensor magnetic resonance imaging tractography assessed using intraoperative subcortical stimulation mapping and magnetic source imaging. J Neurosurg 2007;107:488–94.

63. Pillai JJ. The evolution of clinical functional imaging during the past 2 decades and its current impact on neurosurgical planning. AJNR Am J Neuroradiol 2010;31(2):219–25.

Diffusion Tensor Imaging for Brain Malformations
Does It Help?

Thierry A.G.M. Huisman, MD*,
Thangamadhan Bosemani, MD, Andrea Poretti, MD

KEYWORDS

- Diffusion tensor imaging • Fiber tractography • Children • Neuroimaging • Brain malformations
- Axonal guidance disorders

KEY POINTS

- Diffusion tensor imaging (DTI) is an advanced magnetic resonance (MR) technique that provides qualitative and quantitative information about the microarchitecture of white matter.
- DTI may show important information about the brain microstructure in brain malformations that may go undetected or remains underestimated on conventional MR sequences.
- DTI may better categorize various brain malformations that may look similar on conventional MR imaging, but may be caused by different pathomechanisms.
- Human disorders of axonal guidance result from aberrant axonal wiring and are caused by mutations in genes that code for molecules that guide axons within the brain.
- Much of our knowledge about human disorders of axonal guidance comes from DTI studies of crossing tracts, such as the corpus callosum, optic chiasm, corticospinal tract, and cerebellar peduncles.

INTRODUCTION

Diffusion-weighted imaging (DWI) and in particular diffusion tensor imaging (DTI) have propelled our noninvasive exploration and understanding of many common and rare congenital brain abnormalities, which include malformations as well as disruptions.[1,2] DWI/DTI takes advantage of the preferential mobility and diffusion of water molecules in three-dimensional space within biological tissues with a complex microstructural architecture like the brain. The mobility of water molecules in the brain is dependent on multiple factors, including the microstructural architecture, which is believed to be predominantly determined by the alignment and diameter of fiber tracts and their myelin sheets as well as the three-dimensional distribution and arrangement of neurons. In addition, multiple other spatially organized flow patterns exist within the brain, like blood flow in the arterial and venous networks and the molecular flow of protons, which depend on active and passive transport mechanisms within the brain. Exploring the differential mobility and diffusion of water molecules in the brain gives indirect information about the normal and abnormal internal architecture, networks, and integrity of the pediatric brain.

The differential, three-dimensional direction and magnitude of water mobility can be measured noninvasively, in vivo by adding diffusion-weighted gradients to standard ultrafast magnetic resonance (MR) sequences. Typically, diffusion

Section of Pediatric Neuroradiology, Russell H. Morgan Department of Radiology and Radiological Science, Charlotte R. Bloomberg Children's Center, The Johns Hopkins University School of Medicine, Sheikh Zayed Tower, Room 4174, 1800 Orleans Street, Baltimore, MD 21287-0842, USA
* Corresponding author.
E-mail address: thuisma1@jhmi.edu

Neuroimag Clin N Am 24 (2014) 619–637
http://dx.doi.org/10.1016/j.nic.2014.07.004
1052-5149/14/$ – see front matter © 2014 Elsevier Inc. All rights reserved.

gradients are applied along multiple noncollinear directions in space to resolve the complete diffusion tensor. The more diffusion directions gradients measured, the better is the three-dimensional shape and magnitude of the sampled diffusion tensor. Powerful postprocessing tools subsequently allow reconstructing the course of major fiber tracts within the central nervous system (CNS). DTI has been of invaluable significance to explore common and uncommon brain malformations. Steve Jobs, one of the most influential inventors and entrepreneurs of our time, made a quote that summarizes the goal and value of DTI in brain malformations: "because believing that the dots will connect down the road, will give you the confidence to follow your heart, even when it leads you off the well-worn path." The DTI acquisitions render data sets that have to be postprocessed with an open scientific mind, in which the various dots or seed points have to be connected in a nonbiased mathematical approach to confirm the course of well-known common pathways and networks, which should also allow us to explore and discover unknown or aberrant fiber tracts and anatomic connections. Recognizing these aberrant pathways may be challenging but help us to better understand, classify, or group brain malformations. This approach is similar to high-end brain teasers, in which numbers need to be discovered using a complex mathematical formula

and then connected to uncover or recognize a hidden figure (Fig. 1).

In this article, the basics of DWI/DTI are discussed, including a short historical perspective on the fiber dissection technique, followed by a review of selected brain malformations in which DTI and tractography have contributed to a better understanding of the malformations, and by a clinical case in which DTI showed a disorder of the internal neuroarchitecture that could not be correctly appreciated by conventional anatomic MR imaging.

BASICS OF DIFFUSION-WEIGHTED IMAGING AND DIFFUSION TENSOR IMAGING

DWI generates image contrast based on differences in diffusion characteristics of water molecules within the brain.[1,2] Diffusion represents the random thermal movement of molecules, also known as Brownian motion, within tissues. Diffusion within the brain is determined by a variety of factors, including the type of molecule under investigation, the temperature of the tissue, and most importantly, the microenvironmental architecture in which the diffusion takes place. For example, the rate of diffusion of water molecules within the cerebrospinal fluid (CSF) is higher than the rate of diffusion of water molecules within the brain tissue. By adding diffusion-encoding gradients to standard MR imaging sequences, these

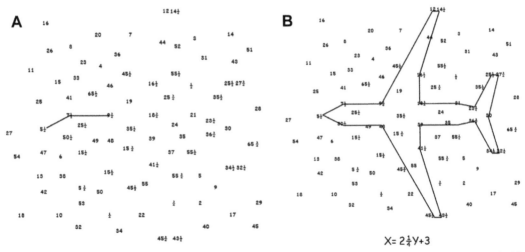

Fig. 1. Connect the dots puzzles are a form of puzzles made of a sequence of dots that have to be connected with a line in the correct order to discover the final picture. Typically, they rely on connecting a row of numbers in ascending order. However, in advanced puzzles, they may go beyond the standard numbering. Identifying, for example, the algebraic sequencing of a group of numbers based on the already connected dots requires analytical skills and an open mind to outline and recognize the figure. In this example, the initial figure (A) shows the starting point of the connect the dots puzzle. Correct analysis of the order of the first 3 numbers allows the discovery of the algebraic formula that connects the sequence of numbers ($x = 2\frac{1}{4}y + 3$). Subsequently, the scientist knows how to connect the numbers, and the outline of an aircraft is discovered (B). This connect the dots puzzle is similar to DTI and fiber tractography in the exploration of normal and anomalous white matter tracts in the brain.

differences in diffusion rates can be translated into and shown as differences in MR signal. These differences in MR signal of the individual imaging voxels can be mapped two-dimensionally as so-called DWI images. Typically, isotropic DWI images are generated (**Fig. 2**). Isotropic DWI images incorporate signal related to both the rate of diffusion and T2-relaxation phenomena. In addition,

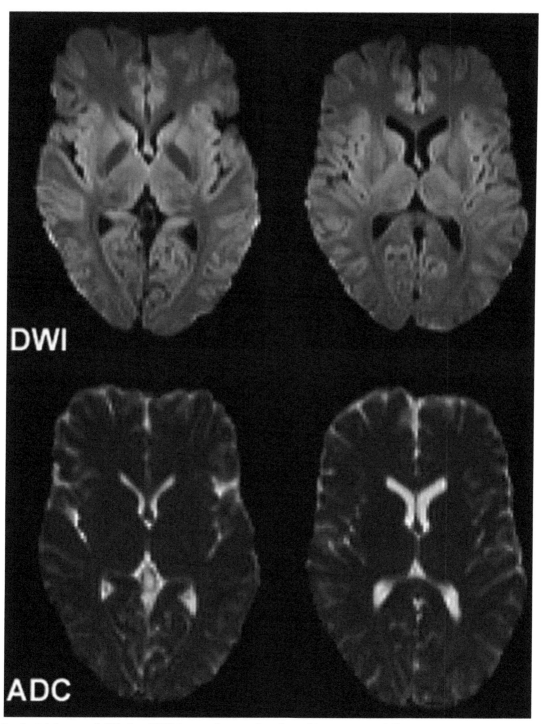

Fig. 2. Axial trace of diffusion (DWI) images (*top row*) and matching apparent diffusion coefficient (ADC) maps (*lower row*) of the brain. CSF with high degree of diffusion is DWI-hypointense and ADC-bright, whereas brain tissue with more restricted diffusion is DWI-hyperintense and ADC-dark.

maps of apparent diffusion can be calculated, also known as apparent diffusion coefficient (ADC). The ADC values are typically displayed as two-dimensional gray-white scale maps, in which the calculated ADC values are translated into brightness maps or so-called ADC maps. Areas with high degrees of diffusion or high ADC values appear bright (eg, CSF), whereas areas with low degrees of diffusion or low ADC values (eg, densely packed white matter tracts) appear darker. The major advantage of ADC is that the T2 contribution of the DWI maps is canceled out, giving a map of the spatial distribution of diffusion in the brain without contamination by the T2-relaxation phenomena (see **Fig. 2**).

DTI takes DWI to the next level of image-based microstructural tissue exploration. The three-dimensional shape and principal direction of diffusion as well as the magnitude of diffusion (diffusion rate) within space differ between the various brain structures. The microstructural architecture as well as physiologic factors determine the diffusion of water molecules within the brain. The effective molecular diffusion in the white matter tracts is, for example, predominantly along the direction parallel to the long axis of white matter tracts and limited in the direction perpendicular to the white matter tracts. The three-dimensional shape of diffusion in white matter tracts resembles an ellipsoid, which is also known as anisotropic

diffusion (**Fig. 3A**). When the degree of diffusion is equal in all directions such as in CSF, in which no barriers limit diffusion, the three-dimensional shape of diffusion resembles a sphere, which is also known as isotropic diffusion (see **Fig. 3B**). The three-dimensional shape of diffusion can be studied by measuring the full tensor of the diffusion (DTI), in which diffusion gradients are applied along at least 6 noncollinear directions in space. Maps of the spatial distribution and magnitude of the anisotropic component of diffusion are generated. Fractional anisotropy (FA) maps are typically calculated, in which the assigned signal intensity is related to the degree of anisotropic diffusion. FA values range between 0 and 1. An FA value of 0 indicates complete isotropic diffusion, and an FA value of 1 indicates complete anisotropic diffusion (**Fig. 4**). These FA values can be mapped topographically, in which voxels with an FA value of 0 are black and voxels with an FA value of 1 are white. In addition, the principal direction of diffusion in three-dimensional space can be color coded (**Fig. 5**) or can be shown as a vector for each voxel (**Fig. 6**). Blue represents a predominantly craniocaudal diffusion, red represents predominantly left to right diffusion, and green represents predominantly anterior-posterior diffusion within the brain. These maps provide information about the architecture and integrity of organized tissues. Finally, by combining the

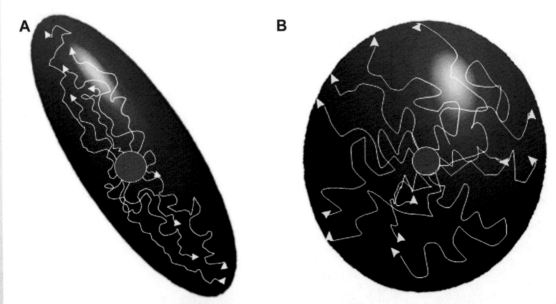

Fig. 3. Anisotropic diffusion (*A*) resembles a three-dimensional ellipsoid in space, with predominant diffusion of molecules along the main axis of the ellipsoid and restricted diffusion perpendicular to the ellipsoid. Isotropic diffusion (*B*) can be represented by a sphere with equal diffusion in all directions in space. The arrows represent the motion of individual molecules. (*From* Huisman TA. Diffusion weighted and diffusion tensor imaging of the brain, made easy. Cancer Imaging 2010;10:S166; with permission.)

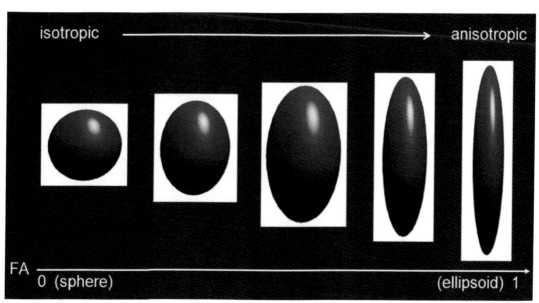

Fig. 4. Range of isotropic toward anisotropic diffusion as can be observed in the various regions of the brain. An FA value of zero represents complete isotropic diffusion (*perfect sphere*), whereas an FA value of 1 represents the hypothetical case of complete anisotropic diffusion (*narrow ellipsoid*). (*From* Huisman TA. Diffusion weighted and diffusion tensor imaging of the brain, made easy. Cancer Imaging 2010;10:S167; with permission.)

magnitude and directional information of anisotropic diffusion of the measured voxels, white matter tracts can be calculated/reconstructed. Voxels with a similar orientation and magnitude of their principal anisotropic diffusion direction are likely to be part of the same white matter tract. Powerful postprocessing mathematical algorithms that connect these voxels (or dots, as mentioned in the quote by Steve Jobs) allow white matter tracts to be studied and visualized in vivo (also known as fiber tractography [FT]) (**Fig. 7**).

WHITE MATTER EXPLORATION FROM ANDREAS VESALIUS TO JOSEF KLINGLER AND BEYOND

The recognition of high-order functionality of the CNS, relying on the complex networking of multiple functional centers by white matter tracts, dates back to the early sixteenth century. Observational and anatomic studies performed by scientists like Andreas Vesalius (1514–1564) and René Descartes (1596–1650), who were anatomists, physicians, and authors of 2 of the most influential books on human anatomy, *De Humani Corporis Fabrica* and *De Homine Figures et Latinitate Donates*, identified and reported white matter tracts within the CNS. The textbook of Descartes was published posthumously by Florant Schuyl in 1662 in Latin and again in 1664 in French by Claude Clerselier, entitled *Le Traité de l'Homme.*[3]

Illustrations in the textbooks show how, for example, heat from a fire close to the foot is transmitted to the brain via a tract extending from the foot via the spinal cord to the brain (**Fig. 8**). In addition, several figures show that the eyes are connected to the brain over the optic nerves, which again appear to extend to the occipital lobes. Several additional early descriptions about white matter tracts exist in the literature. Marcello Malpighi (1628–1694) showed in 1669 that the cerebral white matter is composed of fibers, and Niels Stensen (1638–1686) studied the course of white matter tracts in the brain by following the nerve threads through the brain substance. In the decades and centuries to follow, many more discoveries were made based on the detailed evaluation of the cerebral white matter, partially taking advantage of the scraping method for dissecting cerebral white matter, as suggested by Stensen. The scraping technique allowed studying the branching of white matter tracts in better detail, especially after the brain was prepared by various fixation techniques (eg, injection of alcohol).

White matter tracts were identified, and their branching has been reproduced by many anatomic and histologic studies performed in the early twentieth century. The pioneering work of Santiago Ramón y Cajal (1852–1934), a Spanish pathologist, histologist, and neuroscientist, is considered instrumental in our current understanding of the brain microstructure. Ramón y Cajal believed in

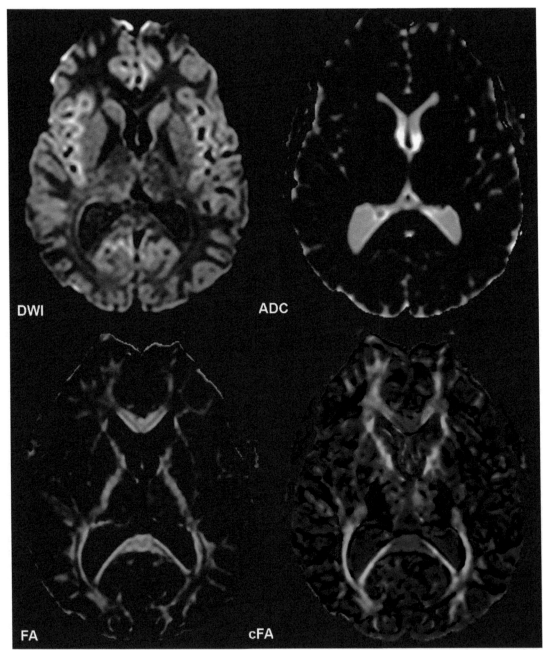

Fig. 5. Sample of matching axial DWI, ADC, FA, and color-coded FA (cFA) images of the brain. The FA map shows high degrees of anisotropic diffusion along white matter tracts in, for example, the corpus callosum and internal capsule. Low degree of anisotropic diffusion is seen in the cortical and central gray matter (areas of less degree of anisotropic diffusion). The color-coded FA maps show the predominant direction of diffusion, with left to right diffusion in the corpus callosum (*red*), superior-inferior diffusion in the internal capsule (*blue*), and anterior-posterior diffusion in the frontal white matter (*green*). (*From* Huisman TA. Diffusion weighted and diffusion tensor imaging of the brain, made easy. Cancer Imaging 2010;10:S167; with permission.)

the neuron or reticular theory, which refers to neural networks in which the relationship between nerve cells is not considered continuous but contiguous.

The scraping technique or fiber dissection technique was again revitalized by Josef Klingler (1888–1963), a laboratory technician and preparator at the Anatomy Institute in Basel, Switzerland.

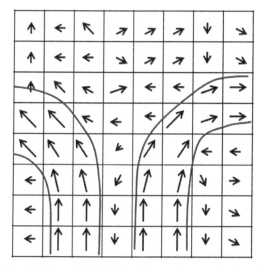

Fig. 6. The principal direction and magnitude of diffusion can be shown by a vector for each voxel. Adjacent voxels with a vector showing a similar magnitude and orientation in three-dimensional space likely cover a white matter tract (*red*).

Under the guidance of Eugen Ludwig, the director of the Institute of Anatomy, Josef Klingler developed a new fiber dissection technique, in which the brain is initially fixed in a 5% formalin solution for 2 to 3 months before the brain is frozen for 8 to 10 days at −10°C. Afterward, the brain is allowed to thaw in water at room temperature. During the freezing process, the formalin solution,

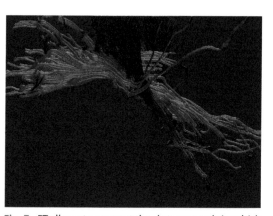

Fig. 7. FT allows to connect the dots or voxels in which the principal direction and magnitude of diffusion are similar, and consequently, three-dimensional displays of the white matter tracts can be calculated. This three-dimensional graph shows a crossing of descending corticospinal tracts (*blue*) and anterior-posterior (*green*) running tracts. The various left to right connecting tracts are seen (*red*). (*From* Huisman TA. Diffusion weighted and diffusion tensor imaging of the brain, made easy. Cancer Imaging 2010;10:S168; with permission.)

which does not penetrate the fibers, expands and consequently loosens up the brain substance, separates white matter tracts, and consequently, facilitates subsequent fiber dissection. This method allowed a detailed analysis of multiple functional systems within the brain, which culminated in a landmark work known as the *Atlas Cerebri Humani*, which was published in 1956 by Ludwig and Klingler as coauthors (**Fig. 9**).

The work of Klingler inspired many neuroscientists, including various influential neurosurgeons like M. Gazi Yasargil, who served as Director of the Department of Neurosurgery at the University Hospital Zurich, Switzerland. Klingler also advised those who wish to learn neuroanatomy that indispensable requirements to be successful are to have a good knowledge of the gross anatomy of the brain and to have patience and perseverance. M. Gazi Yasargil learned as a medical student under the direct guidance and supervision of Klingler starting in 1949; he studied the three-dimensional brain anatomy using Klingler's models for many hours, applied his knowledge in his following career as a neurosurgeon, and even now, many decades later, after his retirement in Zurich, he continues to lecture and publish on the fiber dissection technique. Only recently, a scientific article was published by M. Gazi Yasargil taking advantage of the fiber dissection technique to explore the surgical anatomy of supratentorial midline lesions.[5]

The work of Klingler and Yasargil has regained interest because of the ability of DTI to study the white matter tracts within the brain in vivo. In combination with various functional MR imaging techniques, including functional MR imaging, MR spectroscopy, and perfusion-weighted imaging, the internal neuroarchitecture can be studied in high anatomic and functional detail in vivo (**Fig. 10**).

Two quotes are essential for the future success of DTI in the exploration of complex pediatric brain malformations. First, "The study of history allows us to view the mistakes and successes of the past and is paradoxically the most advanced way to predict the future." DTI of brain malformations should take advantage of and be measured against the knowledge that has been collected over many decades and centuries on brain malformations by macropathology, histology, clinical findings, conventional neuroimaging, and genetics. The second quote involves the statement of Steve Jobs "Because believing that the dots will connect down the road, will give you the confidence to follow your heart, even when it leads you off the well-worn path." Exploration of brain malformations should start with connecting the dots

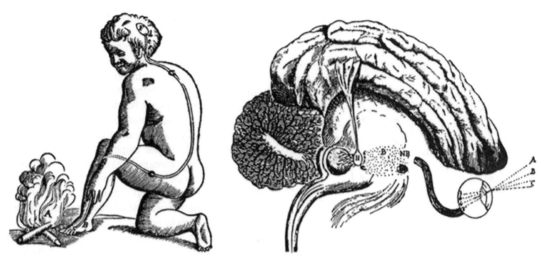

Fig. 8. Two figures out of the textbook of René Descartes, published in 1662, show the early depiction of a white matter tract connecting temperature and pain receptors of the left foot through the spinal cord to the brain, whereas the second illustration shows how Descartes believed that the eyes transmitted visual signal via the optic nerves to the center of the brain, where a third eye was believed to be localized.

or voxels (tractography) to study the well-known white matter tracts, but as neuroscientists, we should also be prepared to get off the well-worn path to identify and understand brain malformations that have remained undetected, unrecognized, or not understood, because conventional anatomic MR imaging showed only the tip of the iceberg of these microstructural brain malformations. DTI may allow transcending MR imaging from basic anatomic imaging toward function and embryology-based anatomic imaging. DTI in combination with our historical data and knowledge should help us to better understand what went wrong during the development of the brain and how to classify brain malformations more accurately.

APPLICATIONS OF DIFFUSION TENSOR IMAGING IN PEDIATRIC BRAIN MALFORMATIONS
Corpus Callosum or Commissural Malformations

Many early DTI studies on brain malformations have focused on the corpus callosum, because this anatomic structure is readily seen on neuroimaging, has a significant size, and is first and foremost a densely packed collection of corticocortical white matter tracts connecting the cortex of both cerebral hemispheres, which is consequently characterized by a high degree of anisotropic diffusion. Corpus callosum malformations are well suited to be studied by DTI (**Fig. 11**).

Depending on the encountered conventional anatomic neuroimaging features, the corpus callosum can be described as hypoplastic or hyperplastic, partial or completely absent (hypogenesis/agenesis), malformed (dysgenesis) or atrophic. These various morphologies may give important hints about the pathogenesis that resulted in the encountered corpus callosum anomaly. The corpus callosum anomaly may be the most prominent neuroimaging finding in the

Fig. 9. Multiple preparations using the fiber dissection technique show the complex architecture of the white matter tracts within the brain.

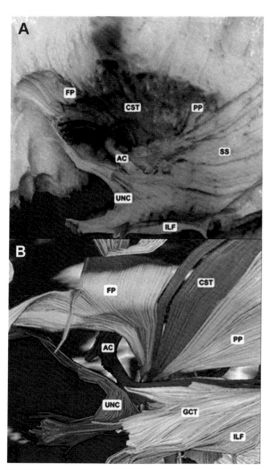

Fig. 10. Comparison between anatomic dissections using the fiber dissection technique and tractography. Qualitative analysis of tract reconstruction using DTI; b0 images of the contralateral hemisphere are used as background for spatial orientation. (*A*) Gross dissection, lateral view; U fibers, SLF, IFO, the nucleus of CL, PT, and GP, as well as part of the UNC were removed. (*B*) Tractographies. AC is divided into anterior and posterior arm. Although, in dissection, it is not possible to identify clear borders between parallel structures and the exposure of a bundle that may require the destruction of a more superficial bundle, tractography enables overlaying of segmented structures using different colors to provide a new view of the relationship between different bundles. AC, anterior commissure; CST, corticospinal tract; FP, fronto-pontine fibers; GCT, geniculocalcarine tract; ILF, inferior longitudinal fasciculus; PP, parietopontine fibers; SS, sagittal stratum; UNC, uncinate fasciculus. (*From* Dini LI, Vedolin LM, Bertholdo D, et al. Reproducibility of quantitative fiber tracking measurements in diffusion tensor imaging of frontal lobe tracts: a protocol based on the fiber dissection technique. Surg Neurol Int 2013;4:51.)

conventional sagittal T1-weighted anatomic image. However, a corpus callosum anomaly is rarely isolated. The corpus callosum belongs to the group of great interhemispheric commissures, which includes the corpus callosum itself as well as the anterior and hippocampal commissures (**Fig. 12**). The development of these commissures depends on complex interacting mechanisms of neuronal migration, cellular and axonal guidance, and successful channeling of the commissural axons across the midline to connect both hemispheres. Because these processes are complex with multiple interactions, henceforth, a corpus callosum anomaly is rarely isolated. If the corpus callosum is malformed, the anterior or hippocampal commissures are frequently also anomalous. Additional gray and white matter abnormalities like, for example, heterotopias or cerebral clefts may coexist (eg, Aicardi syndrome). Charles Raybaud, a renowned pediatric neuroradiologist and an expert on the embryogenesis and pathogenesis of brain malformations, consequently considers commissural agenesis to be a malformative feature rather than a malformation itself.[6]

High-end DTI, including tractography, may give important additional microstructural information about these commissural malformations. These data will advance our knowledge of the commissural anomalies, may allow a better classification of specific patterns of malformation, and accordingly are expected to improve genetic counseling of parents and patients.

The anatomic MR imaging findings in children with a malformed or absent corpus callosum have been extensively reported and include the partial and complete absence of the corpus callosum, parallel coursing, mildly separated lateral ventricles, colpocephaly, and an interhemispheric extension of the third ventricle. Other MR findings include a lack of definition of the cingulate gyrus, separated leaves of the septum pellucidum, malrotation of the hippocampi, and absence of the inferior cingulum. DTI and FT may easily confirm the partial or complete absence of white matter tracts crossing the midline in the expected location of the corpus callosum. In addition, DTI/FT typically shows the Probst bundles, which represent misdirected callosal axons, as large, anterior-posterior oriented intrahemispheric white matter tracts that extend along the medial and superior contour of the lateral ventricles (**Fig. 13**). On DTI/FT, the Probst bundles appear to be continuous with the superior cingulum and fornices, and the microstructure of the right ventral cingulum bundle has been shown to be abnormal as well as reduced in length and volume. Moreover, DTI has also identified that the fornices can be dysplastic and widely

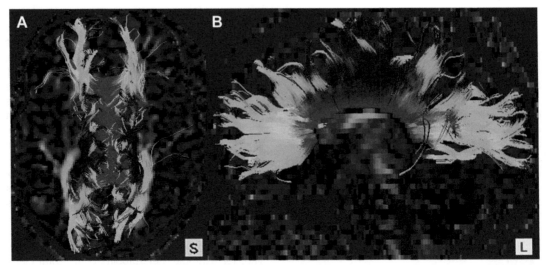

Fig. 11. Axial (*A*) and midsagittal (*B*) FT reconstruction of the corpus callosum superimposed on an axial and midsagittal color-coded FA map, respectively, of a healthy child.

separated. DTI studies have shown a greater diversity of partial callosal connectivity, including several heterotopic tracts that are not present in normally developed, healthy individuals.[7]

DTI/FT may also be helpful in evaluating the full extent of the commissural malformation in very young children. We recently reported on a neonate with a prenatally diagnosed complete corpus callosum agenesis. Postnatal DTI/FT showed a complete commissural malformation with a combined

absence of the corpus callosum, anterior commissure, and hippocampal commissure (**Fig. 14**).[8]

DTI/FT has proved to be helpful in the correct diagnostic workup of children with variant forms of complex corpus callosum dysgenesis. DTI and FT showed, for example, in a case of syntelencephaly, a rare middle interhemispheric variant of holoprosencephaly, that the fibers in the partially developed anterior (genu) and posterior (splenium) segments of the corpus callosum represent true

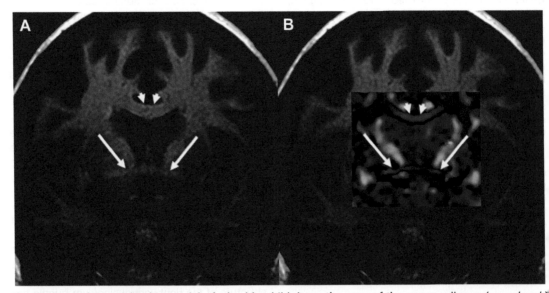

Fig. 12. Coronal T1-weighted image (*A*) of a healthy child shows the genu of the corpus callosum (*arrowheads*) and the anterior commissure (*arrows*). Color-coded FA maps (*B*) of the same child superimposed on a coronal T1-weighted image show the genu of the corpus callosum (*arrowheads*) and the anterior commissure (*arrows*) as structures depicted in red (*left to right course*).

commissural fibers connecting distant cortical regions over the midline, whereas in the fused midline, no fibers could be identified connecting distant functional centers (**Fig. 15**). Detailed analysis of other major white matter bundles and commissures, including the inferior fronto-occipital fasciculus, medial lemniscus, corticospinal tracts (CSTs), and anterior or hippocampal commissure, may help to better classify the type and degree of holoprosencephaly.[9]

With the development of highly advanced MR hardware and software, prenatal or fetal DTI has also become possible. The developing commissures can be studied as early as in the second trimester of pregnancy.[10]

Posterior Fossa Malformations, Including Joubert Syndrome

The classification of the posterior fossa malformations represents a moving target. Vermian hypoplasia with associated cystic dilatation of the fourth ventricle are referred to in the literature as Dandy Walker malformation, Dandy Walker variant, or Dandy Walker spectrum, to mention a few. This Babylonian confusion may have prevented a correct classification of these malformations, impairing parental counseling. In addition, malformations that appeared to be distinct from each other based on the macroanatomic neuroimaging may have more overlapping features than previously believed.

MR imaging, DTI, and FT have played a significant role in the ongoing classification and reclassification of children with Joubert syndrome (JS). For many years, JS was considered to be a well-defined, distinct posterior fossa malformation, with a characteristic clinical presentation (muscular hypotonia, cerebellar ataxia, ocular motor apraxia, irregular neonatal breathing pattern in about 30%–40% of patients and cognitive

impairment). The imaging features were well described. The diagnostic anatomic neuroimaging finding includes the so-called molar tooth sign (MTS), which refers to the shape of the mid-hindbrain, which resembles a molar tooth on axial imaging. The superior cerebellar peduncles are thickened, elongated, course in an axial plane, and the interpeduncular fossa is abnormally deep. In addition, the vermis is hypoplastic, the fastigium of the fourth ventricle is elevated, and the posterior fossa may be enlarged. With the wide availability of MR imaging, many variants of the key findings have been identified, and in addition, many more possibly associated findings like hippocampal malrotation, callosal dysgenesis, migration abnormalities, cephaloceles, and hypothalamic hamartomas have been described in patients with a molar tooth configuration of the mid-hindbrain. Increasing experience with and availability of neuroimaging showed the MTS in other disorders such as Senior-Loken, Dekaban-Arima, Malta, or Varadi-Papp syndromes. These syndromes are not considered as distinct disorders, but as part of JS, and are included in the different phenotypes of JS, depending on the systemic involvement (eg, kidney, eyes, and liver). The Varadi-Papp syndrome or oral-facial-digital (OFD) syndrome type VI represents a rare phenotypic subtype of JS.[11] In the original clinical description, these patients were characterized by polydactyly, oral findings such as tongue hamartomas, intellectual disability, and absence of the cerebellar vermis. The subsequent recognition of the MTS on neuroimaging prompted the inclusion of OFD VI into JS.

Ongoing genetic research has shown that JS belongs to the group of so-called ciliopathies. The 27 genes associated with JS so far encode for proteins of the primary cilium, which plays a key role in the development and functioning of various cells, including retinal photoreceptors, epithelial cells lining the renal tubules and bile ducts and last but not least, neurons itself. These children may present with retinal dystrophy or colobomas, nephronophthisis, or renal cysts. The imaging findings on conventional anatomic T1-weighted and T2-weighted MR imaging underestimate the degree of the underlying malformation. The internal microstructural neuroarchitecture of white matter tracts is expected to be anomalous. Two previous neuropathologic studies[12,13] showed an almost complete absence of pyramidal tract decussation in the caudal medulla and an abnormal or failed decussation of the superior cerebellar peduncles.

An early DTI report published by Charles Raybaud's group[14] confirmed an absence of

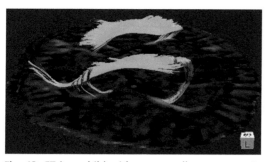

Fig. 13. FT in a child with corpus callosum agenesis. The aberrant course of the Probst fibers is easily recognized by the anterior-posterior course of the tracts. The Probst bundles are shown superimposed on color-coded FA maps.

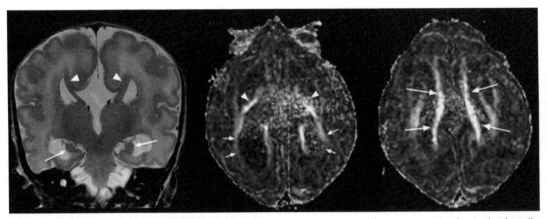

Fig. 14. Coronal T2-weighted MR image in a child with a complete corpus callosum agenesis. The Probst bundles extend along the medial surface of the lateral ventricles (*arrowheads*), hippocampi are malrotated (*small arrows*), and the anterior commissure is absent or significantly hypoplastic. Two matching axial FA maps of the brain show the Probst bundles as tightly packed, FA-hyperintense bands of white matter along the medial surface of the lateral ventricles (*arrows*). The corticospinal tract (*arrowheads*) and the optic tract/radiation (*small arrows*) are also shown as FA-hyperintense bundles. No anterior commissure could be identified on the FA maps.

decussation of the superior cerebellar peduncles on color-coded FA images. A subsequent larger-scale DTI study,[15] which also included FT, confirmed that the fibers of the pyramidal tracts failed to cross/decussate in the lower brainstem and that there was an absence of decussation of the superior cerebellar peduncles (**Fig. 16**).

The value of DTI and FT in the grouping and classification of brain malformations was also shown in patients with a tectocerebellar dysraphism (TCD) with occipital encephalocele (OE). The pathogenesis of TCD-OE is unknown. The pertinent anatomic neuroimaging findings include a severe hypogenesis of the cerebellar vermis, a tectal malformation mimicking a tectal beaking (as may be seen in a Chiari II malformation), and an occipital encephalocele. Additional key imaging findings include an elongated, horizontally oriented superior cerebellar peduncle and a deepened interpeduncular fossa, resulting in an MTS. This finding raises the question whether TCD-OE is a distinct disorder or part of JS. DTI analysis of a 4-year-old child with TCD-OE showed an absence of the decussation of the superior cerebellar peduncles, supporting the hypothesis that TCD-OE may belong to JS.[16]

Recently, the spectrum of conventional neuroimaging findings in JS has been systematically evaluated in a large cohort of 75 patients.[17] No neuroimaging-genotype correlation could be found, which supports the notion that significant variability and heterogeneity exist in JS. An intrafamilial heterogeneity could also be seen in affected siblings. DTI and FT may possibly help to improve the microstructural imaging

genotype classification of these posterior fossa malformations.

Anomalous Decussations in Many Malformations

Vulliemoz and colleagues[18] published a review article on the normal and anomalous crossing of nerve tracts from 1 hemisphere in the brain to the contralateral sense organ or limb (**Fig. 17**). These investigators reported that evolutionary and teleologic arguments suggest that midline crossing emerged in response to distinct physiologic and anatomic constraints. In several genetic and developmental disorders, including Klippel-Feil syndrome, X-linked Kallmann syndrome, essential mirror movements, horizontal gaze palsy and progressive scoliosis (HGPS), pontine tegmental cap dysplasia (**Fig. 18**), and Chiari II syndrome, anomalous decussations and commissures have been described. Crossed pathways may also be involved in the recovery and compensatory brain rewiring after brain injury. DTI and FT seem well suited to explore these neuroarchitectural disorders.

Recognition of an anomalous or absent decussation of the superior cerebellar peduncles has been shown in HGPS, pontine tegmental cap dysplasia, and JS. In addition, failure of the pyramidal tracts to cross in the medulla has also been suggested in Chiari II syndrome. This finding may be of significance for the better understanding of children who present with a non–skin-covered, open spinal dysraphia and associated Chiari II syndrome and may influence the prenatal treatment options and parental counseling.

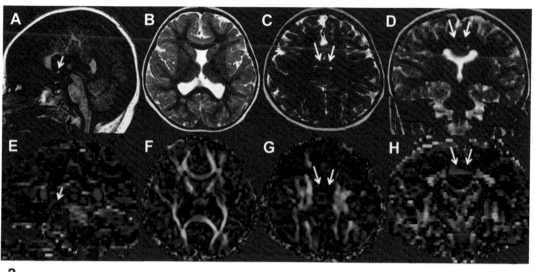

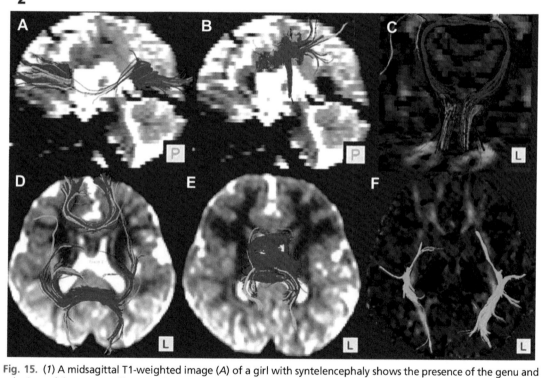

Fig. 15. (*1*) A midsagittal T1-weighted image (*A*) of a girl with syntelencephaly shows the presence of the genu and splenium of the corpus callosum, whereas the body of the corpus callosum is completely lacking. The anterior commissure is present (*white arrow*). Axial T2-weighted image (*B*) shows the presence of the genu and splenium of the corpus callosum. The basal ganglia and thalami are well separated. Axial T2-weighted image at a higher level (*C*) and coronal T2-weighted image (*D*) show absence of the body of the corpus callosum and fusion of the posterior frontal lobes and part of the parietal regions with continuation of both the gray and white matter across the midline (*arrows* in *C, D*). Midsagittal (*E*) axial (*F, G*) and coronal (*H*) color-coded FA maps confirm the presence of the genu and splenium, absence of the body of the corpus callosum, presence of the anterior commissure (*white arrow* in [*E*]), and fusion of the posterior frontal lobes and part of the parietal regions with continuation of the white matter across the midline as a thick bundle of red (*arrows* in *G, H*). (*2*) FT data superimposed to midsagittal (*A, B*) and axial (*D, E*) T2-weighted b0 images and to axial and coronal (*C*) and axial (*F*) color-coded FA maps shows that fibers running through the genu and the splenium of the corpus callosum project to the anterior frontal and occipitotemporal lobes, respectively (*A, D*), whereas the white matter fibers included within the fused regions project to the posterior frontal and parietal lobes (*B, E*). The corticospinal and medial lemniscal tracts are present and not fused at the level of the brain stem, project to the precentral and postcentral gyri, but show interhemispheric connection at the level of the fused hemispheres (*C*). The inferior fronto-occipital fasciculi are easy to be indentified (*F*) and partially connect the fibers projecting to the occipitotemporal lobes with those projecting to the anterior frontal lobes (*A, D*). (*From* Verschuuren S, Poretti A, Meoded A, et al. Diffusion tensor imaging and fiber tractography in syntencephaly. Neurographics 2013;3:165, 166; with permission.)

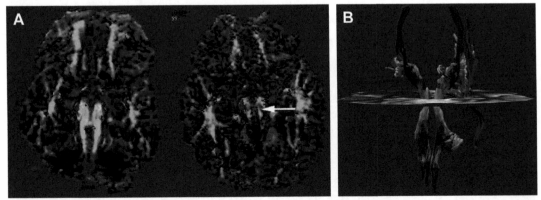

Fig. 16. (*A*) Child with JS (*first image*) shows on axial color-coded FA maps at the level of the pontomesencephalic junction the characteristic green encoded horizontal orientation of the superior cerebellar peduncles and the absence of the red dot within the midbrain representing the failure of the superior cerebellar peduncle to decussate. A matching color-coded FA map (*second image*) of a healthy individual is seen on the left with the normal red dot in the midbrain (*arrow*). (*B*) Combined three-dimensional FT and axial T2-weighted image shows the course of the CST without identifiable crossing fibers at the level of the lower medulla oblongata. A group of noncrossing fibers of the superior cerebellar peduncle is also shown on the left side (*green encoded*). (*From Poretti A, Boltshauser E, Loenneker T, et al. Diffusion tensor imaging in Joubert syndrome. AJNR Am J Neuroradiol 2007;28:1930, 1932; with permission.*)

The association of an open, non–skin-covered spinal dysraphia and hindbrain herniation (Chiari II malformation) is well known. Various randomized trials have shown that early, intrauterine surgical closure of the nonneurulated spinal cord may arrest the progressive traumatic and degenerative damage of the spinal cord while exposed to the amniotic fluid in utero, resulting in improved postnatal spinal cord function.[19,20] The Chiari II malformation is believed to be secondary to a chronic CSF leakage out of the nonneurulated spinal cord into the amniotic cavity, which prevents an

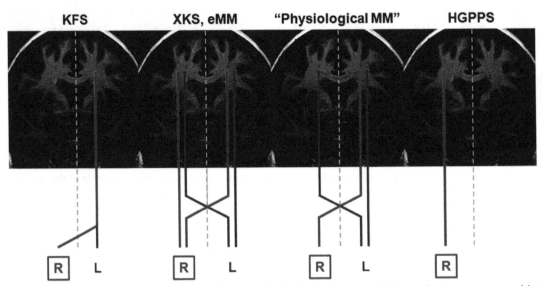

Fig. 17. Anomalous decussations in various disorders. Red indicates tracts mediating voluntary movement; blue indicates tracts involved in mirror movements (MM). In Klippel-Feil syndrome (KFS), pyramidal decussation is absent, and axons may branch in the spinal cord. In X-linked Kallmann syndrome (XKS) and essential MM (eMM) neurons in the left motor cortex with ipsilateral and contralateral projections are coactivated, and there is activation of the right motor cortex. In physiologic MM of childhood, coactivation of both motor cortices occur because of insufficient transcallosal inhibition of the right motor cortex (*dashed red line*). The ipsilateral left CST may also be involved. In horizontal gaze palsy and progressive scoliosis (HGPPS), the right motor cortex controls right-sided muscles.

A

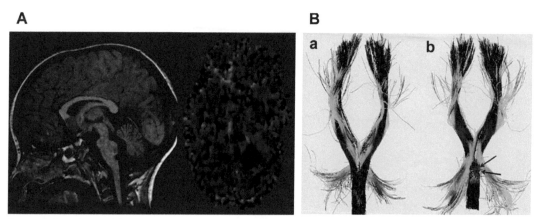

B

Fig. 18. (A) Midsagittal T1-weighted image in a child with pontine tegmental cap dysplasia shows the pontine tegmental cap protruding into the fourth ventricle combined with a flat profile of the ventral pons. Axial color-coded FA map presents the ectopic bundle of fibers (cap) as a red tract at the dorsal aspect of the pons. (B) Anterior (a) and posterior (b) projection of a three-dimensional FT of the same patient shows the absence of the normally ventrally located transverse pontine fibers, whereas the ectopic bundle of fibers (cap) are seen along the dorsal aspect of the pons (black arrows). The decussation of the superior cerebellar peduncles is absent. (From Poretti A, Meoded A, Rossi A, et al. Diffusion tensor imaging and fiber tractography in brain malformations. Pediatr Radiol 2013;43:45; with permission.)

adequate expansion of the developing rhomben-cephalic vesicle, which is again associated with a small posterior fossa. Early in utero closure of the defect has also been shown to limit or resolve the hindbrain herniation, often within weeks after fetal surgery. This rather simplistic explanation for the Chiari II malformation cannot explain the additional findings in the supratentorial brain like, for example, corpus callosum malformations or migrational disorders. Likely multiple genetic or epigenetic factors play a role in the development of a Chiari II malformation. DTI and FT have

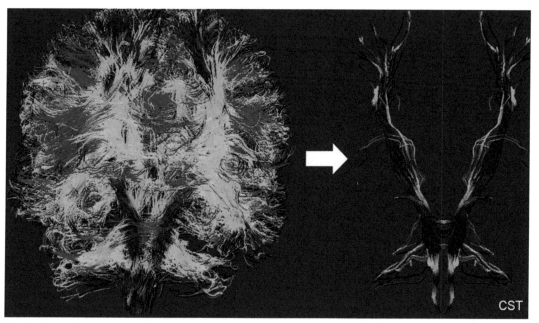

Fig. 19. Three-dimensional FT of all fibers within the brain. If all fibers are simultaneously reconstructed, individual white matter tracts cannot be studied because they are obscured. If the seed points for FT reconstruction are carefully positioned, individual white matter tracts (eg, CST) can be extracted from the complete data set and are consequently amenable for evaluation.

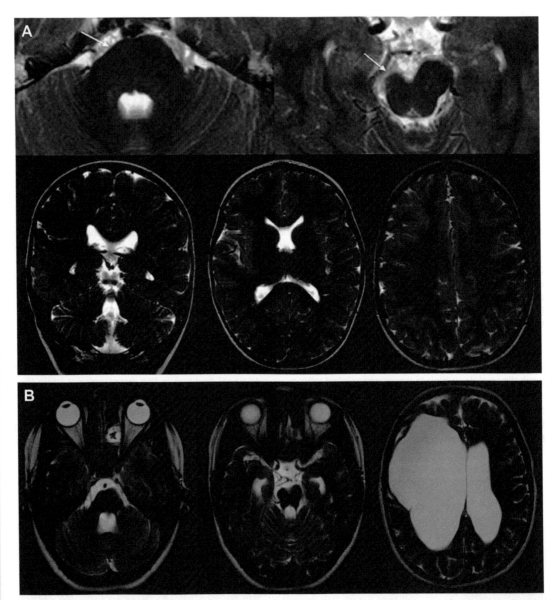

Fig. 20. (A) Axial and coronal T2-weighted images of a 3-year-old boy (child 1) with headache and mild left-sided muscular hypotonia since birth. The imaging shows a high-grade volume loss of the right pons and right cerebral peduncle (arrows). No focal lesion is noted within the supratentorial brain to match the unilateral brain stem volume loss. (B) Second child for comparison with a similar volume loss of the right pons and right cerebral peduncle. A large porencephalic cyst is noted within the ipsilateral hemispheric white matter, which matches and explains the ipsilateral brain stem volume loss. (C) Axial color-coded FA maps of child 1 show the normal blue/violet color-coded CST on the left in the pons and cerebellar peduncle. The contralateral right CST is obviously missing; in particular, no blue/violet CST is seen in the expected location in the pons and cerebellar peduncle (white arrows), suggesting absence of the right CST. The color-coded image on the level of the internal capsule shows blue-encoded CST in the expected location bilaterally. These findings suggest that the CST may be intact but follow an aberrant course in the brainstem. Axial color-coded FA maps of child 2 show a similar absence of the blue-encoded descending CST at the right anterior pons; however, also no blue-encoded CST are noted in the ipsilateral internal capsule. (D) FT superimposed on color-coded FA maps show the complete aberrant course of the right CST extending through the dorsal brain stem in the expected location of the ML in child 1. The left CST shows a normal course through the ventral brainstem at the level of the pons. For comparison, FT shows a highly atrophic almost absent right CST in typical location (anterior pons) in the second child with the large porencephalic cyst. ([A, C, D] From Meoded A, Poretti A, Dzirasa L, et al. Aberrant course of the corticospinal tracts in the brain stem revealed by diffusion tensor imaging/tractography. Neurographics 2012;2:140, 141; with permission.)

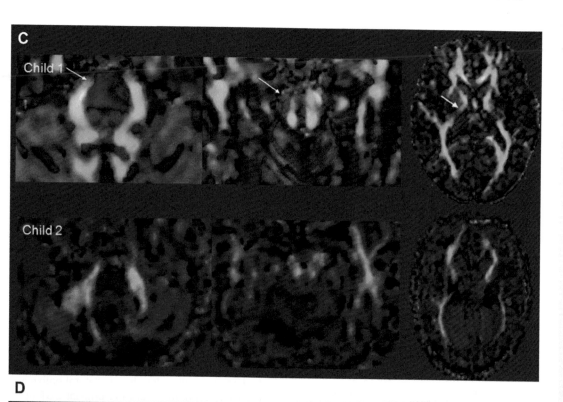

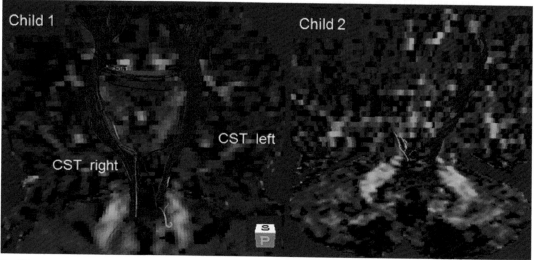

Fig. 20.

identified various microstructural anomalies, like aberrant crossing white matter tracts in the cingulum, a reduction in the number of transverse pontine fibers, reduced FA values in the corpus callosum, increased FA values in the anterior commissure, which remain undetected on conventional MR imaging.[7] These additional data may help to predict functional outcome and subclassify patients and can possibly serve to monitor treatment results.

FINAL REMARKS AND 2 ILLUSTRATIVE CASES TO THINK ABOUT
It Is All About Connecting the Dots

As mentioned earlier, it is all about connecting the dots. However, this task may not be simple in complex brain malformations. Powerful postprocessing software programs may identify hundreds or thousands of white matter tracts within the sampled brain (Fig. 19). However, too many reconstructed fibers may obscure the relevant aberrant,

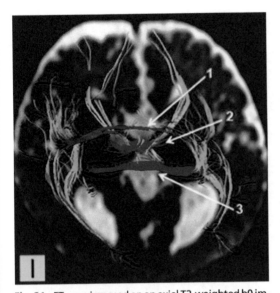

Fig. 21. FT superimposed on an axial T2-weighted b0 image of a child with agenesis of the corpus callosum show in addition to the anterior commissure (1) 2 unclassified, unknown white matter tracts (2, 3), which appear to connect the nonfused thalami across the midline. (*From* Poretti A, Meoded A, Rossi A, et al. Diffusion tensor imaging and fiber tractography in brain malformations. Pediatr Radiol 2013;43:49; with permission.)

maldeveloped, or missing white matter tracts. To study the normal and abnormal brain neuro-architecture, one needs (1) a good guidance (post-processing tools, eg, deterministic or probabilistic, and which thresholds to use), (2) to know where to start and possibly end the fiber reconstruction (start and end seed point), and (3) as mentioned almost 100 years ago by Josef Klingler, those wishing to learn the neuroanatomy need to have a good knowledge of the brain anatomy, as well as patience and perseverance. This way, one can extract the correct and relevant information out of the complete three-dimensional tractography reconstruction (see **Fig. 19**).

Illustrative Case

One puzzling case should show the significance of DTI and FT in the diagnostic workup of puzzling findings. A 3-year-old boy was referred for a brain MR imaging study because of headache and a minimal left-sided muscular hypotonia since birth. The clinical examination showed a mildly decreased coordination on the left. The anatomic MR images showed a significant reduction in size of the right brainstem and mesencephalon (**Fig. 20**A). This finding is typically encountered when a large white matter lesion (eg, porencephalic) is present in the ipsilateral cerebral hemisphere (see **Fig. 20**B). However, in this child, the

supratentorial brain appeared unremarkable on anatomic T1-weighted and T2-weighted MR imaging. However, the color-coded FA maps showed a surprising finding. The blue-encoded descending CST appeared absent at its expected location in the right anterior pons, although it was present and symmetric at the level of the internal capsule. A matching child with a large porencephalic cyst in the right cerebral hemisphere is shown in **Fig. 20**C. In this second patient, the CST appear absent or significantly diminished both at the level of the pons and internal capsule. Three-dimensional FT allowed us to better understand the findings. FT showed that the descending CST did run through the internal capsule bilaterally as expected, but that the more caudal extension of the right CST follows an aberrant course and is located more posteriorly in the pons, likely following the course of the ascending medial lemniscus (ML) (see **Fig. 20**D). For comparison, in the child with the large porencephalic cyst, FT shows some small, residual CST in the expected location of the anterior, atrophic right brainstem. An aberrant course of the CST is an uncommon, but not unknown finding. It usually refers to a collateral pathway of the CST, separated from the original CST at the level of the midbrain, descends through the ML within the pons, and reenters the original CST at the upper medulla.[21] Previous DTI studies had shown that aberrant CST may be seen in approximately 18% of healthy brains, suggesting that aberrant CST may represent a physiologic anomaly or variation.[21] In our patient, DTI and FT helped to identify the present pathology in much better detail. This finding may be of significance for future treatment options and more specific classifications of malformations.

Nonsolved Case

One final case shows that anatomic and microstructural DTI/FT imaging should go hand in hand and may help to identify unknown white matter tracts that have not yet been described or cannot be explained by our current knowledge of brain development. **Fig. 21** shows the neuroimaging findings of a 4-month-old child with a prenatal diagnosis of corpus callosum agenesis. Conventional imaging showed the classical imaging features of a corpus callosum agenesis.[7] However, 2 white matter tract–like connections between the thalami were identified on axial T2-weighted imaging immediately posterior to the intact anterior commissure. FT showed 2 matching white matter tracts or connections crossing the midline. The significance of this finding remains unclear; it is arguable that these fibers represent true commissural fibers, which may represent a confusing artifact; future research may show that this is real.

SUMMARY

DTI and FT allow us to study the microstructure of the CNS in vivo and are consequently a valuable tool for the better understanding of the normal and abnormal brain development. The collected data will help to better classify malformations and may give important hints to the genetic bases of the encountered findings. To answer the question of the title of this article: DTI and FT are helpful for brain malformations.

REFERENCES

1. Huisman TA. Diffusion weighted imaging: basic concepts and application in cerebral stroke and head trauma. Eur Radiol 2003;13:2283–97.
2. Huisman TA. Diffusion weighted and diffusion tensor imaging of the brain, made easy. Cancer Imaging 2010;10:S163–71.
3. Legée G. L'Homme de René Descartes (editions de 1662 et 1664): physiologie et macansime. Histoire des Sciences Médicales 1987;4:381–98.
4. Agrawal A, Kapfhammer JP, Kress A, et al. Josef Klingler's models of white matter tracts: influences on neuroanatomy, neurosurgery, and neuroimaging. Neurosurgery 2011;69:238–54.
5. Yasargil MG, Ture U, Yasargil DC. Surgical anatomy of supratentorial midline lesions. Neurosurg Focus 2005;18(6B):E1.
6. Raybaud C. The corpus callosum, the other great forebrain commissures, and the septum pellucidum: anatomy, development, and malformation. Neuroradiology 2010;52:447–77.
7. Poretti A, Meoded A, Rossi A, et al. Diffusion tensor imaging and fiber tractography in brain malformations. Pediatr Radiol 2013;43:28–54.
8. Smith T, Tekes A, Boltshauser E, et al. Commissural malformations: beyond the corpus callosum. J Neuroradiol 2008;35:301–3.
9. Verschuuren S, Poretti A, Meoded A, et al. Diffusion tensor imaging and fiber tractography in syntencephaly. Neurographics 2013;3:164–8.
10. Meoded A, Poretti A, Tekes A, et al. Prenatal MR diffusion tractography in a fetus with complete corpus callosum agenesis. Neuropediatrics 2011; 42:122–3.
11. Poretti A, Vitiello G, Hennekam RC, et al. Delineation and diagnostic criteria of oral-facial-digital syndrome type IV. Orphanet J Rare Dis 2012;7:4.
12. Friede RL, Boltshauser E. Uncommon syndromes of cerebellar vermis aplasia. I: Joubert syndrome. Dev Med Child Neurol 1978;20:758–63.
13. Yachmis AT, Rorke LB. Neuropathology of Joubert syndrome. J Child Neurol 1999;14:655–9.
14. Widjaja E, Blaser S, Raybaud C. Diffusion tensor imaging of midline posterior fossa malformations. Pediatr Radiol 2006;36:510–7.
15. Poretti A, Boltshauser E, Loenneker T, et al. Diffusion tensor imaging in Joubert syndrome. AJNR Am J Neuroradiol 2007;28:1929–33.
16. Poretti A, Singhi S, Huisman TA, et al. Tecto-cerebellar dysraphism with occipital encephalocele: not a distinct disorder, but part of the Joubert syndrome spectrum. Neuropediatrics 2011;42:170–4.
17. Poretti A, Huisman TA, Scheer I, et al. Joubert syndrome and related disorders: spectrum of neuroimaging findings in 75 patients. AJNR Am J Neuroradiol 2011;32:1459–63.
18. Vulliemoz S, Raineteau O, Jabaudon D. Reaching beyond the midline: why are human brains cross wired? Lancet Neurol 2005;4:87–99.
19. Adzick NS, Thoam EA, Spong CY, et al. A randomized trial of prenatal versus postnatal repair of myelomeningocele. N Engl J Med 2011;364: 993–1004.
20. Meuli M, Moehrlen E. Fetal surgery for myelomeningocele: a critical appraisal. Eur J Pediatr Surg 2013; 23:103–9.
21. Meoded A, Poretti A, Dzirasa L, et al. Aberrant course of the corticospinal tracts in the brain stem revealed by diffusion tensor imaging/tractography. Neurographics 2012;2:139–43.

Pretherapeutic Functional Magnetic Resonance Imaging in Children

Lucie Hertz-Pannier, MD, PhD[a,b,*],
Marion Noulhiane, PhD[a,b], Sebastian Rodrigo, MD, PhD[a,b],
Catherine Chiron, MD, PhD[a,b]

KEYWORDS

- Functional magnetic resonance imaging • Child • Cortical mapping • Motor • Language • Memory
- Reading • Brain development

KEY POINTS

- Blood-oxygen-level-dependent contrast may be negative in babies and infants.
- Simple block paradigms are the most robust for clinical applications in children; passive tasks can be used.
- Brain plasticity is maximal in children, with a possibility of efficient right organization of language in early left hemisphere lesions.
- Contralateral motor reorganization is also possible in early prenatal lesions (persistence of ipsilateral corticospinal tract).
- Resting state functional magnetic resonance imaging may be a promising tool for pretherapeutic mapping in children in the future.

INTRODUCTION

In children, like in adults, the main (if not only) clinical application of functional magnetic resonance imaging (fMRI) is to provide reliable mapping of eloquent cortices (mostly, motor and language areas), and of their relationship with the planned resection in case of tumor or epilepsy surgery, to select patients, tailor resection, and avoid postoperative deficits. When combined with clinical, neuropsychological and neurophysiologic data, anatomofunctional magnetic resonance (MR) imaging techniques (MR imaging, diffusion tensor imaging [DTI], and fMRI) offer the possibility of a noninvasive presurgical workup, which has tremendous consequences for children's management not only by reducing the need for invasive techniques but also by making many more children amenable to presurgical exploration, thus affecting patient management. In that context, all methods implemented must reach high sensitivity for detecting activated areas at the individual level, especially in young children. Therefore, most teams use validated tasks amenable to patients with variable abilities, in robust block paradigms, with individual analyses involving adapted statistical methods. Still most needed here are further validation and standardization of the whole process across clinical teams.

The mere comparison between the explosive number of fMRI studies in adults and the still limited studies in children, especially in clinical applications, highlights the intrinsic difficulties of studying children. Recently, the possibility of studying brain functional connectivity with fMRI during rest (resting state functional connectivity

[a] UMR 1129, INSERM, Paris Descartes University, CEA-Saclay, Gif sur Yvette, France; [b] UNIACT/Neurospin, I2BM, DSV, CEA-Saclay, Gif sur Yvette, France
* Corresponding author. U1129/UNIACT/Neurospin, Bat 145, PC 156, 91191 Gif sur Yvette, France.
E-mail address: Lucie.hertz-pannier@cea.fr

Neuroimag Clin N Am 24 (2014) 639–653
http://dx.doi.org/10.1016/j.nic.2014.07.002
1052-5149/14/$ – see front matter © 2014 Elsevier Inc. All rights reserved.

MR imaging) may make it possible to overcome several of those limitations in the future, to assess the development of neuronal networks from birth on, in health and in disease, and to map eloquent cortex before surgery even in uncooperative or deficient patients.

In this article, some specificities of fMRI in children (eg, blood-oxygen-level-dependent [BOLD] response and brain maturation, paradigm design, technical issues, feasibility, data analysis) are reviewed, then the main knowledge on presurgical cortical mapping in children (motor, language, reading, memory) is summarized, and the emergence of resting state fMRI in presurgical cortical mapping is discussed.

HOW TO PERFORM FUNCTIONAL MR IMAGING IN CHILDREN
Blood-Oxygen-Level-Dependent Contrast in the Developing Brain

The developing brain is characterized by a succession of progressive and regressive events, with intense synaptic growth from birth on leading to synaptic overproduction and redundancy in the primary school years, and then, slow progressive synaptic pruning with stabilization of efficient networks during adolescence and young adulthood.[1] This triphasic process occurs earlier in primary systems, and later into the second decade for the associative networks, and is accompanied by changes in glucose consumption and blood flow.[2,3]

In the recent years, fMRI has emerged as a unique tool to study the exquisite plasticity of the immature brain, which sustains both normal learning and memory acquisition, and recovery after a focal insult or abnormality with an incomparably better functional outcome compared with adults with similar condition. The general pattern of functional maturation of a specific network has been shown as regional specialization of activated clusters with age, starting from a more widespread activation in earlier ages,[4,5] and associating progressive and regressive changes in different regions.[6] These focal changes are associated with changes in short-range and long-range connectivity, as recently discovered by functional connectivity studies (see later discussion).

These combined biological events in immature networks, associated with changes in vascular reactivity during neuronal firing, may contribute to the negative BOLD response during visual and sensorimotor stimulations described in neonates and infants.[7–9] However, part of this negative response might also be attributed to sedation, which is commonly used at this age. Beyond the first weeks of life, BOLD hemodynamic response is stable across ages, although with possible increase in amplitude until adulthood,[10] and some variations across tasks.[11]

Which Paradigm Design?

Block or event?
So far, all fMRI clinical applications in children have used block paradigms, in which the patient performs the tasks repeatedly over activation and reference periods (usually 20 to 40 seconds each), repeated several times in a single trial. This approach is the most robust and reproducible, because of good statistical power per unit time, and therefore is used in clinical applications such as individual presurgical motor or language mapping. It can also be usefully applied in clinical research programs in which children are to be pooled in groups for comparing activation differences according to a clinical marker.

More sophisticated single-event paradigms, which allow monitoring brain response during processing of a single stimulus, may prove useful in patients, because they avoid using a control task (thus reducing a possible confounding factor), they permit accounting for interstimulus response variability, and they offer extended possibilities of experimental designs eg, in memory studies. However, their implementation remains difficult in clinical environments (especially in children), because of long acquisition times, lower sensitivity, large data volumes, and the need for customized and time-consuming analyses.

Choosing tasks adapted to the child's age and performance
The most critical part of fMRI studies resides in the choice of activation and reference tasks, because data analysis most often relies on cognitive subtraction (ie, the resulting activated areas are believed to sustain the components that are involved in the activated state but not in the reference one). For example, the comparison of an auditorily cued semantic decision task and a simple tone discrimination task shows mainly regions involved in semantic processes.[12] On the other hand, the comparison of a more global language task (eg, sentence generation to a given noun) compared with simple rest shows a larger functional network, which includes numerous modules of receptive and expressive language (phonemic discrimination, phonology, lexical and semantic processing, syntax, verbal working memory and prearticulatory processing). In motor paradigms, global hand movements like grasping or clutching compared with rest show the hand primary sensorimotor region with a few associated regions (supplementary sensorimotor area), whereas

alternating complex sequential finger movements activates a larger network, including the premotor cortex.

fMRI experimental constraints are particularly demanding for children, because paradigms are designed in a rigid manner, according to a priori models of BOLD contrast time course. In addition, the intrinsically low BOLD contrast/noise ratio requires the repetition of events to gain statistical power. In that context, task complexity is critical in children, in terms of cognitive/attentional demands. According to the age and cognitive level of the patients, block paradigms with simple tasks are most often suited, such as, for example, alternating hand movements with rest for motor mapping. Tasks can almost always be adapted to the performance level (even in motor paradigms, from complex sequential finger tapping to simple grasp movement, or passive wrist flexion-extension). In cognitive clinical studies, such as language studies, tasks with explicit demands are most often used, and adapted to the patient's abilities and performance. In children, this means using tasks adapted from age-validated neuropsychological tests and appropriately testing them before MR imaging.

Strictly passive tasks can also be used in particular cases, such as passive movements in patients with motor deficits, or presentation of auditory stimuli in neonates, and asleep infants and toddlers.[13,14] Although these tasks may show interesting activation often grossly comparable with that of active ones, they may not provide the same level of functional assessment in cognitive studies. Sedation can be occasionally used to assess basic functions for clinical purposes (eg, auditory stimulation before cochlear implantation,[15] motor mapping[16]), but with a careful choice of anesthetic drugs and dosages.[16,17]

The use of rest as a reference task is being debated because of the uncertainty regarding what children do while resting. In all cases, giving clues to the child on rest instruction (eg, listening to the scanner noise, concentrating on their own breathing) may help them to comply. On the one hand, it has the advantage of simplicity for very young or disabled children, who have difficulties in rapidly alternating different tasks. On the other hand, children may involuntarily not stop the activation task (resulting in falsely negative results, especially in language tasks), and there are no means of controlling ongoing cognitive activity during rest. Some experimenters therefore use very simple task like tone listening as references in children with sufficient mental flexibility.

Multiple tasks are required when testing complex cognitive functions such as language[18] to increase the robustness of lateralization assessment by combining the different tasks[19] and to show the whole network. In some instances, lateralization may vary according to the type of task, either as a normal pattern (eg, left semantic vs right prosody) or related to mixed language representation secondary to left focal epilepsy or lesion (eg, with left dominance for expressive language and right dominance for receptive one) (see later discussion).

Controlling performances

Monitoring of task performance is desirable for fully analyzing and interpreting activation maps, because the latter reflect what has been done during scanning. This analysis may be obtained by monitoring responses of the patient pressing on joystick or buttons. In case of unilateral responses, balancing the side of the responding hand may be useful to avoid systematic bias in brain activation. However, this right-left balance may complicate the paradigm for young children not fully acquainted with their own right and left sides. In motor studies, because BOLD signal depends on both movement frequency and strength, these parameters may be controlled for by cuing movements with a metronome, and monitoring them by video recordings, buttons, and so forth. However, in language fMRI studies, most tasks are performed silently, producing similar activation to overt ones, but avoiding artifacts caused by face movements. Not only does this situation preclude any performance control but it may also not be amenable to deficient children. Some experimenters have used oral responses (with online response recording), associated with adapted MR sequences with no image acquisition during the response interval to avoid articulation-related motion artifacts, taking benefit from the delayed hemodynamic response. Eye-tracking devices are being increasingly used to monitor eye movements during cognitive tasks, but the experimental setup is demanding for children and remains largely beyond the possibilities of a clinical environment.

Technical Issues

Hardware

High field MR imaging is being considered by the US Food and Drug Administration as minimal risk procedure up to 8 T for adults and children, and up to 4 T for neonates younger than 1 month. Three-Tesla fMRI has become standard in babies and children as in adults, including in healthy individuals for research protocols. The increased sensitivity of BOLD contrast at higher field strength can be used to either shorten acquisition time or increase spatial resolution to improve localization of activated clusters, which can be valuable in young children with small heads, all while maintaining adequate signal-to-noise ratio.

Multichannel coils with parallel imaging further improve the signal-to-noise ratio but make it even more critical to use coils adapted to the head size. In neonates and infants, smaller coils such as knee coils provide better signal and improve the sensitivity of fMRI. MR-compatible incubators are needed to prevent hypothermia in neonates (especially premature babies), but they are expensive and cumbersome.

Acoustic noise

One issue often neglected in fMRI is the acoustic noise created by Lorentzian forces secondary to gradient switching in echo planar images (EPI) (in functional imaging as well as in DTI). Not only may noise prevent children from remaining still because of anxiety or difficulty in sleeping but the risk of acoustic trauma must also not be underestimated, because functional MR imaging sequences often reach 110-db levels at peak frequencies. Because noise level depends on multiple sequence parameters (eg, type of sequence, spatial and temporal resolutions, parallel imaging), acoustic measurements should be ideally performed for each sequence, whenever possible. Careful prevention must always be undertaken, including in asleep or sedated infants and children, with a variety of devices (eg, earplugs, headphones, foams). Some manufacturers offer hardware options reducing acoustic noise of various sequences by modifying gradients, shape, and strength.

Temporal and spatial resolution

Temporal resolution of fMRI mainly depends on the shape of the hemodynamic response, which is comparable with adults after the first few months of life (see earlier discussion). Shortening repetition time from standard 3 to 5 seconds to 2 to 2.5 seconds provides better sampling of subtle variations of the hemodynamic response and increases statistical power (beware of acoustic noise).

Spatial resolution can strongly benefit from higher fields, and it is standard practice to acquire 3-T EPI data with $3 \times 3 \times 3$ mm^3 voxels. Although this nominal resolution is not clearly reflected in the results because of numerous steps of spatial filtering, it permits better localization of activated clusters in small anatomic regions by reducing partial volume effects. On the other hand, motion artifacts are more conspicuous and problematic in highly resolved scans.

Real-time fMRI may be of particular value in clinical studies in children, because it provides continuous monitoring of the acquisition, by reconstructing and analyzing the images online, and providing a constant update of the quality of the functional study. This factor is especially relevant when paradigms are being kept simple, with reasonable data sets and standard statistical analyses. However, this might prove a challenge in more sophisticated studies with event-related paradigms, large data sets, and analyses requiring heavy postprocessing.

Feasibility of Fuctional MR Imaging in Children

Cooperation

In fMRI activation studies, the child's cooperation is critical. However, MR imagers remain child unfriendly, and strict immobility is mandatory to avoid motion artifacts. Obtaining compliance to the tasks is therefore a challenge in young or deficient children and requires extra time and resources, with at best a dedicated visit before the study with the child and the parents. This visit with the experimenter(s) who will perform the fMRI study (eg, radiologist, neurologist, neuropsychologist) is necessary to show the child the imager and explain the tasks, to train them to remain still in a mock scanner if available, and to practice the fMRI tasks. It also makes it possible to adapt the paradigm in case of poor compliance to optimize feasibility of clinical studies, and sometimes, to cancel the study, when sufficient compliance cannot be obtained, thus optimizing scanner occupancy. During scanning, many adaptations can be implemented to improve the child's comfort and quietness, such as having the experimenter and the parents in the magnet room, interacting often with the child through intercom, playing movies on a screen during anatomic scans, monitoring the child's movements through an MR-compatible camcorder and providing them with feedback during scanning. In all cases, good head immobilization is necessary to discourage movements. Providing the child with visual inputs also decreases head motion artifacts.[20]

Scan duration

Statistical power depends directly on the number of scan repetitions and thus, on scanning duration. On the one hand, paradigms are to be made long enough to obtain reliable contrast to noise; on the other hand, attentional resources and compliance of children cannot be maintained during scans that are too long. Higher field acquisitions (3 T) do contribute to alleviate these constraints. Still, unlike in adults, in whom 10-minute to 15-minute runs are commonly acquired, in most children, the whole acquisition is preferably segmented in shorter runs of 2 to 4 minutes. It is advisable to repeat similar runs during a single session, given the high rate of poor-quality data in younger children. A whole study (including anatomic images, diffusion-weighted images with a sufficient number of directions to perform reliable tractography, and fMRI) must be completed in 20 minutes in babies or poorly compliant children, and in a maximum of 1 hour in older school-age children with no significant cognitive or behavioral impairments. In some instances, additional sequences may be needed (eg, gadolinium-enhanced perfusion MR, MR angiography, arterial spin labeling). Acquisition may then be split or repeated in 2 or more sessions separated by a break, even on separate days, because there are no limitations, given the absence of known side effects. In that case, images from different sessions must be coregistered during analysis.

Cooperation can be obtained for adapted paradigms from children with a developmental age of around 5 to 6 years or IQs around 60, if there are no behavioral disorders. Passive tasks can be used in sleeping or quiet neonates, infants, and children (either with or without sedation), using receptive language tasks, sensory stimulations, and so forth. Overall, the attrition rate of fMRI studies in children is higher than in adults, especially in activation studies.

Data Analysis

Head motion remains a critical limiting factor, especially in uncooperative, young, or debilitated patients, and is more frequent and pronounced in boys than in girls.[20] The use of dedicated registration algorithms is most often necessary, but the choice of registration method is empirical, depending on the type and amplitude of movements, and does not significantly influence the results.[21] Motion parameters can be introduced as regressors of noninterest in the analysis to reduce variance. Some algorithms are based on data interpolation to replace heavily corrupt images; others take into account discarded, and thus missing, data. Overall, the resulting corrected images must be checked carefully, because many registered data may be discarded because of insufficient correction.

Statistical analysis of pediatric data sets follows the same rules and constraints as in adults and strongly depends on the goal of the study: in presurgical studies of patients, the main goal is to optimize at the individual level the sensitivity of the detection of activated areas; resection of these

areas results in postoperative deficits, which may depend on multiple factors (eg, age, efficiency, attention, disease, medications). In such circumstances, testing multiple thresholds and taking into account the performance level are likely to increase the sensitivity of detection of activated networks, especially in children. On the other hand, a threshold that is too lenient leads to widespread activation, which may overestimate the risk of lesioning an eloquent cortex and, thus, lead to unjustified denial of surgery. Overall, in presurgical studies, thresholding and interpretation of activation maps still depend heavily on the expertise of the investigator, especially for data sets containing residual motion artifacts.

MAPPING ELOQUENT CORTEX IN FOCAL EPILEPSIES AND BRAIN TUMORS IN CHILDREN

Clinical fMRI activation studies in children are basically limited to presurgical mapping, to select patients for surgery and avoid postoperative deficits, by planning the resection according to the spatial relationship between eloquent cortices and the epileptogenic zone or the tumor. In addition, DTI can be obtained during the same MR examination, to show the anatomic connectivity of involved regions, by tracking the main fascicles (eg, corticospinal tracts, arcuate and uncinate fasciculi). When combined with clinical, neuropsychological, and neurophysiologic data, fMRI offers the possibility of reducing the need for invasive techniques and extends the range of patients amenable to presurgical explorations.[22] However, fMRI highlights regions that are activated by, but not always critical to, the tasks (ie, resection would not necessary lead to functional deficit), depending on the type of contrast that has been designed in the paradigm. This situation is to be contrasted with electrostimulation methods, in which transient induced functional deficits are supposed to reproduce those that result from the (undesirable) resection of the stimulated region. However, numerous studies[23] have shown the good correspondence of both methods when appropriate methodologies are being used, and their complementarities, in children as in adults.

fMRI has also shown that some malformations of the cortical development (eg, heterotopias, polymicrogyrias) may retain functional cortical organization (eg, vision, motor, language) with a risk of postoperative deficit in case of a resection of the malformed cortex (**Fig. 1**).[24] By contrast, it seems that Taylor-type focal cortical dysplasias may not retain functional activity within the area containing balloon cells (hypersignal on fluid-attenuated

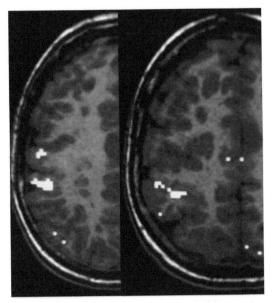

Fig. 1. Hand motor activation within a malformation of cortical development (polymicrogyria) in a child with rolandic epilepsy.

inversion recovery or T2 images,[25] although this is debated.[26]

Motor Mapping

fMRI mapping of the primary motor cortex has been probed in several series of pediatric patients with tumors, epilepsy foci, or perinatal lesions located in the central region and represents the most common and robust clinical application of fMRI in children, using various hand movements depending on the child's age and condition (Figs. 2–4), with fair reproducibility of activation between active and passive movements (see Fig. 3). These studies have shown consistent activation in regions predicted by the

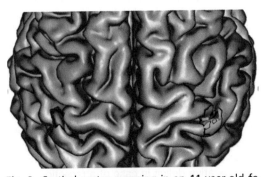

Fig. 2. Cortical motor mapping in an 11 year-old female with a right precentral focal cortical dysplasia (red). Left-hand and right-hand motor activation (rainbow and blue, respectively), showing the normal functional anatomy of the hand.

electrophysiologic data (Penfield homonculus), even when the lesion is close to the functional areas (see Fig. 4). Plastic changes of the cortical organization could also be shown in cases of early lesions within the motor cortex, in excellent agreement with the results of cortical stimulation. For example, motor plasticity has been extensively studied with fMRI and transcranial magnetic stimulation in children with unilateral spastic cerebral palsy (congenital hemiplegia), showing that the central and precentral cortex contralateral to the lesion can take over the impaired function and that the presumed date of the prenatal injury is critical to the development of functional compensation and plasticity.[27] Those children with earlier insults (first trimester) had the best motor recovery, sustained by the persistence of the ipsilateral corticospinal tract. However, this type of reorganization was observed less in children with later lesions (around birth). Functional reorganization after surgery in infancy was documented by preoperative and postoperative fMRI using passive motor tasks in young sedated infants with rolandic epilepsies caused by dysplastic lesions in the central region, showing (1) the contribution of fMRI to the delineation of eloquent cortex even in difficult conditions and (2) the posterior reorganization of the motor cortex, associated with complete or partial motor recovery.[16] Overall, these results confirm that motor fMRI can be performed efficiently and with good data quality in toddlers and children.[28] Together with other clinical considerations, motor fMRI results with good localizing power contribute to the decision-making process for children with epilepsy caused by brain lesions close to the central sulcus (see Fig. 4).[29]

Language Mapping in Children

How to perform language fuctional MR imaging in children

Expressive tasks such as verbal fluency or verb generation are associated with more lateralized networks and have a better correlation with invasive methods like the Wada test (see later discussion) than do receptive tasks.[30] Moreover, sentence-level tasks have been shown to carry significant advantages in terms of frontal and temporal activation, which is valuable for mapping perisylvian areas,[31] and they are also easier to perform for children than single word tasks (Figs. 5 and 6). For example, generating sentences from a concrete noun activates a large left perisylvian network, comprising both expressive and receptive language areas as well as the usual cortical areas

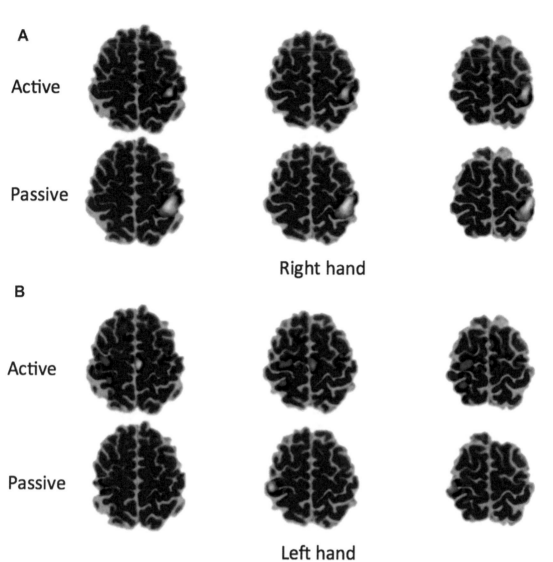

Fig. 3. Comparison of active and passive movement in a right-handed child. (*A*) Right hand: excellent reproducibility with slightly larger activated region during passive movements caused by increased sensory inputs. (*B*) Left hand: active movements are less efficient (nondominant hand), with more bilateral activation and more movement artifacts.

found to be coactivated in language tasks (supplementary sensorimotor area, dorsolateral prefrontal cortex, and basal temporal regions, see **Figs. 5** and **6**). Semantic decision tasks have also proved efficient for activating Broca and Wernicke areas in patients with epilepsy and for studying the different patterns of language reorganization.[32]

Laterality indices are commonly calculated from the number of activated regions on each hemisphere or more precisely in homologous regions of interest on each side, but they are sensitive to both the language tasks and the statistical thresholds.[33] Alternatively, bootstrap methods over a range of statistical thresholds[34] may help better characterize the lateralization. Altogether, multiple

validated language tasks, adapted to the child's level, combining at least perceptive components with semantic processing, and expressive components with language production, are necessary, along with careful correction of head movements and multithreshold analysis to optimize the reliability of language mapping in children.

Language dominance
In healthy right-handed individuals, language is predominantly represented in the left hemisphere. Anatomic brain asymmetries in the perisylvian regions are present from fetal life on, and recent fMRI studies have shown that the leftward asymmetry of language networks is present in early

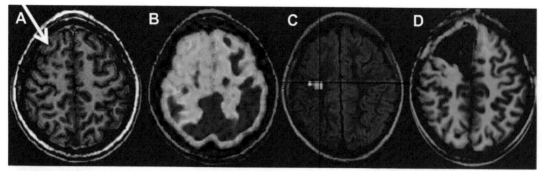

Fig. 4. Cortical mapping in a 6-year-old child with precentral cortical dysplasia (Taylor type) with subcontinuous tonic and clonic seizures of the left upper limb. (*A*) T1 images shows slight blurring of the gray-white interface in the prefrontal region (*arrow*). (*B*) Positron emission tomography scan show deep hypometabolism of the precentral cortex, just abutting the precentral gyrus. (*C*) fMRI during hand clutching, compared with rest (with a seizure during fMRI), confirms the localization of the primary motor cortex in the precentral gyrus, just at the limit of the hypometabolic zone, which was confirmed by corticography. (*D*) Surgery was tailored with intraoperative monitoring (Ste Anne Hospital, Paris, France). The child is seizure free without postoperative deficit.

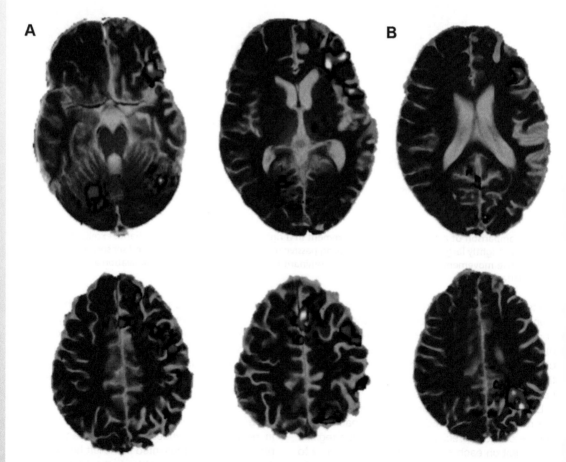

Fig. 5. Left language dominance in a child with left hemisphere epilepsy and progressive atrophy. (*A*) Sentence generation compared with rest. Activation is clearly predominant on the left side and on frontal areas including the Broca area, precentral and prefrontal cortex, presupplementary motor area, and contralateral cerebellar activation. (*B*) Sentence listening activates the Broca area along with the parietal cortex (angular gyrus).

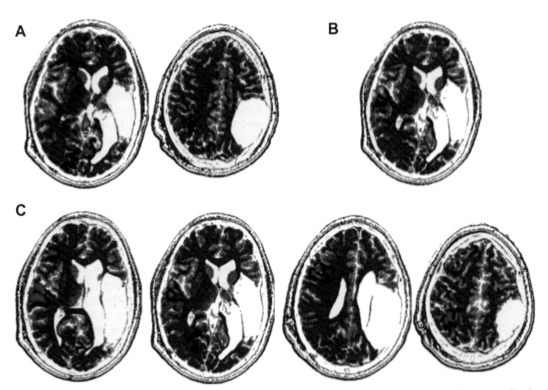

Fig. 6. Right dominance in a child with a large left prenatal stroke and candidate for a hemispherotomy (Rothschild Foundation, Paris). (*A*) Sentence generation shows activation in the right homolog of the Broca areas (inferior frontal gyrus) and right presupplementary motor area. (*B*) Word repetition activates the superior temporal gyrus. (*C*) Listening to a sentence shows the combination of the frontal and temporal activations seen in the previous tasks.

infancy, before oral language has started,[13,35] but asymmetry remains weaker in early childhood[14,36] than later, and strengthens over the years toward the adult left dominant pattern.[36–38]

Atypical (right or bilateral) representation of language may occur in 4% to 6% of right-handed individuals and 22% to 24% of left-handed healthy individuals. In adults with left hemisphere injury, tumor, or epilepsy, the capacity of language networks to reorganize either by interhemispheric shift[39] or by intrahemispheric displacement of eloquent areas[40] depends on many variables, such as handedness, type and location of the lesion, age at onset and duration of epilepsy, baseline of cognitive status. Atypical language dominance is more frequent in early left lesions, because brain plasticity is maximal during childhood: networks may reorganize in the contralateral hemisphere and language networks tend to be more fuzzy and less robust compared with healthy children (see Fig. 6).[41,42] In adults with early left temporal lobe epilepsy (LTLE), for example, this proportion can reach up to 33%.[43] In children with LTLE, atypical expressive (but not receptive) language organization depends on handedness and epilepsy duration. Right-handed children

usually retain left dominance, by contrast to adults (personal data, paper in review). Early LTLE seems to hamper the normal progression of left hemispheric specialization of expressive, but not receptive, language during childhood, especially in left-handers, in line with a long-term effect of epilepsy on language network organization, strongly correlated with the plasticity of the motor system. However, functional reorganization of language networks is not costless: children with atypical language tend to have lower levels of cognitive efficiency, especially for visuospatial skills.[44] Electrical stimulation in children has shown that developmental lesions and early onset seizures do not displace language cortex from prenatally determined sites, whereas lesions acquired before the age of 5 years may cause language to relocate to the opposite hemisphere only when language cortex is destroyed.[45]

The Wada test (intracarotid amytal test) has long been considered the gold standard to assess language lateralization before surgery, but its localizing power is limited to the determination of hemispheric dominance, it carries significant limitations, and it is invasive and stressful for children. fMRI is a good noninvasive alternative that provides clinically relevant information in children for the assessment of language dominance.[46] However, even although fMRI assessment of language dominance is now everyday practice in adults, fMRI is not yet fully accepted as a standard of care in pediatric epilepsy, because of the limited number of published studies validating the method in children.[46–48] In a series of 100 adults,[49] the discordance between Wada test and fMRI in terms of language dominance remained low (9%). Because the only gold standard for testing the function of a specific cortical area would be an unexpected postoperative deficit, which is rare, it is most often impossible to conclude on language dominance in such cases. In both tests, results depend on the nature and multiplicity of language tasks and of the individual's compliance, in addition to amytal distribution in the Wada test and to statistical issues and head movement artifacts in fMRI.

Language mapping in children

Presurgical language cortical mapping may be needed when surgery is to be performed in the dominant hemisphere, but it carries significant risks and is particularly difficult to perform in children. Direct intraoperative cortical stimulation, considered the gold standard in adults, is not feasible in most children. More recently, perioperative stimulation using subdural grids and depth electrodes has been challenged because of insufficient sensitivity in children, which may result from reorganized language distribution, limited testing capacity, and incomplete myelination with high stimulation thresholds. Colocalization between intraoperative stimulations and fMRI activations has been assessed in both isolated cases and case series in adults and children[19,23,50–52] and shown to lie within 1 to 2 cm in several preliminary reports. Overall, in these studies, the sensitivity of fMRI varied from 38% to 100% and the specificity from 65% to 97% (Fig. 7).[23] However, strict comparison of both techniques remains difficult, because cortical stimulation discloses only limited regions critical to language functions, whereas fMRI does not provide hierarchical information on the numerous activated regions, which may not all be essential to language (low specificity). These techniques may be seen as complementary: in children with epilepsy, fMRI during sentence generation enabled the detection of all critical regions shown by cortical stimulation within a large perisylvian language network, at the expense of relatively weak specificity,[23] suggesting that fMRI would be useful for optimizing the placement of intracranial electrodes when language mapping is necessary (see Fig. 7).

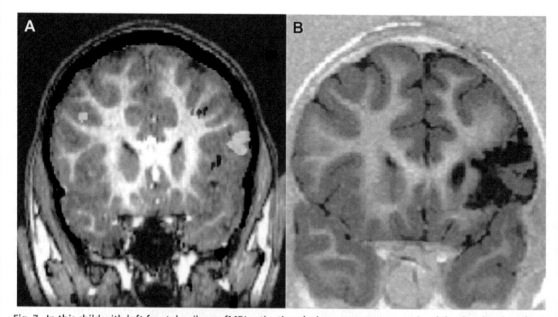

Fig. 7. In this child with left frontal epilepsy, fMRI activation during sentence generation (A) colocalized perfectly with electrostimulation, which allowed the resection to be tailored, as shown in (B) (Rothschild Foundation, Paris), with the child seizure free and with no language deficit postoperatively. (Adapted from de Ribaupierre S, Fohlen M, Bulteau C, et al. Presurgical language mapping in children with epilepsy: clinical usefulness of functional magnetic resonance imaging for the planning of cortical stimulation. Epilepsia 2012;53:73; with permission.)

Reading

The presurgical assessment of reading is critical in surgery of the inferotemporal lobe and occipital lateral region, because postoperative reading deficits may severely compromise schooling. The visual word form area (VWFA), which lies in the midportion of the left occipitotemporal sulcus, encodes the identity of visual letters and supports literacy.[53] This system specializes from the cortical area dedicated to face processing during reading acquisition, and matures until the age of 10 years, although it is already left lateralized at the time of reading acquisition. After this letter-decoding phase in the ventral temporo-occipital pathway, children translate letter strings into phonologic and lexical representations in the left perisylvian language areas. We showed[54] a dissociated reorganization of both components in a child who had early left inferotemporal epilepsy caused by pial angioma before reading acquisition, who maintained a left perisylvian language network, with an elective contralateral plasticity of the VWFA, allowing resection of the left epileptic focus without creating any postoperative reading deficit. This unique developmental pattern might be caused by first early surgery before reading acquisition. By contrast, in another child with temporo-occipital epilepsy starting at age 5 years and operated at age 12 years of a gliotic lesion, clear postoperative regression of reading abilities was observed, despite preservation of left VWFA (Fig. 8), which was just contiguous to the resection cavity, and with a stronger involvement of the left perisylvian language network (Fig. 9). At 2 years after surgery, the child had recovered his preoperative level, and at 4 years postoperatively, he was reading with persisting difficulties (corresponding to a 4-year delay), concomitant with late epilepsy relapse, suggesting the persistence of epileptic cortex in the occipitotemporal region.

Memory

Temporal lobe epilepsy can cause specific memory deficits in children with distinct patterns of deficits according to the lateralization of seizure onset.[48,55–57] Children with LTLE are mostly impaired on verbal episodic memory, whereas children with right temporal lobe epilepsy (RTLE) are mostly impaired on visuospatial episodic memory. After surgery, children tend to recover from memory deficits better than adults, suggesting that the developing brain may benefit from compensatory cognitive and neurofunctional mechanisms.[56]

Whereas exploration of episodic memory with fMRI is just emerging in pediatric temporal lobe epilepsy (TLE), and preliminary data suggest that a frontohippocampoparietal network may be bilaterally impaired in left TLE, studies in adults with TLE show that mesiotemporal structures are asymmetrically impaired: activations are greater contralaterally to the epilepsy, in good concordance with individual results of the memory Wada test.[58] However, fMRI is not commonly used as clinical pretherapeutic tool for memory assessment in children, whether in temporal lobe epilepsy or in patients with tumor, because the investigation of the role of medial temporal lobe structures in the development of episodic memory is just beginning, and the effect of mesial developmental pathologies remains largely unknown.

Resting State Fuctional MR Imaging: An Emerging Technique for Pretherapeutic Mapping in Children: A Bright Future?

Resting state fMR imaging (rsfMR imaging) has emerged as a novel way for investigating the development of large-scale organization of developing networks, by measuring functional connectivity (ie, the temporal coherence between measurements of activity in different connected neural ensembles, such as spontaneous high-amplitude low frequency [<0.1 Hz] BOLD signal fluctuations during rest [ie, in individuals performing no explicit task]).[59] Using spontaneous activity, resting state maps can be generated that closely reflect the activation maps computed from an fMRI activation study (eg, motor, language, visual, activation).

The advantages of rsfMR imaging in pediatric populations are that functional brain organization can be examined independently of task performance, in deficient, asleep, or even sedated

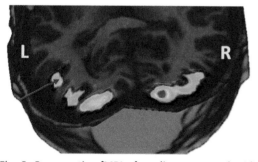

Fig. 8. Preoperative fMRI of reading compared with checkerboards in an 11-year-old boy with occipitotemporal epilepsy related to a gliotic lesion. Activation of the primary and secondary visual cortex and of the VWFA (arrow) on the left side. P<.05 false discovery rate.

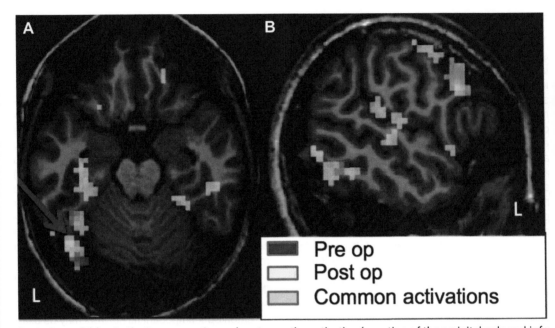

Fig. 9. Same child as in **Fig. 8**: preoperative and postoperative activation (resection of the occipital pole and inferior aspect of the calcarine fissure). (*A*) Despite the preservation of the VWFA (*red arrow*), the child experienced a durable decrease in reading abilities. (*B*) Note the increased engagement of the perisylvian language network postoperatively.

children, and that a full data set can be collected in as little as 5 minutes.[60] rsfMR imaging data are collected as participants lie in the MR imaging scanner, typically with eyes closed or fixating gaze on a cross-hair, without any specific cognitive demand, or even sleeping. Thus, data can be collected from low-functioning and very young populations. However, the patients must remain still, because data corrupted by head motion cannot be properly analyzed, even after motion correction. Different analysis approaches are being evaluated in this emerging field; the application in clinics is preliminary.

The commonly used hypothesis-driven seed-based approach typically involves choosing 1 or more region of interest (ROI) to investigate the whole-brain functional connectivity, often using a regression or correlation model. However, it can be biased by the selection of the ROI, especially in distorted anatomies (tumors, malformations) and is time consuming. Unlike ROI-based analysis, various model-free data-driven approaches (such as independent component analysis), whereby four-dimensional fMRI data are decomposed into a set of independent one-dimensional time series and associated three-dimensional spatial maps, describing the temporal and spatial characteristics of the underlying signal[61] are widely used for analyzing rsfMR imaging data. Within-subject and between-subject measures computed from rsfMR imaging are consistent and reproducible.[62,63]

However, the methods are constantly evolving, and their presurgical application is just nascent in adults[64,65] but has not been tested in children. In a recent study, Mitchell and colleagues[66] used a supervised neural network technique form rsfMR imaging data to identify functional networks in adult patients with brain tumors, showing encouraging sensitivity and specificity for motor and language mapping compared with corticography. However, at the individual level, the method lacked precision in labeling specific networks and missed a few critical regions, thus leading to potential surgical morbidity if not correctly identified. However, it shows the potential of such approaches for the presurgical planning of those patients, if thorough validation on larger series is performed.

The benefit of such approaches is likely to be at least equivalent in children, in whom results suggest that resting state networks driven by spontaneous signal fluctuations are present already in the infant brain.[67] Studies have reported that this intrinsic organization can be shown in awake, asleep, sedated, and event anesthetized patients. Beyond infancy, multiple studies agree that by age 7 to 9 years, children manifest a similar small world type of functional architecture to adults,[68,69] although the organizations of individual functional subnetworks as well as their interactions have a protracted developmental course.

Beyond the unique clinical application of presurgical mapping, fMRI (combined with DTI and other MR modalities) is helpful in unraveling the neural correlates of various cognitive developmental diseases (eg, learning disorders, attention-deficit/hyperactivity disorder, autism), of brain plasticity in children with brain lesions, such as motor plasticity in cerebral palsy, or language plasticity in focal epilepsies, and of different therapeutic approaches (eg, drugs, rehabilitation methods). One exquisite advantage of fMRI, drawn from its noninvasiveness, rests in the possibility to repeat studies longitudinally during normal child development, during disease progression or disease resolution, or during a specific treatment. These clinical research imaging studies, which involve homogeneous populations of children (patients and controls), with increased statistical power, but usually lower sensitivity at the individual level, pave the way for future therapeutic approaches and plead for the continuous development of transdisciplinary research in pediatric neuroimaging.

ACKNOWLEDGMENTS

The authors would like to thank Dr S. Lippe, K. Monzalvo, and G. Dehaene, Neurospin, CEA-Saclay, C. Bulteau and G. Dorfmuller, Rothschild Foundation, and F Chassoux, and B Devaux, Ste Anne Hospital, Paris, for their contribution.

REFERENCES

1. Huttenlocher PR, Dabholkar AS. Regional differences in synaptogenesis in human cerebral cortex. J Comp Neurol 1997;387:167–78.
2. Chiron C, Raynaud C, Maziere B, et al. Changes in regional cerebral blood flow during brain maturation in children and adolescents. J Nucl Med 1992;33:696–703.
3. Chugani HT, Phelps ME, Mazziotta JC. Positron emission tomography study of human brain functional development. Ann Neurol 1987;22:487–97.
4. Gaillard WD, Balsamo LM, Ibrahim Z, et al. fMRI identifies regional specialization of neural networks for reading in young children. Neurology 2003;60: 94–100.
5. Gaillard WD, Hertz-Pannier L, Mott SH, et al. Functional anatomy of cognitive development: fMRI of verbal fluency in children and adults. Neurology 2000;54:180–5.
6. Brown TT, Lugar HM, Coalson RS, et al. Developmental changes in human cerebral functional organization for word generation. Cereb Cortex 2005; 15:275–90.
7. Marcar VL, Strassle AE, Loenneker T, et al. The influence of cortical maturation on the BOLD response: an fMRI study of visual cortex in children. Pediatr Res 2004;56:967–74.
8. Morita T, Kochiyama T, Yamada H, et al. Difference in the metabolic response to photic stimulation of the lateral geniculate nucleus and the primary visual cortex of infants: a fMRI study. Neurosci Res 2000;38:63–70.
9. Heep A, Scheef L, Jankowski J, et al. Functional magnetic resonance imaging of the sensorimotor system in preterm infants. Pediatrics 2009;123(1): 294–300.
10. Shapiro KL, Johnston SJ, Vogels W, et al. Increased functional magnetic resonance imaging activity during nonconscious perception in the attentional blink. Neuroreport 2007;18:341–5.
11. Brauer J, Neumann J, Friederici AD. Temporal dynamics of perisylvian activation during language processing in children and adults. Neuroimage 2008;41:1484–92.
12. Humphries C, Binder JR, Medler DA, et al. Syntactic and semantic modulation of neural activity during auditory sentence comprehension. J Cogn Neurosci 2006;18:665–79.
13. Dehaene-Lambertz G, Dehaene S, Hertz-Pannier L. Functional neuroimaging of speech perception in infants. Science 2002;298:2013–5.
14. Redcay E, Kennedy DP, Courchesne E. fMRI during natural sleep as a method to study brain function during early childhood. Neuroimage 2007;38: 696–707.
15. Altman NR, Bernal B. Brain activation in sedated children: auditory and visual functional MR imaging. Radiology 2001;221:56–63.
16. Barba C, Montanaro D, Frijia F, et al. Focal cortical dysplasia type IIb in the rolandic cortex: functional reorganization after early surgery documented by passive task functional MRI. Epilepsia 2012;53(8): e141–5.
17. Heinke W, Koelsch S. The effects of anesthetics on brain activity and cognitive function. Curr Opin Anaesthesiol 2005;18:625–31.
18. Wilke M, Holland SK, Altaye M, et al. Template-O-Matic: a toolbox for creating customized pediatric templates. Neuroimage 2008;41:903–13.
19. Rutten GJ, Ramsey NF, van Rijen PC, et al. FMRI-determined language lateralization in patients with unilateral or mixed language dominance according to the Wada test. Neuroimage 2002;17:447–60.
20. Yuan W, Altaye M, Ret J, et al. Quantification of head motion in children during various fMRI language tasks. Hum Brain Mapp 2009;30:1481–9.
21. Oakes TR, Johnstone T, Ores Walsh KS, et al. Comparison of fMRI motion correction software tools. Neuroimage 2005;28:529–43.
22. Petrella JR, Shah LM, Harris KM, et al. Preoperative functional MR imaging localization of language and motor areas: effect on therapeutic decision making

in patients with potentially resectable brain tumors. Radiology 2006;240:793–802.

23. de Ribaupierre S, Fohlen M, Bulteau C, et al. Presurgical language mapping in children with epilepsy: clinical usefulness of functional magnetic resonance imaging for the planning of cortical stimulation. Epilepsia 2012;53:67–78.

24. Liegeois F, Connelly A, Cross JH. Language reorganization in children with early onset lesions of the left hemisphere: an fMRI study. Brain 2004;127:1229–36.

25. Marusic P, Najm IM, Ying Z, et al. Focal cortical dysplasias in eloquent cortex: functional characteristics and correlation with MRI and histopathologic changes. Epilepsia 2002;43:27–32.

26. Chassoux F, Devaux B, Landré E, et al. Stereoelectroencephalography in focal cortical dysplasia: a 3D approach to delineating the dysplastic cortex. Brain 2000;123(Pt 8):1733–51.

27. Staudt M, Pavlova M, Bohm S, et al. Pyramidal tract damage correlates with motor dysfunction in bilateral periventricular leukomalacia (PVL). Neuropediatrics 2003;34:182–8.

28. De Tiège X, Connelly A, Liégeois F, et al. Influence of motor functional magnetic resonance imaging on the surgical management of children and adolescents with symptomatic focal epilepsy. Neurosurgery 2009;64(5):856–64.

29. Staudt M, Gerloff C, Grodd W, et al. Reorganization in congenital hemiparesis acquired at different gestational ages. Ann Neurol 2004;56(6):854–63.

30. Lehericy S, Cohen L, Bazin B, et al. Functional MR evaluation of temporal and frontal language dominance compared with the Wada test. Neurology 2000;54:1625–33.

31. Barnett A, Marty-Dugas J, McAndrews MP. Advantages of sentence-level fMRI language tasks in presurgical language mapping for temporal lobe epilepsy. Epilepsy Behav 2014;32:114–20. http://dx.doi.org/10.1016/j.yebeh.2014.01.010.

32. Berl MM, Zimmaro LA, Khan OI, et al. Characterization of atypical language activation patterns in focal epilepsy. Ann Neurol 2014;75(1):33–42. http://dx.doi.org/10.1002/ana.24015.

33. Seghier M. Laterality index in functional MRI: methodological issues. Magn Reson Imaging 2008;26:594–601.

34. Wilke M, Schmithorst VJ. A combined bootstrap/histogram analysis approach for computing a lateralization index from neuroimaging data. Neuroimage 2006;33(2):522–30.

35. Dehaene-Lambertz G, Montavont A, Jobert A, et al. Language or music, mother or Mozart? Structural and environmental influences on infants' language networks. Brain Lang 2010;114:53–65.

36. Szaflarski JP, Holland SK, Schmithorst VJ, et al. fMRI study of language lateralization in children and adults. Hum Brain Mapp 2006;27:202–12.

37. Holland SK, Plante E, Weber Byars A, et al. Normal fMRI brain activation patterns in children performing a verb generation task. Neuroimage 2001;14(4):837–43.

38. Ressel V, Wilke M, Lidzba K, et al. Increases in language lateralization in normal children as observed using magnetoencephalography. Brain Lang 2008;106:167–76.

39. Rasmussen T, Milner B. The role of early left-brain injury in determining lateralization of cerebral speech functions. Ann N Y Acad Sci 1977;299:355–69.

40. Ojemann G, Ojemann J, Lettich E, et al. Cortical language localization in left, dominant hemisphere. An electrical stimulation mapping investigation in 117 patients. J Neurosurg 1989;71:316–26.

41. Yuan W, Szaflarski JP, Schmithorst VJ, et al. fMRI shows atypical language lateralization in pediatric epilepsy patients. Epilepsia 2006;47(3):593–600.

42. Springer JA, Binder JR, Hammeke TA, et al. Language dominance in neurologically normal and epilepsy subjects: a functional MRI study. Brain 1999;122(Pt 11):2033–46.

43. Thivard L, Hombrouck J, du Montcel ST, et al. Productive and perceptive language reorganization in temporal lobe epilepsy. Neuroimage 2005;24(3):841–51.

44. Lidzba K, Staudt M, Wilke M, et al. Lesion-induced right-hemispheric language and organization of nonverbal functions. Neuroreport 2006;17(9):929–33.

45. Duchowny M, Harvey AS. Pediatric epilepsy syndromes: an update and critical review. Epilepsia 1996;37(Suppl 1):S26–40.

46. Hertz-Pannier L, Gaillard WD, Mott SH, et al. Noninvasive assessment of language dominance in children and adolescents with functional MRI: a preliminary study. Neurology 1997;48:1003–12.

47. Hertz-Pannier L, Chiron C, Jambaque I, et al. Late plasticity for language in a child's non-dominant hemisphere: a pre- and post-surgery fMRI study. Brain 2002;125:361–72.

48. Liegeois F, Cross JH, Gadian D-. Role of fMRI in the decision-making process: epilepsy surgery for children. J Magn Reson Imaging 2006;23:933–40.

49. Woermann FG, Jokeit H, Luerding R, et al. Language lateralization by Wada test and fMRI in 100 patients with epilepsy. Neurology 2003;61:699–701.

50. FitzGerald DB, Cosgrove GR, Ronner S, et al. Location of language in the cortex: a comparison between functional MR imaging and electrocortical stimulation. AJNR Am J Neuroradiol 1997;18:1529–39.

51. Roux FE, Boulanouar K, Lotterie JA, et al. Language functional magnetic resonance imaging in preoperative assessment of language areas: correlation

with direct cortical stimulation. Neurosurgery 2003; 52:1335–45 [discussion: 1345–7].

52. Ruge MI, Victor J, Hosain S, et al. Concordance between functional magnetic resonance imaging and intraoperative language mapping. Stereotact Funct Neurosurg 1999;72:95–102.

53. Dehaene S, Cohen L. The unique role of the visual word form area in reading. Trends Cogn Sci 2011; 15(6):254–62.

54. Cohen L, Lehéricy S, Henry C, et al. Learning to read without a left occipital lobe: right-hemispheric shift of visual word form area. Ann Neurol 2004;56(6):890–4.

55. Jambaque I, Dellatolas G, Dulac O, et al. Verbal and visual memory impairment in children with epilepsy. Neuropsychologia 1993;31:1321–37.

56. Jambaque I, Dellatolas G, Fohlen M, et al. Memory functions following surgery for temporal lobe epilepsy in children. Neuropsychologia 2007;45: 2850–62.

57. Mabbott DJ, Smith ML. Memory in children with temporal or extra-temporal excisions. Neuropsychologia 2003;41:995–1007.

58. Detre JA, Maccotta L, King D, et al. Functional MRI lateralization of memory in temporal lobe epilepsy. Neurology 1998;50:926–32.

59. Fox MD, Raichle ME. Spontaneous fluctuations in brain activity observed with functional magnetic resonance imaging. Nat Rev Neurosci 2007;8: 700–11.

60. Van Dijk KR, Hedden T, Venkataraman A, et al. Intrinsic functional connectivity as a tool for human connectomics: theory, properties, and optimization. J Neurophysiol 2009;103:297–321.

61. Beckmann CF, DeLuca M, Devlin JT, et al. Investigations into resting-state connectivity using independent component analysis. Philos Trans R Soc Lond B Biol Sci 2005;360:1001–13.

62. Damoiseaux JS, Rombouts SA, Barkhof F, et al. Consistent resting-state networks across healthy subjects. Proc Natl Acad Sci U S A 2006;103: 13848–53.

63. Shehzad Z, Kelly AM, Reiss PT, et al. The resting brain: unconstrained yet reliable. Cereb Cortex 2009;19:2209–29.

64. Zhang D, Johnston JM, Fox MD, et al. Preoperative sensorimotor mapping in brain tumor patients using spontaneous fluctuations in neuronal activity imaged with functional magnetic resonance imaging: initial experience. Neurosurgery 2009;65(6 Suppl):226–36.

65. Shimony JS, Zhang D, Johnston JM, et al. Resting-state spontaneous fluctuations in brain activity: a new paradigm for presurgical planning using fMRI. Acad Radiol 2009;16(5):578–83. http://dx. doi.org/10.1016/j.acra.2009.02.001.

66. Mitchell TJ, Hacker CD, Breshears JD, et al. A novel data-driven approach to preoperative mapping of functional cortex using resting-state functional magnetic resonance imaging. Neurosurgery 2013;73(6):969–82 [discussion: 982–3].

67. Fransson P, Skiöld B, Engström M, et al. Spontaneous brain activity in the newborn brain during natural sleep–an fMRI study in infants born at full term. Pediatr Res 2009;66(3):301–5.

68. Fair DA, Cohen AL, Dosenbach NU, et al. The maturing architecture of the brain's default network. Proc Natl Acad Sci U S A 2008;105:4028–32.

69. Supekar K, Musen M, Menon V. Development of large-scale functional brain networks in children. PLoS Biol 2009;7:e1000157. http://dx.doi.org/10. 1371/journal.pbio.1000157.

Resting-State Blood Oxygen Level–Dependent Functional Magnetic Resonance Imaging for Presurgical Planning

Mudassar Kamran, MD, PhD[a], Carl D. Hacker, BA[b],
Monica G. Allen, PhD[c], Timothy J. Mitchell, PhD[c],
Eric C. Leuthardt, MD[d], Abraham Z. Snyder, MD, PhD[e],
Joshua S. Shimony, MD, PhD[a],*

KEYWORDS

- Functional MR imaging • Resting-state functional MR imaging • rsfMR imaging
- Resting-state networks • RSNs • Multilayered perceptron • MLP • Eloquent cortex

KEY POINTS

- Resting-state functional MR imaging (rsfMR imaging) is a promising technique for presurgical planning with the objective of decreasing morbidity while maximizing complete resection of pathologic tissue. However, the methodology is still in early stages of development.
- Further research is necessary to make these tools more accurate and available in the operating room.
- Additional research is needed to explore the differences between rsfMR imaging, task fMR imaging, and electrocortical stimulation mapping, and to better understand the consequences of disrupted resting-state networks outside the motor and language systems.
- Related engineering development should incorporate the presurgical MR imaging results into intraoperative neuronavigation systems, including the rsfMR imaging results in conjunction with white matter fiber bundle anatomy derived from diffusion tensor imaging.

INTRODUCTION
Background

Functional MR imaging (fMR imaging) detects changes in the blood oxygen level–dependent (BOLD) signal that reflect the neurovascular response to neural activity. Traditionally, fMR imaging has been used to localize function within the brain by presenting a stimulus or imposing a task (eg, presenting a flashing checkerboard pattern or generating verbs from nouns) to elicit neuronal responses.[1,2] This type of experiment has been very effective at localizing functionality within the brain, as evidenced by the many thousands of publications using task-based fMR imaging.

The human brain consumes a disproportionate amount of energy relative to its weight. The brain constitutes approximately 2% of the body's weight but consumes 20% of the body's energy use.[3] Performance of a task only minimally increases

[a] Mallinckrodt Institute of Radiology, Washington University School of Medicine, 4525 Scott Avenue, St Louis, MO 63110, USA; [b] Medical Student Training Program, Washington University School of Medicine, 4525 Scott Avenue, St Louis, MO 63110, USA; [c] Department of Neurological Surgery, Mallinckrodt Institute of Radiology, Washington University School of Medicine, 4525 Scott Avenue, St Louis, MO 63110, USA; [d] Department of Neurological Surgery, Washington University School of Medicine, 4525 Scott Avenue, St Louis, MO 63110, USA; [e] Department of Neurology, Mallinckrodt Institute of Radiology, Washington University School of Medicine, 4525 Scott Avenue, St Louis, MO 63110, USA
* Corresponding author.
E-mail address: shimonyj@mir.wustl.edu

Neuroimag Clin N Am 24 (2014) 655–669
http://dx.doi.org/10.1016/j.nic.2014.07.009

energy expenditure.[4] Thus, task-based experiments ignore most of the brain's activity, which is largely devoted to signaling.[4–8]

Biswal and colleagues[9] were the first to demonstrate that spontaneous fluctuations in the BOLD signal in the resting state correlated within the somatomotor system. Before this observation, spontaneous fluctuations in the BOLD signal in the resting state were regarded as noise and generally averaged out over many trials or task blocks.[10,11] More recent studies have shown that these spontaneous fluctuations reflect the brain's functional organization.[12] Correlated intrinsic activity is currently referred to as functional connectivity MR imaging or resting-state fMR imaging (rsfMR imaging). The development of these methods has opened up many exciting possibilities for future neurocognitive research as well as clinical applications. This article focuses on the application of rsfMR imaging to presurgical planning. **Table 1** summarizes key features of both task-based fMR imaging and rsfMR imaging. Snyder and Raichle[12] give a historical review of the resting state.

Resting-State Networks

Correlated intrinsic activity defines functional connectivity. Functionally connected regions are known as resting-state networks (RSNs); equivalently, intrinsic connectivity networks.[13] The rsfMR imaging scans generally are acquired while the subject is in a state of quiet wakefulness.[14] The importance of RSNs is that their topography closely corresponds to the topography of responses elicited by a wide variety of sensory, motor, and cognitive tasks.[15] Intrinsic activity persists, albeit in somewhat modified form, during sleep[16,17] or even under sedation.[18] The persistence of the spontaneous fluctuations during states of reduced awareness suggests that intrinsic neuronal activity plays an important role in the maintenance of the brain's functional integrity.[19] Spontaneous BOLD activity has been detected in all mammalian species investigated thus far,[20–22] which reinforces the notion that this phenomenon is important from a physiologic and evolutionary point of view. However, the precise physiologic functions of intrinsic activity remain unknown. Examples of important RSNs follow and are summarized in **Table 2**.

Default mode network

Perhaps the most fundamental RSN is the default mode network (DMN) (**Fig. 1A**), first identified by a meta-analysis of task-based functional neuroimaging experiments performed with positron emission tomography.[23,24] The defining property of the DMN is that it is more active at rest than during performance of goal-directed tasks. The DMN was first identified using rsfMR imaging by Greicius and colleagues.[25] This finding has since been replicated many times over using a variety of analysis methods.[15,26–32] Some investigators have hypothesized that there are two large anticorrelated systems in the brain,[33,34] one anchored by the DMN and the other composed of systems controlling executive and attentional mechanisms. This dichotomy has been variously referred to as task-positive versus task-negative[28,32,33,35,36] and intrinsic versus extrinsic.[34,37] Although the nomenclature associated with the DMN remains controversial,[38,39] the topography of the DMN is remarkably consistent across diverse analysis strategies.

Sensory and motor resting-state networks

The somatomotor network, first identified by Biswal and colleagues,[9] encompasses primary and higher order motor and sensory areas (see **Fig. 1B**). The visual network spans much of the occipital cortex (see **Fig. 1C**).[15,26–29] The auditory network includes Heschl gyrus, the superior temporal gyrus, and the posterior insula.[15] The language network includes Broca and Wernicke areas but also extends to prefrontal, temporal, parietal, and subcortical regions (see **Fig. 1D**).[40–42]

Table 1
Key features of task-based fMR imaging and rsfMR imaging

Task-Based fMR Imaging	rsfMR Imaging
Neuronal activity is studied while performing a well-defined task (eg, finger tapping or object naming).	Neuronal activity is studied in the absence of a task (when the subject in the scanner is in a state of quiet wakefulness).
Maps a single functional system at a time	Maps all functional systems simultaneously
Task-related changes in the BOLD signal are measured. Regions in the brain associated with a given task are localized.	Spontaneous fluctuations in the BOLD signal are measured. Correlated intrinsic activity defines functional connectivity.
Immune to spurious variance in the BOLD signal (eg, P_{CO_2} levels, head motion)	Vulnerable to contamination and requires denoising to remove sources of spurious variance

Table 2 rsfMR imaging networks	
1. Default mode network	Most robust RSN More active at rest than during performance of goal-directed tasks
2. Somatomotor network	Includes primary and higher order motor and sensory areas
3. Auditory network	Includes Heschl gyrus, superior temporal gyrus, and posterior insula
4. Visual network	Includes most of the occipital cortex
5. Language network	Includes Broca, Wernicke, and multiple other language-related areas Extends to prefrontal, temporal, parietal, and subcortical regions
6. Dorsal attention network	Tasks requiring spatial attention Includes intraparietal sulcus and frontal eye field
7. Ventral attention network	Involved in detection of environmentally salient events Includes temporal-parietal junction
8. Frontoparietal control network	Associated with working memory and control of goal-directed behavior Includes lateral prefrontal cortex and inferior parietal lobule
9. Cingulo-opercular network	Associated with performance of tasks requiring executive control Medial superior frontal and anterior prefrontal cortices, anterior insula

Attention and cognitive-control resting-state networks

RSNs involved in attentional and cognitive control include the dorsal attention network and the ventral attention network.[13,28,29,43,44] The dorsal attention network (see **Fig. 1E**) includes the intraparietal sulcus and the frontal eye fields and is recruited by tasks requiring control of spatial attention. The ventral attention network (see **Fig. 1F**), which includes the temporal-parietal junction and ventral frontal cortex, is involved in the detection of environmentally salient events.[43–45] The frontoparietal control network (see **Fig. 1G**), which includes the

lateral prefrontal cortex and the inferior parietal lobule, is associated with working memory and control of goal-directed behavior.[46,47] Finally, the cingulo-opercular network, also known as the salience network[13] or the core control network,[48] includes the medial superior frontal cortex, anterior insula, and anterior prefrontal cortex. The cingulo-opercular network is thought to enable the performance of tasks requiring executive control.[28,47,48]

APPLICATION TO PRESURGICAL PLANNING
Review of the Literature

Multiple studies have demonstrated that maximal resection of a brain tumor while sparing nearby eloquent cortex leads to improved outcomes with reduced morbidity.[49–53] Similar considerations apply to surgical resections for intractable epilepsy. Historically, neurosurgeons have been concerned with localization of the motor and language system because these parts of the brain instantiate critical functionality (eloquent cortex). However, a broader understanding of brain function suggests that all parts of the brain contribute to important functionality.[29,32,34,42] Thus, improved functional mapping of multiple RSNs beyond motor and language systems could lead to further improvements in patient outcomes.

Several publications have explored the use of rsfMR imaging for use in presurgical planning. An early case report described use of rsfMR imaging to localize the motor cortex in a patient with a brain tumor.[54] Kokkonen and colleagues[55] similarly compared motor task-based fMR imaging data to resting-state data and showed that the motor functional network could be localized based on resting-state data in eight subjects with tumor, as well as 10 healthy control subjects. In surgery for epilepsy, the higher spatial resolution afforded by rsfMR imaging over electroencephalography could provide a distinct advantage in mapping epileptic foci or networks. Seed-based methods were used by Liu and colleagues[56] to successfully locate sensorimotor areas by using rsfMR imaging in subjects with tumors or epileptic foci close to sensorimotor areas. They found agreement between rsfMR imaging and task-based fMR imaging, as well as intraoperative cortical stimulation data. In another study from the same laboratory, Stufflebeam and colleagues[57] were able to localize areas of increased functional connectivity in five of six subjects that overlapped with epileptogenic areas identified by invasive encephalography. Zhang and colleagues[58] used graph methods and a pattern classifier applied to rsfMR imaging data to identify subjects as either having medial temporal lobe epilepsy or as normal controls.

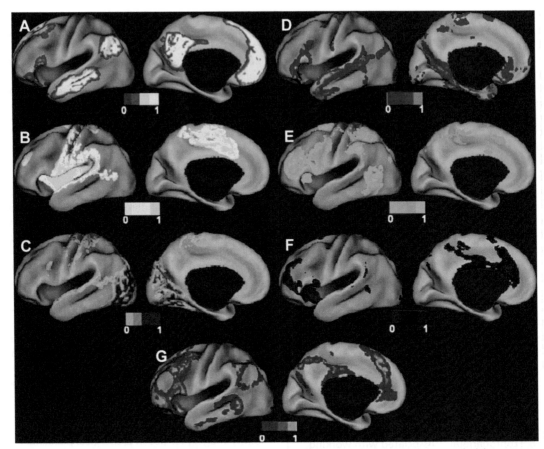

Fig. 1. Surface plots of RSNs as derived from fuzzy c-means algorithm. (*A*) Default mode network. (*B*) Somatomotor network. (*C*) Visual network. (*D*) Language network. (*E*) Dorsal attention network. (*F*) Ventral attention network. (*G*) Frontoparietal control network. (*From* Lee MH, Hacker CD, Snyder AZ, et al. Clustering of resting state networks. PLoS One 2012;7(7):e40370.)

Using data from 16 subjects with intractable medial temporal lobe epilepsy and 52 normal controls, they achieved an average classification sensitivity of 77.2% and a specificity of 83.86%. Bettus and colleagues[59] reported that increases in basal functional connectivity were a specific marker of the location of the epileptogenic zone in 22 subjects with mesial temporal lobe epilepsy. Weaver and colleagues[60] studied four subjects with nonlesion, focal epilepsy along with 16 control subjects to determine whether the seizure focus could be found using the functional patterns near the epileptogenic zone. By averaging voxel homogeneity across regions of interest and comparing that with other regions, they were able to accurately identify the epileptic focus. Tie and colleagues[61] used spatial independent component analysis (sICA) on a training group of 14 healthy subjects to identify the language network based on rsfMR imaging. The result of that analysis was then used to identify the language network in a second group of 18 healthy subjects at the individual level. They further proposed an automated system for localizing the language network in individual patients using sICA. A more detailed presentation of the authors' experiences using rsfMR imaging for presurgical mapping with both seed-based and multilayer perceptron (MLP) approaches follows.

Overview of Processing Methods

rsfMR imaging methodology currently is dominated by two complementary strategies: spatial sICA[26] and seed-based correlation mapping.[9] Both strategies depend on spontaneous neural activity being correlated (phase coherent) within widely distributed regions of the brain. Both strategies yield highly reproducible results at the group level.[30,62] sICA decomposes rsfMR imaging data into a sum of components, each component corresponding to a spatial topography and a time course. In contrast, seed-based correlation mapping is computed by voxel-wise evaluation of the

Pearson correlation between the time courses in a targeted region of interest and all other voxels in the brain.[63]

The principal advantage of sICA is that it provides a direct means of separating artifact from BOLD signals of neural origin, although this separation typically requires observer expertise. The results obtained using sICA may vary substantially depending on processing parameters (eg, number of requested components). Thus, sICA can be difficult to use in the investigation of targeted RSNs, especially in single subjects. In contrast, targeting of selected RSNs is built into seed-based correlation mapping. However, the principal difficulty in using seed-based correlation mapping is exclusion of nonneural artifact, which is typically accomplished using regression techniques.[63–65]

sICA and seed-based correlation mapping both represent strategies for assigning RSN identities to brain voxels. Because sICA makes no a priori assumptions regarding the topography of the obtained components, this method exemplifies unsupervised classification. In contrast, seed-based correlation mapping depends on previous knowledge, and so exemplifies supervised classification. Hacker and colleagues[42] discuss the distinction between supervised and unsupervised methodologies.

Hacker and colleagues[42] recently described a technique for mapping the topography of known RSNs in individuals using MLP. Perceptrons are machine learning algorithms that can be trained to associate arbitrary input patterns with discrete output labels.[66] An MLP was trained to associate seed-based correlation maps with particular RSNs. Running the trained MLP on correlation maps corresponding to all voxels in the brain generates voxel-wise RSN membership estimates. Thus, RSN mapping using a trained MLP exemplifies supervised classification. An example of the RSN produced by the MLP algorithm in three subjects is presented in **Fig. 2**.

Hacker and colleagues[42] demonstrated that the MLP accurately generates RSN topography estimates in individuals consistent with previous studies, even in brain regions not represented in the training data. These findings are important to future applications because they demonstrate that this approach can reliably and effectively map multiple RSNs in individual subjects.

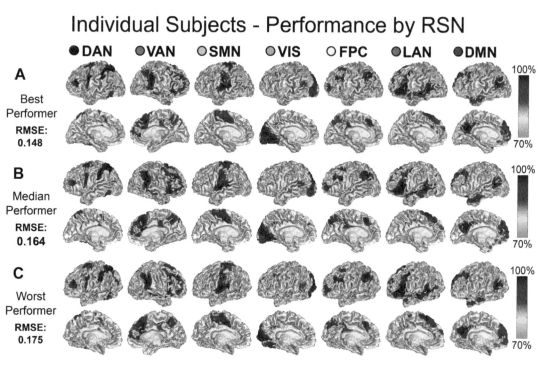

Individual Subjects - Performance by RSN

● DAN   ● VAN   ○ SMN   ○ VIS   ○ FPC   ● LAN   ● DMN

A Best Performer RMSE: 0.148 — 100% / 70%

B Median Performer RMSE: 0.164 — 100% / 70%

C Worst Performer RMSE: 0.175 — 100% / 70%

Fig. 2. Single-subject, voxel estimation of RSNs using the trained MLP in three subjects. The results are from the (A) best, (B) median, and (C) worst performers as determined by root mean square classification error. MLP output was converted to a percentile scale and sampled onto each subject's cortical surface. DAN, dorsal attention network; DMN, default mode network; FPC, frontoparietal control network; LAN, language network; SMN, somatomotor network; VAN, ventral attention network; VIS, visual network. (*From* Hacker CD, Laumann TO, Szrama NP, et al. Resting state network estimation in individual subjects. Neuroimage 2013;82:622; with permission.)

Preoperative Sensorimotor Mapping in Brain Tumor Patients Using Seed-Based Approach

Zhang and colleagues[67] describe the initial experiences in using rsfMR imaging brain mapping for presurgical planning of tumor resections in four subjects with tumors. The tumors were all adjacent to the motor and sensory cortices, thus necessitating accurate localization before surgery to minimize postoperative deficits. Each of the subjects was scanned using rsfMR imaging and task-based fMR imaging while performing a block design finger-tapping task. fMR imaging in each subject included four 7-minute runs (28 minutes total). rsfMR imaging data previously acquired from a group of normal controls (N = 17) was also used for comparison.

In the subjects with tumor, the seed was placed in the hemisphere contralateral to the tumor at coordinates taken from an independent group of subjects who performed button-press tasks.[68,69] Electrocortical stimulation (ECS) mapping was performed on three of the four subjects with tumor and these data, in addition to task-based fMR imaging, were used for comparison with the resting-state data. Compared with the task-based fMR imaging, the results of rsfMR imaging analysis were more consistent with the intraoperative ECS findings. Given that rsfMR imaging does not depend on task performance by the patient this outcome suggests that rsfMR imaging may be more reliable for purposes of presurgical planning.

The following is a discussion of two of the four subjects from this study:

Case 1: A glioblastoma was diagnosed in the right hemisphere of a 45-year-old man. ECS during the surgery found that motor cortex was shifted anteriorly. **Fig. 3**A shows the results of the task-based fMR imaging, which confirmed the anterior displacement of motor cortex. However, the task-based result was unreliable because one of the runs showed likely artifactual activation in the posterior part of the tumor (see **Fig. 3**B). rsfMR imaging was more consistent and also demonstrated anterior shifting of motor cortex ipsilateral to the tumor.

Case 2: A 64-year-old man developed focal motor seizures secondary to mass in the left hemisphere (**Fig. 4**A). Finger-tapping fMR imaging showed atypical response topography, including activation in right parietal cortex, in addition to the expected activation of the somatomotor area (see **Fig. 4**B). Seed-based (see **Fig. 4**C) correlation mapping rsfMR imaging showed the somatomotor RSN without parietal involvement. Correlation mapping with a seed in the right parietal cortex matched the topography of the dorsal attention network (see **Fig. 4**D). The authors' interpretation of this result is that, during the task-based fMR imaging, the subject had to strongly focus his attention to complete the task, which accounts for the activation in the attentional network. This case illustrates the potential increased specificity of the rsfMR imaging method. The findings of the

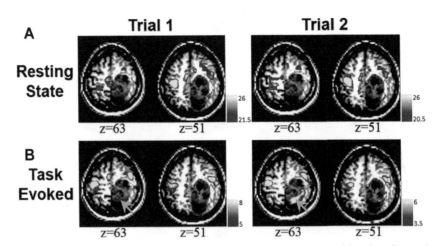

Fig. 3. Comparison of resting state and task-related fMRI mapping in a 45-year-old with a diagnosis of Glioblastoma (case 1). (*A*) Resting state correlation mapping × 2 shows anterior displacement of the motor cortex by the tumor. (*B*) Finger-tapping fMRI × 2 shows similar distribution but with activity within the tumor (*blue arrows*) as seen in trial 2 but not in trial 1. z, Talairach coordinate. (*From* Zhang D, Johnston JM, Fox MD, et al. Preoperative sensorimotor mapping in brain tumor patients using spontaneous fluctuations in neuronal activity imaged with functional magnetic resonance imaging: initial experience. Neurosurgery 2009;65(6 Suppl):229; with permission.)

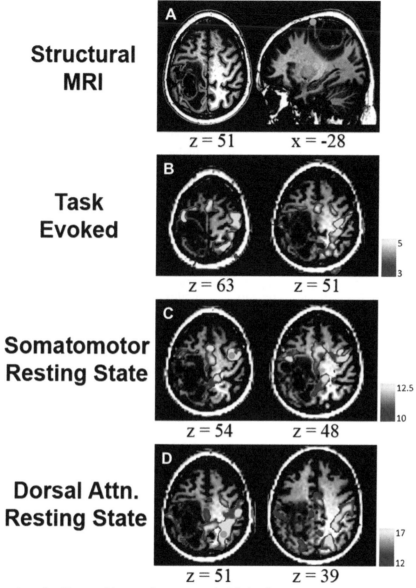

Fig. 4. MR imaging of a 64-year-old man who presented with focal motor seizures (case 2). (A) Structural MR imaging revealed a tumor in left parietal cortex that invades territory near the central sulcus (neurologic convention). The green circle represents the location of ipsilateral hand response to cortical stimulation. (B) Task-related activity was seen bilaterally in frontal lobe. In addition, a large band of activity appeared in right parietal cortex, not consistent with the pattern of activity from the sensorimotor network. (C) Resting-state correlation mapping using a seed in the right (unaffected) hemisphere (blue circle) showed ipsilateral correlations anterior to the tumor as well as a region of activity in midline parietal cortex. Note absence in the correlation mapping results of parietal activity seen in the task-related map. (D) Parietal activation seen during task-evoked scan is revealed to be a separate RSN, the dorsal attention network that is normally dissociated from the sensorimotor network using a seed (blue circle). x, Talairach coordinate; z, Talairach coordinate. (From Zhang D, Johnston JM, Fox MD, et al. Preoperative sensorimotor mapping in brain tumor patients using spontaneous fluctuations in neuronal activity imaged with functional magnetic resonance imaging: initial experience. Neurosurgery 2009;65(6 Suppl):230; with permission.)

rsfMR imaging were consistent with the intraoperative ECS.

Preoperative Mapping of Functional Cortex Using Multilayered Perceptron

Mitchell and colleagues[70] reported application of MLP-based RSN mapping to presurgical planning in six subjects with intractable epilepsy and seven subjects with brain tumors. Subjects with epilepsy underwent electrocorticographic monitoring to localize the epileptogenic zone of seizure onset and to perform functional mapping with ECS. Subjects with tumors underwent intraoperative ECS mapping before resection of the tumor mass. This article focuses only on the results in the subjects with epilepsy.

Preoperative resting-state functional MR imaging analysis

MLP analysis was performed in all subjects as previously described. To determine the probability that an electrode covers a portion of an RSN, electrode MR imaging coregistration was used with the results of the MLP analysis; gray matter voxels located within 30 mm of the electrode were averaged with a weight inversely proportional to the square of their distance from the electrode.

Electrode MR imaging coregistration in subjects monitored for seizure

Electrodes were segmented based on a CT image coregistered to the subject's MR imaging using methodology similar to that previously described.[71,72] Electrodes imaged in the postgrid implantation CT typically are displaced inward relative to the cortical surface imaged on preoperative MR imaging because of traction from dural oversewing and postsurgical edema. This inward displacement was corrected by projecting electrode coordinates outwards to the brain surface along a path normal to the plane of the grid.

Electrocortical stimulation mapping

Electrodes were classified as over eloquent cortex using ECS mapping. Motor regions were defined by the presence of induced involuntary motor movements. Language sites were defined by speech arrest during stimulation.

Comparison of multilayer perceptron–based resting state network mapping to electrocortical stimulation mapping

An electrode was classified as positive or negative in the MLP results according the probability of its belonging to the appropriate RSN (motor or language). These probabilities were then plotted against the ECS results to generate receiver operating characteristic (ROC) curves.

These ROC curves were averaged and the area under the curve (AUC) was used as a measure of the agreement between the MLP and ECS methods.

Results in subjects with epilepsy

Fig. 5 demonstrates a high degree of qualitative overlap between the location of the motor and language networks compared with the ECS results in the subjects with epilepsy. The positive motor ECS electrodes were centered in the precentral gyrus. The MLP-mapped motor areas encompassed both the precentral and postcentral gyri. The positive language ECS electrodes were centered in the pars opercularis of the inferior frontal gyrus, approximately in Brodmann area (BA) 44. The MLP language positive regions were in pars triangularis of the inferior frontal gyrus, which corresponds to BA 45. The anteriorly shifted MLP-based localization of language cortex (BA 45 vs 44) demonstrates expected differences between the two methods related to methodology and suggests the possibility that the definition of eloquent cortex should be expanded. Quantitative comparisons were performed with an ROC analysis, which yielded an average AUC of 0.89 for the motor network and an average AUC of 0.76 for the language network. These findings demonstrate that MLP-based mapping can identify RSNs in the presence of distorted anatomy.

Minimization of false negatives

Loci in MLP maps outside the appropriate RSN but eloquent as determined by ECS are defined as MLP false negatives. Minimization of MLP false negatives is critical to reduce surgical morbidity because resection of a false negative area could lead to a clinical deficit. Fig. 6 illustrates the results of an analysis undertaken to minimize MLP motor false negatives. This analysis showed that the probability of an MLP false negative could be reduced to less than 2% by expanding the no-cut zone by 15 mm around the contour corresponding to 85% likelihood of belonging to the motor RSN.

In summary, MLP-based RSN mapping robustly identified all networks in all subjects, including those with distorted anatomy attributable to mass effect. When the ECS-positive sites were analyzed, rsfMR imaging had AUCs of 0.89 and 0.76 for motor and language identification, respectively. MLP false negatives were minimized by including a 15 mm safety margin around the edge of the motor RSN. These findings demonstrate that the MLP-defined RSNs are able to identify eloquent cortex.

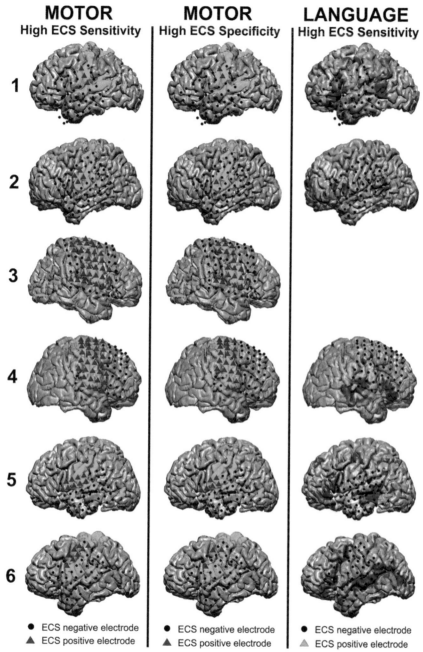

Fig. 5. Comparison of ECS and MLP results for the motor and language cortex in six epilepsy patients. Red triangles are ECS positive and black circles are ECS negative. In the left column, the high ECS sensitivity method was used to classify motor electrodes as ECS positive (*red triangles*) and compared with the MLP results displayed in light blue. In the middle column, the high ECS specificity method was used to classify motor electrodes. In the right column, the high ECS sensitive method was used to classify language electrodes as ECS-positive (*green triangles*) with the MLP results displayed in orange. (*From* Mitchell TJ, Hacker CD, Breshears JD, et al. A novel data-driven approach to preoperative mapping of functional cortex using resting-state functional magnetic resonance imaging. Neurosurgery 2013;73(6):975 [discussion: 982–83]; with permission.)

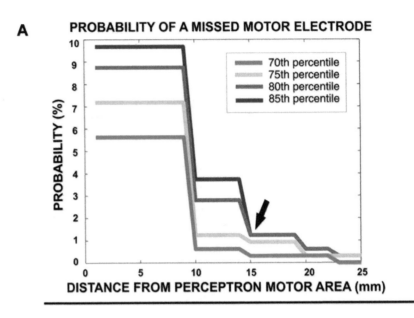

A PROBABILITY OF A MISSED MOTOR ELECTRODE

Legend:
- 70th percentile
- 75th percentile
- 80th percentile
- 85th percentile

Y-axis: PROBABILITY (%)
X-axis: DISTANCE FROM PERCEPTRON MOTOR AREA (mm)

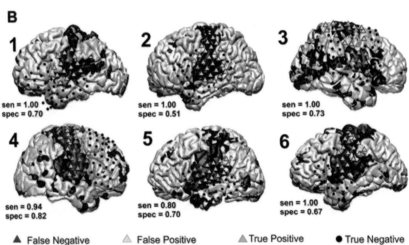

B

1 sen = 1.00 spec = 0.70

2 sen = 1.00 spec = 0.51

3 sen = 1.00 spec = 0.73

4 sen = 0.94 spec = 0.82

5 sen = 0.80 spec = 0.70

6 sen = 1.00 spec = 0.67

▲ False Negative   △ False Positive   ▲ True Positive   ● True Negative

Fig. 6. The method used to define a no-cut area in epilepsy patients, in which the probability of damage to motor cortex is substantial. (*A*) To define the area, several MLP thresholds (70th, 75th, 80th, and 85th percentiles) were used to classify electrodes as covering motor cortex, and the no-cut zone was expanded around each of the motor electrodes. The probability of a missed motor electrode, which could result in motor deficits, was plotted against the radius of expansion. The *black arrow* points to an optimal no-cut zone of 15 mm. (*B*) A visualization of the method performed at the 85% and at a radius of expansion of 15 mm. Red triangles (false negative) mark the motor cortex as determined by ECS that were missed by the MLP method. Yellow triangles are false positive, green triangles are true positive, and black circles are true negative. (*From* Mitchell TJ, Hacker CD, Breshears JD, et al. A novel data-driven approach to preoperative mapping of functional cortex using resting-state functional magnetic resonance imaging. Neurosurgery 2013;73(6):978 [discussion: 982–83]; with permission.)

A summary of key points in the application of rsfMR imaging in presurgical planning is presented in **Box 1**. Following are cases illustrating the integration of rsfMR imaging in neurosurgical planning for patients with brain tumors, particularly when the application of ECS may be limited.

Illustrative Cases

Case example 1
A 57 year-old-man with distant history of rectal adenocarcinoma presented with persistent headache and blurred vision. Brain MR imaging examination demonstrated an enhancing left frontoparietal

mass, initially favored to represent a high-grade primary glial neoplasm.

Preoperative rsfMR imaging showed the left motor activation center was located anterior superior to the tumor, abutting the peritumor edema with minimal displacement (Fig. 7A). The Broca area was located anterior to the peritumor edema, whereas the Wernicke area abutted the inferior portion of left frontoparietal junction mass (see Fig. 7B). Given the close proximity of the mass to the motor and language centers, it was decided that an awake-craniotomy would be performed with ECS.

In the operating room, following administration of the circumferential field block, the patient was noted to have significant aspiration, with the gastric contents appearing at the patient's nose and mouth. Proceeding with an awake-craniotomy and brain mapping was thought to be of considerable risk given the aspiration. Surgical options at this stage included: (1) perform a biopsy alone or (2) proceed with surgical resection based on the preoperative fMR imaging that would offer therapeutic benefit; however, at an increased risk of permanent speech or motor deficits. After consultation with the family, it was decided to continue with surgical resection given the preoperative rsfMR imaging findings that helped characterize the spatial relationship between the motor and language centers and the frontoparietal mass, suggesting a potential corridor through the parietal lobe for tumor resection.

A standard craniotomy was then performed. Continued stereotactic navigation was used to visualize the optimal gyrus for surgical approach. This surgical corridor was posterior and oblique relative to the tumor and nonintuitive based on anatomy landmarks alone. Along this deeper track the tumor was gross totally resected. This resection of the tumor was confirmed with intraoperative MR imaging.

The patient's postoperative course was unremarkable with no new speech or motor deficits. Surgical pathologic results were consistent with glioblastoma multiforme, World Health Organization grade 4. Following the frontoparietal tumor resection, the patient experienced complete resolution of headache and blurred vision.

Case example 2
A 47 year-old man with left frontal lobe anaplastic oligodendroglioma undergoing chemotherapy treatment, status after partial surgical resection and after fractionated radiation treatment, was noted to have a new mass-like nodular area of enhancement at the tumor resection site on the 1-year follow-up brain MR imaging examination. These imaging findings were concerning for tumor recurrence. The patient had profound expressive aphasia at the time of presentation and could not perform task-based fMR imaging.

rsfMR imaging demonstrated regions related to motor tasks (see Fig. 7C) and the Wernicke area were not in close proximity to the recurrent tumor and were, therefore, of less concern from a neurosurgical standpoint. However, the Broca area was less than 1 cm from the edge of the previous resection cavity and abutting the edematous parenchyma surrounding the new foci of enhancement (see Fig. 7D).

The consensus decision based on the clinical picture and the imaging findings was to perform a repeat awake-craniotomy with surgical resection of the recurrent tumor. This was discussed with the patient. A standard awake craniotomy was performed; however, once the brain was exposed and the patient was roused, the patient was combative and could not adequately follow the commands despite repeated attempts of mild sedation using narcotics to reduce the patient's pain and discomfort. Given the patient's condition, mapping could not be accomplished. A 2 × 2 cm block of tissue corresponding to the enhancing mass noted on the previous MR imaging examination was resected furthest away from the speech and motor areas identified on preoperative rsfMR imaging.

Postoperatively, there was no worsening of patient's speech or motor function. Biopsy results

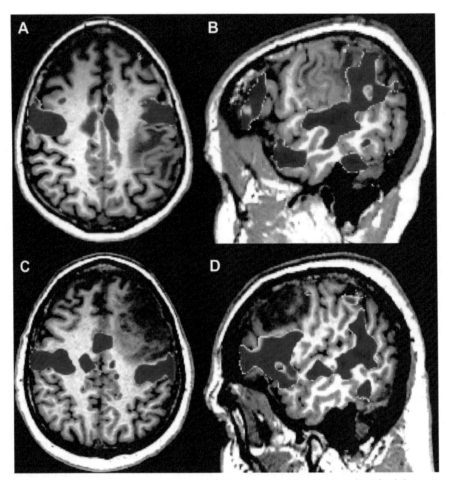

Fig. 7. Examples of RSN (*red*) superposed on T1-weighted images in two case examples. The (*A*) somatomotor and (*B*) language RSNs are shown for case example 1. Similarly, the (*C*) somatomotor and (*D*) language RSNs are shown for case example 2.

for the resected tissue were consistent with radiation necrosis with no evidence of tumor recurrence.

Case example 3

A 41-year-old man with a history of grade III anaplastic astrocytoma, status after awake-craniotomy, was noted to have a new enhancing lesion in the superior temporal gyrus on routine follow-up brain MR imaging examination, 3 years after the initial surgery.

Preoperative rsfMR imaging demonstrated a distinct gap between the site of recurrence and the language network. Wernicke area localized 2 cm posterior to the recurrent tumor. Given concern for recurrence, the patient was considered for minimally invasive laser ablation treatment. The alternative of a standard awake craniotomy with brain mapping and surgical resection was discussed. However the patient chose the less invasive laser ablation treatment, which was believed

to be optimal given the confidence in the preoperative rsfMR imaging findings. The laser interstitial thermal ablation involves the stereotactic placement of a laser probe into the tumor for MR imaging–guided heating of the lesion.

Preoperatively, the planned trajectory took into account the RSNs for language, thus allowing successful penetration of the tumor without disrupting language associated sites.

The patient's postoperative course was unremarkable and he was discharged from the hospital 2 days following the minimally invasive laser ablation treatment without complications.

Case example 4

A 29-year-old multilingual man developed grade IV glioblastoma multiforme, status after biopsy and chemoradiation treatment. On the most recent 1-year follow-up MR imaging examination, a new focus of enhancement was identified in the white matter of the left frontal lobe.

The preoperative rsfMR imaging showed close proximity between the suspected tumor recurrence and the language network, with the tumor located deep to the activation corresponding to the Broca area. The new focus of enhancement was located several centimeters anterior to the motor strip and less than a centimeter distant from the supplementary motor area. Given these findings, awake-craniotomy and resection of tumor was planned.

During the awake-craniotomy, once the brain was exposed, stereotactic navigation was used to localize the site of the recurrent tumor. ECS mapping was performed at the tumor site and adjacent regions with multiple iterations using various speech paradigms, with no speech arrest. Of note, these negative sites included regions identified with task-based and rsfMR imaging as belonging to the language network. Subsequently, subpial dissection and resection of the inferior fontal gyrus affected by the tumor was performed while the patient was maintained in conversation without any difficulty.

During the postoperative hospital stay and at the time of discharge, the patient's sensory and motor components of speech did not demonstrate any worsening. Contrary to illustrative case numbers 1 to 3, this example illustrates that the rsfMR imaging, though useful for operative planning, should be used in conjunction with ECS when possible because it remains the gold standard technique for functional mapping of the brain during neurosurgery.

SUMMARY

This article provided a brief overview of rsfMR imaging and its applications in neurosurgical practice. RSN imaging methods and the common analysis techniques were discussed with limited literature review. Finally, several cases using the MLP-based technique in patients with brain tumors were presented. This experience suggests how MLP-based RSN mapping can be applied to assist in presurgical planning.

As these results demonstrate, rsfMR imaging is a promising technique for presurgical planning with the objective of decreasing morbidity while maximizing complete resection of pathologic tissue. However, the methodology is still in early stages of development. Further research is necessary to make these tools more accurate and available in the operating room. Additional research is needed to explore the differences between rsfMR imaging and ECS mapping, and to better understand the consequences of disrupted RSNs outside the motor and language systems. Related

engineering development should incorporate the presurgical MR imaging results into intraoperative neuronavigation systems, including the rsfMR imaging results in conjunction with white matter fiber bundle anatomy derived from diffusion tensor imaging.

ACKNOWLEDGMENTS

The authors wish to thank the National Institutes of Health for its generous support of this project via NIH R21 CA159470. Dr Snyder is supported by National Institute of Mental Health Grant P30 NS048056.

REFERENCES

1. Posner MI, Raichle ME. Images of mind. New York: Scientific American Library: Distributed by W.H. Freeman and Co; 1997.
2. Spitzer M, Kwong KK, Kennedy W, et al. Category-specific brain activation in fMRI during picture naming. Neuroreport 1995;6(16):2109–12.
3. Clarke DD, Sokoloff L. Circulation and energy metabolism of the brain. 1999. [Online]. Available at: http://www.ncbi.nlm.nih.gov/books/NBK20413/. Accessed April 8, 2014.
4. Raichle ME, Mintun MA. Brain work and brain imaging. Annu Rev Neurosci 2006;29(1):449–76.
5. Shulman RG, Rothman DL, Behar KL, et al. Energetic basis of brain activity: implications for neuroimaging. Trends Neurosci 2004;27(8):489–95.
6. Attwell D, Laughlin SB. An energy budget for signaling in the grey matter of the brain. J Cereb Blood Flow Metab 2001;21(10):1133–45.
7. Ames A 3rd, Li YY, Heher EC, et al. Energy metabolism of rabbit retina as related to function: high cost of Na+ transport. J Neurosci 1992;12(3): 840–53.
8. Lennie P. The cost of cortical computation. Curr Biol 2003;13(6):493–7.
9. Biswal B, Yetkin FZ, Haughton VM, et al. Functional connectivity in the motor cortex of resting human brain using echo-planar MRI. Magn Reson Med 1995;34(4):537–41.
10. Purdon PL, Weisskoff RM. Effect of temporal autocorrelation due to physiological noise and stimulus paradigm on voxel-level false-positive rates in fMRI. Hum Brain Mapp 1998;6(4):239–49.
11. Triantafyllou C, Hoge RD, Krueger G, et al. Comparison of physiological noise at 1.5 T, 3 T and 7 T and optimization of fMRI acquisition parameters. Neuroimage 2005;26(1):243–50.
12. Snyder AZ, Raichle ME. A brief history of the resting state: the Washington University perspective. Neuroimage 2012;62(2):902–10.

13. Seeley WW, Menon V, Schatzberg AF, et al. Dissociable intrinsic connectivity networks for salience processing and executive control. J Neurosci 2007;27(9):2349–56.

14. Fox MD, Raichle ME. Spontaneous fluctuations in brain activity observed with functional magnetic resonance imaging. Nat Rev Neurosci 2007;8(9):700–11.

15. Smith SM, Fox PT, Miller KL, et al. Correspondence of the brain's functional architecture during activation and rest. Proc Natl Acad Sci U S A 2009;106(31):13040–5.

16. Sämann PG, Tully C, Spoormaker VI, et al. Increased sleep pressure reduces resting state functional connectivity. MAGMA 2010;23(5–6):375–89.

17. Larson-Prior LJ, Zempel JM, Nolan TS, et al. Cortical network functional connectivity in the descent to sleep. Proc Natl Acad Sci U S A 2009;106(11):4489–94.

18. Mhuircheartaigh RN, Rosenorn-Lanng D, Wise R, et al. Cortical and subcortical connectivity changes during decreasing levels of consciousness in humans: a functional magnetic resonance imaging study using propofol. J Neurosci 2010;30(27):9095–102.

19. Pizoli CE, Shah MN, Snyder AZ, et al. Resting-state activity in development and maintenance of normal brain function. Proc Natl Acad Sci U S A 2011;108(28):11638–43.

20. Hutchison RM, Gallivan JP, Culham JC, et al. Functional connectivity of the frontal eye fields in humans and macaque monkeys investigated with resting-state fMRI. J Neurophysiol 2012;107(9):2463–74.

21. Schwarz AJ, Gass N, Sartorius A, et al. Anti-correlated cortical networks of intrinsic connectivity in the rat brain. Brain Connect 2013;3(5):503–11.

22. Nasrallah FA, Tay HC, Chuang KH. Detection of functional connectivity in the resting mouse brain. Neuroimage 2014;86:417–24.

23. Shulman GL, Fiez JA, Corbetta M, et al. Common blood flow changes across visual tasks: II. Decreases in cerebral cortex. J Cogn Neurosci 1997;9(5):648–63.

24. Gusnard DA, Raichle ME, Raichle ME. Searching for a baseline: functional imaging and the resting human brain. Nat Rev Neurosci 2001;2(10):685–94.

25. Greicius MD, Krasnow B, Reiss AL, et al. Functional connectivity in the resting brain: a network analysis of the default mode hypothesis. Proc Natl Acad Sci U S A 2003;100(1):253–8.

26. Beckmann CF, DeLuca M, Devlin JT, et al. Investigations into resting-state connectivity using independent component analysis. Philos Trans R Soc Lond B Biol Sci 2005;360(1457):1001–13.

27. De Luca M, Beckmann CF, De Stefano N, et al. fMRI resting state networks define distinct modes of long-distance interactions in the human brain. Neuroimage 2006;29(4):1359–67.

28. Power JD, Cohen AL, Nelson SM, et al. Functional Network Organization of the Human Brain. Neuron 2011;72(4):665–78.

29. Yeo BT, Krienen FM, Sepulcre J, et al. The organization of the human cerebral cortex estimated by intrinsic functional connectivity. J Neurophysiol 2011;106(3):1125–65.

30. Damoiseaux JS, Rombouts SA, Barkhof F, et al. Consistent resting-state networks across healthy subjects. Proc Natl Acad Sci U S A 2006;103(37):13848–53.

31. van den Heuvel M, Mandl R, Hulshoff Pol H. Normalized cut group clustering of resting-state fMRI data. PLoS One 2008;3(4):e2001.

32. Lee MH, Hacker CD, Snyder AZ, et al. Clustering of resting state networks. PLoS One 2012;7(7):e40370.

33. Fox MD, Snyder AZ, Vincent JL, et al. The human brain is intrinsically organized into dynamic, anti-correlated functional networks. Proc Natl Acad Sci U S A 2005;102(27):9673–8.

34. Golland Y, Golland P, Bentin S, et al. Data-driven clustering reveals a fundamental subdivision of the human cortex into two global systems. Neuropsychologia 2008;46(2):540–53.

35. Chai XJ, Castañón AN, Ongür D, et al. Anticorrelations in resting state networks without global signal regression. Neuroimage 2012;59(2):1420–8.

36. Zhang Z, Liao W, Zuo XN, et al. Resting-state brain organization revealed by functional covariance networks. PLoS One 2011;6(12):e28817.

37. Doucet G, Naveau M, Petit L, et al. Brain activity at rest: a multiscale hierarchical functional organization. J Neurophysiol 2011;105(6):2753–63.

38. Jack AI, Dawson AJ, Begany KL, et al. fMRI reveals reciprocal inhibition between social and physical cognitive domains. Neuroimage 2012;66C:385–401.

39. Spreng RN. The fallacy of a 'task-negative' network. Front Psychol 2012;3:145.

40. Tomasi D, Volkow ND. Resting functional connectivity of language networks: characterization and reproducibility. Mol Psychiatry 2012;17(8):841–54.

41. Lee MH, Smyser CD, Shimony JS. Resting-state fMRI: a review of methods and clinical applications. AJNR Am J Neuroradiol 2013;34(10):1866–72.

42. Hacker CD, Laumann TO, Szrama NP, et al. Resting state network estimation in individual subjects. Neuroimage 2013;82:616–33.

43. Corbetta M, Shulman GL. Control of goal-directed and stimulus-driven attention in the brain. Nat Rev Neurosci 2002;3(3):201–15.

44. Fox MD, Corbetta M, Snyder AZ, et al. Spontaneous neuronal activity distinguishes human dorsal and ventral attention systems. Proc Natl Acad Sci U S A 2006;103(26):10046–51.

45. Astafiev SV, Shulman GL, Corbetta M. Visuospatial reorienting signals in the human temporo-parietal junction are independent of response selection. Eur J Neurosci 2006;23(2):591–6.

46. Vincent JL, Kahn I, Snyder AZ, et al. Evidence for a frontoparietal control system revealed by intrinsic functional connectivity. J Neurophysiol 2008; 100(6):3328–42.

47. Power JD, Petersen SE. Control-related systems in the human brain. Curr Opin Neurobiol 2013;23(2): 223–8.

48. Dosenbach NU, Visscher KM, Palmer ED, et al. A core system for the implementation of task sets. Neuron 2006;50(5):799–812.

49. Keles GE, Lamborn KR, Berger MS. Low-grade hemispheric gliomas in adults: a critical review of extent of resection as a factor influencing outcome. J Neurosurg 2001;95(5):735–45.

50. Keles GE, Chang EF, Lamborn KR, et al. Volumetric extent of resection and residual contrast enhancement on initial surgery as predictors of outcome in adult patients with hemispheric anaplastic astrocytoma. J Neurosurg 2006;105(1):34–40.

51. Lacroix M, Abi-Said D, Fourney DR, et al. A multivariate analysis of 416 patients with glioblastoma multiforme: prognosis, extent of resection, and survival. J Neurosurg 2001;95(2):190–8.

52. McGirt MJ, Chaichana KL, Gathinji M, et al. Independent association of extent of resection with survival in patients with malignant brain astrocytoma. J Neurosurg 2009;110(1):156–62.

53. Sanai N, Mirzadeh Z, Berger MS. Functional outcome after language mapping for glioma resection. N Engl J Med 2008;358(1):18–27.

54. Shimony JS, Zhang D, Johnston JM, et al. Resting-state spontaneous fluctuations in brain activity: a new paradigm for presurgical planning using fMRI. Acad Radiol 2009;16(5):578–83.

55. Kokkonen SM, Nikkinen J, Remes J, et al. Preoperative localization of the sensorimotor area using independent component analysis of resting-state fMRI. Magn Reson Imaging 2009;27(6):733–40.

56. Liu H, Buckner RL, Talukdar T, et al. Task-free presurgical mapping using functional magnetic resonance imaging intrinsic activity. J Neurosurg 2009;111(4):746–54.

57. Stufflebeam SM, Liu H, Sepulcre J, et al. Localization of focal epileptic discharges using functional connectivity magnetic resonance imaging. J Neurosurg 2011;114(6):1693–7.

58. Zhang X, Tokoglu F, Negishi M, et al. Social network theory applied to resting-state fMRI connectivity data in the identification of epilepsy networks with iterative feature selection. J Neurosci Methods 2011;199(1):129–39.

59. Bettus G, Bartolomei F, Confort-Gouny S, et al. Role of resting state functional connectivity MRI in presurgical investigation of mesial temporal lobe epilepsy. J Neurol Neurosurg Psychiatry 2010; 81(10):1147–54.

60. Weaver KE, Chaovalitwongse WA, Novotny EJ, et al. Local functional connectivity as a pre-surgical tool for seizure focus identification in non-lesion, focal epilepsy. Front Neurol 2013;4:43.

61. Tie Y, Rigolo L, Norton IH, et al. Defining language networks from resting-state fMRI for surgical planning—a feasibility study. Hum Brain Mapp 2014; 35(3):1018–30.

62. Shehzad Z, Kelly AM, Reiss PT, et al. The resting brain: unconstrained yet reliable. Cereb Cortex 2009;19(10):2209–29.

63. Fox MD, Zhang D, Snyder AZ, et al. The global signal and observed anticorrelated resting state brain networks. J Neurophysiol 2009;101(6):3270–83.

64. Jo HJ, Saad ZS, Simmons WK, et al. Mapping sources of correlation in resting state FMRI, with artifact detection and removal. Neuroimage 2010;52(2): 571–82.

65. Vincent JL, Snyder AZ, Fox MD, et al. Coherent spontaneous activity identifies a hippocampal-parietal memory network. J Neurophysiol 2006; 96(6):3517–31.

66. Rumelhart DE, Hinton GE, Williams RJ. Learning representations by back-propagating errors. Nature 1986;323(6088):533–6.

67. Zhang D, Johnston JM, Fox MD, et al. Preoperative sensorimotor mapping in brain tumor patients using spontaneous fluctuations in neuronal activity imaged with functional magnetic resonance imaging: initial experience. Neurosurgery 2009;65(6 Suppl):226–36.

68. Fox MD, Snyder AZ, Zacks JM, et al. Coherent spontaneous activity accounts for trial-to-trial variability in human evoked brain responses. Nat Neurosci 2006; 9(1):23–5.

69. Zacks JM, Braver TS, Sheridan MA, et al. Human brain activity time-locked to perceptual event boundaries. Nat Neurosci 2001;4(6):651–5.

70. Mitchell TJ, Hacker CD, Breshears JD, et al. A novel data-driven approach to preoperative mapping of functional cortex using resting-state functional magnetic resonance imaging. Neurosurgery 2013; 73(6):969–82 [discussion: 982–3].

71. He BJ, Snyder AZ, Vincent JL, et al. Breakdown of functional connectivity in frontoparietal networks underlies behavioral deficits in spatial neglect. Neuron 2007;53(6):905–18.

72. Hermes D, Miller KJ, Noordmans HJ, et al. Automated electrocorticographic electrode localization on individually rendered brain surfaces. J Neurosci Methods 2010;185(2):293–8.

Applications of Blood-Oxygen-Level-Dependent Functional Magnetic Resonance Imaging and Diffusion Tensor Imaging in Epilepsy

CrossMark

Umair J. Chaudhary, MBBS, MSc, PhD[a,b,*],
John S. Duncan, MA, DM, FRCP, FMedSci[a,b,c]

KEYWORDS

- Epilepsy • Blood-oxygen-level-dependent • Functional magnetic resonance imaging • Language
- Memory • Electroencephalography-fMRI • Diffusion tensor imaging • Tractography

KEY POINTS

- Language-related networks can be mapped noninvasively using functional magnetic resonance imaging (fMRI). Verbal fluency paradigms can provide lateralization of the Broca area; however, further paradigm development is needed to predict naming difficulties after temporal lobe resection.
- Functional imaging can map memory-related networks noninvasively, and word encoding shows promise for detecting verbal memory decline after temporal lobe resection.
- Simultaneous electroencephalography (EEG)-fMRI can localize interictal and seizure-related blood-oxygen-level-dependent networks noninvasively, in concordance with intracranial EEG-based localization, which may be helpful in surgical planning.
- Tractography can be used to minimize visual field defects in patients undergoing temporal lobe resection.
- Multimodal image integration can combine fMRI and diffusion tensor imaging maps for visual display, which can be helpful in reducing the risk of surgical damage to the eloquent cortex.

APPLICATIONS OF FUNCTIONAL MAGNETIC RESONANCE IMAGING IN EPILEPSY

The life time prevalence of epilepsy ranges from 2.7 to 12.4 per 1000 in western countries.[1] Around 30% of patients with epilepsy remain refractory to antiepileptic drugs and continue to have seizures.[2,3] Over the last decade, non-invasive imaging techniques such as functional magnetic resonance imaging (fMRI) and diffusion tensor imaging (DTI) have helped to better understand mechanisms of seizure generation and propagation, and to localize epileptic, eloquent and cognitive networks.[4] This review considers the clinical applications of fMRI and DTI, for mapping

Disclosures: Research funding from Wellcome Trust grant 97914 and Department of Health's grant HICF T4-275 NIHR UCLH Biomedical Research Centre funding scheme. Programme grant: Novel multimodality imaging techniques for neurosurgical planning and stereotactic navigation in epilepsy surgery UCLH/UCL and BRC grant.
a Department of Clinical and Experimental Epilepsy, UCL Institute of Neurology, Queen Square, London WC1N 3BG, UK; b MRI Unit, Epilepsy Society, Chesham Lane, Chalfont St Peter, Buckinghamshire SL9 0RJ, UK; c Queen Square Division, UCLH NHS Foundation Trust, Queen Square, London WC1N 3BG, UK
* Corresponding author. MRI Unit, Epilepsy Society, Chesham Lane, Chalfont St Peter, Buckinghamshire SL9 0RJ, UK.
E-mail address: umair.chaudhary@ucl.ac.uk

cognitive and epileptic networks and organization of white matter tracts in individuals with epilepsy.

Increased neuronal activity secondary to a task performance causes variations in the cerebral blood flow, blood volume, and blood oxygenation. This situation results in changes in the ratio of oxyhemoglobin and deoxyhemoglobin concentrations in brain, which is detected as blood-oxygen-level-dependent (BOLD) effect by functional magnetic resonance imaging (fMRI) in specific brain areas that are recruited during the task. Therefore, fMRI provides an indirect measure of neuronal activity. Functional MR imaging has been used to map language and memory networks before and after surgery with high spatial resolution. Simultaneous recording of electroencephalography (EEG) and fMRI can map BOLD networks associated with interictal epileptiform discharges (IED) and seizures in focal and generalized epilepsy.[5]

Language-Related Blood-Oxygen-Level-Dependent Networks in Epilepsy

fMRI can map language networks in patients with refractory epilepsy undergoing epilepsy surgery for research and clinical purposes. Various language paradigms to activate anterior (Broca area: expressive language) and posterior (Wernicke area: comprehension; anterior temporal lobe: semantic integration) language areas[6–14] have been used to lateralize typical and atypical language representation. Verbal fluency, verb generation, and semantic decision tasks are commonly used tasks for language evaluation in a clinical context, providing complementary information.[15,16] Verb generation causes more discrete activation, whereas verbal fluency activates language-related areas that are not found with the former.[15] Language lateralization via fMRI has been compared with neuropsychological evaluation, cortical stimulation, or Wada test. Real-time fMRI analysis can improve the processing speed of fMRI data analysis and has good concordance of language localization with conventional general linear model–based analysis or cortical stimulation.[17,18]

Statistical threshold
Lateralization index (LI) is calculated to detect hemispheric dominance for language networks on fMRI maps, comparing activations in the left and right hemispheres.[19–22] Choice of details (eg, selecting whole brain or prespecified regions or excluding midline structures for calculating LI) may affect lateralization.[9] Choosing appropriate statistical thresholds is an important issue when evaluating language dominance using fMRI, because the extent and thus localization of fMRI activation depends on the former. Conventional

threshold, adaptive threshold, and bootstrap techniques have been used to assess the laterality of language-related fMRI maps.[6,19,21] The bootstrap technique is particularly advantageous in that it is more specific and accurately identifies outliers.[19,21] To avoid dependence of language lateralization on arbitrarily selected statistical thresholds and LI, threshold-independent scores[23,24] have been used and compared with the Wada test, providing language lateralization at individual level. Data-driven approaches have been used to localize language networks in patients with focal epilepsy and have shown significant differences in language organization, as an effect of epilepsy, which were not seen previously with conventional fMRI analysis.[25–28] Pattern classifying algorithms have also been used to classify language-related fMRI maps automatically, corroborating with existing LI and visual rating classification methods.[29,30] For most purposes, comparing left and right activations using the bootstrap method is most satisfactory.

Localization of language networks
Patients with left hemisphere[31] or left temporal lobe epilepsy (TLE)[32] have a higher likelihood of atypical language lateralization than patients with an epileptic focus in the right hemisphere or right temporal lobe. Patients with left TLE with hippocampal sclerosis (HS) and left language dominance have increased recruitment of homologous right hemisphere in addition to left hemisphere language areas for language processing, suggesting widespread language representation[33,34] and greater cognitive effort performed compared with controls.[31,35] There is an increase and posterior shift of language-related activation in the right inferior frontal gyrus (IFG) after left hemisphere injury. However, activations in left IFG remain in the same location.[36] Compared with patients with frontal lobe epilepsy (FLE), patients with TLE have more atypical language in the Wernicke area, whereas a frontal focus affects anterior language areas more.[37] In comparison, patients with nonlesional TLE and right TLE show left lateralized language.[32,34] There is coupling between functional and structural measures for left language lateralization in the patients with right TLE, and decoupling between the functional and structural indices of the patients with left TLE, suggesting complex language networks in left TLE.[38] Language areas activated for abstract and concrete words are also different for patients with TLE, with or without HS, suggesting that HS is associated with altered functional organization of cortical networks involved in lexical and semantic processing.[33] Atypical language representation

may also occur in patients with normal structural MR imaging, mesial temporal sclerosis, focal cortical lesions, and stroke.[39,40]

Language lateralization deduced from fMRI concurs with the Wada test in 80% to 90% of patients when using conjunction analysis of 3 language paradigms or semantic decision paradigm, suggesting the clinical usefulness of the test.[7,9,41,42] Concordance between fMRI and Wada test is the highest for patients with right TLE with left language dominance and for frontal language areas; and the lowest for patients with left TLE with left language dominance.[41] Atypical language dominance on fMRI[42,43] and interhemispheric language dissociation[44] are correlated with Wada/fMRI discordance. This finding suggests that fMRI may be more sensitive than Wada or cortical stimulation to map the whole network involved in language processing but is less specific at individual level compared with cortical stimulation.[45] fMRI language localization can replace Wada test in most patients. However, Wada test may still be required when a patient cannot perform the fMRI task, for example, because of having a pacemaker or suffering claustrophobia, for validation of atypical language representation on fMRI or for the evaluation of selective language areas near structural abnormalities.[46]

Also, functional connectivity is reduced and reorganized in patients with TLE or intractable epilepsy within the language network.[47,48] More specifically, functional connectivity is decreased in the left hemisphere irrespective of the epileptogenic focus[49] and frontotemporal network,[48] which is associated with impaired performance on language assessment.[48] Performance on language tasks is also correlated to networks in posterior temporal regions showing increased functional connectivity for both patients with left and right medial TLE.[50]

Language lateralization decreases,[51] and reorganization in frontal, temporal and parietal language networks increases,[35] with earlier age of seizure onset[39] but is not associated with type and location of lesion (acquired or developmental), symptoms, and gender.[52,53] However, others have not found any association between language lateralization and age of seizure onset[37] but have found an association between language lateralization and handedness, location and nature of pathologic substrate, and duration of epilepsy.[39,54,55] Verbal memory performance on neuropsychological evaluation is also found to be associated with language lateralization, suggesting a link between inferior frontal cortex and hippocampus.[56,57] Gray matter in language networks increases in the hemisphere contralateral to the epileptic focus,[58]

and recruitment of the contralateral hemisphere in language processing in patients with atypical language representation may suggest compensatory reorganization mechanisms.[32]

A relative decrease in cerebral blood flow in the left Wernicke area is correlated with decreased activation in the left IFG and LI, suggesting distributed but interconnected language networks.[8] γ Activity in higher frequency range increases and is positively correlated with BOLD responses in the inferior frontal and middle temporal gyri. This γ activity lasts longer in the frontal lobe and declines quickly in the temporal lobe, which may explain difficulties in detecting BOLD in the temporal lobe.[59]

Language fMRI activations of polymicrogyric cortex over Broca area suggest that it retains functionality, and surgical resection should be considered with caution.[60] In patients with generalized epilepsy, fMRI has shown that language function is impaired, as represented by reduced suppression of the default mode network, an inadequate suppression of activation in the left anterior temporal lobe and the posterior cingulate cortex, and an aberrant activation in the right hippocampal formation.[61] Children with benign epilepsy with centrotemporal spikes (BECTS) and other epilepsy types also show bihemispheric language networks, which may represent a compensatory response for ongoing epileptic activity in brain.[62,63] Also, anterior language networks are affected more in BECTS, resulting in language difficulties for functions dependent on the integrity of anterior language regions (eg, sentence production).[64]

Prognostic value

Language mapping using fMRI is more accurate than Wada test in predicting naming postoperatively.[65] Activation in the left hippocampus during verbal fluency task, in patients with right TLE, is associated with preserved naming function. In contrast, patients with left TLE, who are more proficient in naming, involve left frontal lobe, suggesting compensatory responses caused by ongoing epileptic activity in the left hippocampus.[13] Preoperative language fMRI activation with verbal fluency in the left middle frontal gyrus (MFG) can be used to predict significant naming decline in patients with left TLE, with good sensitivity but suboptimal specificity (**Fig. 1**).[66] Auditory and visual naming paradigms may give more specific prediction of naming difficulties after anterior temporal lobe resection (ATLR).[67]

Postoperative findings

In postoperative patients with left TLE with left hemispheric language dominance, language representation is more bihemispheric than in controls

(i)

A

Left temporal lobe epilepsy

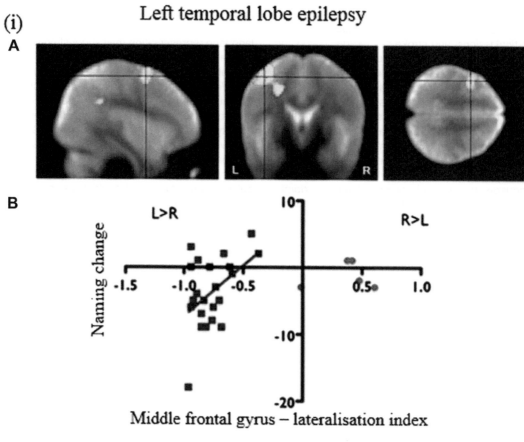

B

Middle frontal gyrus – lateralisation index

(ii)

A   Clinically significant naming decline

B   No significant naming decline

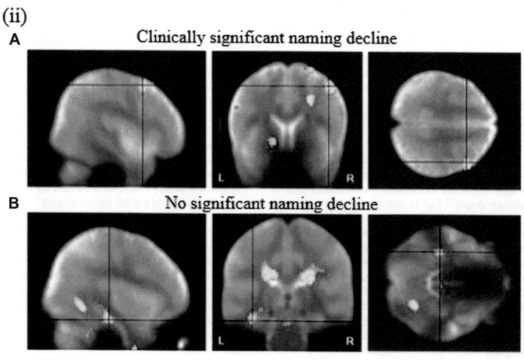

and patients with right TLE, suggesting that redistribution of language to temporofrontal and interhemispheric areas represent reorganization of language function.[11] Postoperative activation in the right MFG and remaining left posterior hippocampus was correlated with better naming for patients with and without significant naming decline, respectively, again suggesting reorganization in language networks after surgery (see **Fig. 1**).[66] Proficient reading skills after left ATLR depend on integration between normal systems involving the left middle temporal, right hippocampus, and anterior superior temporal sulcus, and recruitment of the right IFG, which is not activated in controls.[68]

Effect of epileptic activity and antiepileptic drugs
Antiepileptic drugs can affect cognitive processing.[40] Topiramate has an effect on activation in the basal ganglia, anterior cingulated, and posterior visual cortex and can cause reduced deactivation of the default mode network-related areas during a language task, suggesting interference in cognitive processing.[69,70] There has also been some evidence suggesting that atypical language reorganization/dominance may be affected by the presence and absence of ongoing epileptic activity. Chronic frequent interictal epileptic activity in left temporal lobes may be associated with a left-right shift of language representation.[71,72] Also, atypical language lateralization in the right hemisphere may shift back to the left hemisphere in seizure-free patients after left selective amygdalohippocampectomy.[73]

Memory-Related Blood-Oxygen-Level-Dependent Networks in Epilepsy

Memory impairment is common in patients with epilepsy. Working and long-term memory (autobiographical memory [AM], verbal, visual memory) may become affected, in a material-specific way, based on the site of lesion in TLE and FLE. Functional imaging can show memory networks noninvasively and reliably and also the effect of surgery on these networks.[74–76] Anatomic localization of memory-related networks as well as LIs has been applied to study the effects of epilepsy and epilepsy surgery on memory,[77–79] as discussed later.

Autobiographical memory-related networks
This network, including the hippocampus, medial prefrontal cortex, temporal poles, retrosplenial and lateral parietal cortex, shows reduced activation in patients with left HS and transient epileptic amnesia.[80,81] The connectivity of a sclerosed left hippocampus is reduced, whereas connections between extrahippocampal nodes are increased.[81] In patients with transient epileptic amnesia, there is reduced activation of the right hemisphere, more specifically of the posterior parahippocampal gyrus, temporoparietal junction, and the cerebellum, for midlife and recent memories. In addition, there is reduced effective connectivity between the right posterior parahippocampal gyrus and the right middle temporal gyrus.[81] These findings suggest that there is functional reorganization and connectivity of the neural network supporting AM retrieval in patients with TLE and transient epileptic amnesia.[80,81]

Episodic memory-related networks
Verbal memory encoding recruits a bilateral network, including parietal, temporal, and frontal cortices, lateralized to the hemisphere contralateral to the epileptic focus, in patients with TLE.[82,83] Greater left hippocampal activation for word encoding is correlated with better verbal memory in patients with left TLE.[84–86] Frontal lobe involvement is more bilateral in left TLE and lateralized in right TLE.[87] Also, greater fMRI activation in the contralateral hippocampus is correlated with worse memory performance, suggesting that reorganization of memory to the healthy medial temporal lobe is an inefficient process.[86]

Fig. 1. (*i*) Prediction of naming decline using preoperative verbal fluency fMRI in patients with left TLE. (*A*) Whole-brain voxel by voxel analysis. Left MFG activation for verbal fluency correlates with change in naming scores after left ATLR, characterized by greater naming decline in patients with greater preoperative fMRI activation. (*B*) Prediction of naming decline in individual patients—language LI for verbal fluency in the MFG. Strongly left lateralized MFG activation for verbal fluency correlates with clinical significant naming decline after left ATLR ($r^2 = 0.21$, $P = .03$). For comparison, 5 patients with left TLE and atypical language representation are indicated by green circles; these patients were not included in this study. (*ii*) Efficiency of postoperative language networks. (*A*) Left TLE with clinically significant decline in naming. Greater postoperative right MFG fMRI activation for verbal fluency correlates with better postoperative naming scores, characterized by greater, but inefficient, recruitment of the contralateral frontal lobe. (*B*) Left TLE without clinically significant naming decline. Greater postoperative left posterior hippocampal fMRI activation for verbal fluency correlates with better postoperative naming scores, characterized by efficient recruitment of the remaining ipsilateral posterior hippocampal structures. (*Modified from* Bonelli SB, Thompson PJ, Yogarajah M, et al. Imaging language networks before and after anterior temporal lobe resection: results of a longitudinal fMRI study. Epilepsia 2012;53:645, 647; with permission.)

Visual memory encoding recruits a more widespread bilateral cortical network, also lateralized to the hemisphere contralateral to the epileptic focus in patients with right HS. Lateralization of visual memory encoding to the contralateral hemisphere is associated with decreased and increased verbal memory performance in patients with left and right TLE, respectively.[82,88,89] Greater right hippocampal activation for face encoding is correlated with better visual memory in patients with right TLE.[84,86] Functional connectivity is reduced between the posterior cingulate and the epileptogenic hippocampus and increased between the posterior cingulate and the contralateral hippocampus.[90,91] Functional reorganization of networks involving extratemporal (orbitofrontal cortex, anterior cingulum [left TLE] and insula [right TLE]), and temporal structures (parahippocampus and fusiform gyrus) for verbal, visual and nonmaterial specific memory encoding suggests compensatory mechanisms to mitigate the failure of the sclerosed hippocampus.[82,92–94]

Verbal and visual memory immediate recall shows less activation in patients with HS compared with controls.[82] Patients tend to use the opposite hippocampus and parahippocampal gyrus on the same side, suggesting adaptation or functional reorganization.[92]

Working memory-related networks

Working memory is also affected in patients with TLE with HS, showing variable connectivity between brain regions.[95] Stronger functional connectivity between superior parietal lobe (BOLD activation) and sclerosed hippocampus (BOLD deactivation) is associated with worse performance, suggesting that the segregation of the task-positive and task-negative functional networks is disrupted, resulting in working memory dysfunction in TLE.[96] There is reduced right superior parietal lobe activity; and hippocampal activity from the healthy hippocampus is progressively suppressed as the working memory load increases with maintenance of good performance in patients with TLE.[97] Patients with FLE recruit more widely distributed networks for memory encoding compared with controls, particularly the frontal lobe contralateral to the seizure focus, which is associated with performance, suggesting a compensatory response of brain.[76] Moreover, pediatric patients with FLE show decreased frontal lobe connectivity, which is associated with cognitive impairment, despite intact fMRI activation pattern for working memory. This decreased frontal lobe connectivity may explain the cognitive problems encountered in children with FLE.[98] A higher number of secondary generalized seizures may induce functional reorganization of working memory–related network (eg, increased activation and reduced functional connectivity of prefrontal cortex), explaining working memory dysfunction in patients with focal epilepsy.[99,100] In contrast to focal epilepsy, patients with juvenile myoclonic epilepsy (JME) do not show a difference in working memory–related BOLD network compared with controls.[101]

Prognostic value

Verbal memory or visual memory may decline in up to one-third of patients undergoing left or right ATLR, respectively. Preoperative memory performance, age at onset of epilepsy, language lateralization, and asymmetry of activation on fMRI for verbal and visual memory can predict verbal memory decline in left ATLR but are less able to predict visual memory decline in right ATLR.[77,84] The variability of fMRI BOLD signal in the left hippocampus can predict verbal retention, suggesting that variability in brain signals may reflect functional integrity of the area and can be used as a possible clinical tool to predict memory.[102] Preoperatively, verbal and visual memory depend on the damaged left and right hippocampus respectively, as well as contralateral hippocampus.[84] Greater BOLD activation of the diseased left hippocampus and its connectivity to ipsilateral posterior cingulate leads to stronger verbal memory decline after left ATLR.[90,103–105] On the other hand, greater BOLD activation of the diseased right hippocampus is associated with more visual memory decline after right ATLR.[104] Conversely, reduced activation of the medial temporal region ipsilateral to the epileptogenic region is correlated with a favorable memory outcome after surgery.[106]

Postoperative findings

After surgery, patients with left TLE show different pattern of recruitment of frontal lobes for verbal memory encoding.[87] It is suggested that there is effective preoperative reorganization of verbal memory function to the ipsilateral posterior medial temporal lobe as greater preoperative than postoperative activation of this area for word encoding is correlated with better verbal memory outcome after left ATLR, and postoperative reorganization is ineffective (**Fig. 2**).[78] Others have suggested that postoperative visual and verbal memory performance is positively associated with the activation of contralateral medial temporal lobe and its connectivity to posterior cingulate cortex ipsilateral to the sclerosed hippocampus after temporal lobe resection.[85,90,107]

A   Left temporal lobe epilepsy – verbal memory (word encoding)
Efficiency of preoperative reorganisation

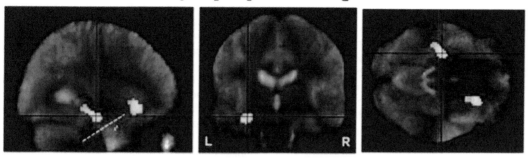

B   Efficiency of postoperative reorganisation

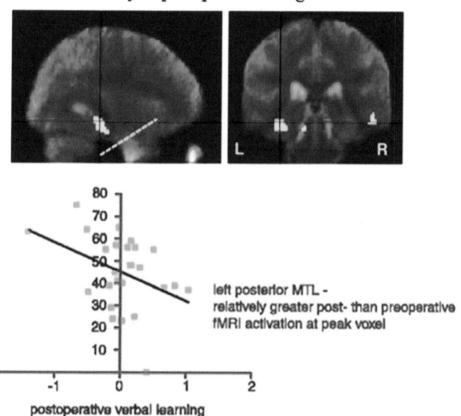

left posterior MTL -
relatively greater post- than preoperative
fMRI activation at peak voxel

postoperative verbal learning

Fig. 2. (A) Efficiency of preoperative reorganization of verbal memory function in left TLE. Correlational analysis: greater preoperative than postoperative activation on encoding words in the left posterior medial temporal lobe is associated with better verbal learning outcome. Yellow line indicates the estimated hippocampal resection margin for the left TLE group. (B) Efficiency of postoperative reorganization of verbal memory function in left TLE. Correlational analysis: greater postoperative than preoperative left posterior medial temporal lobe functional MR imaging activation for word encoding correlates with worse postoperative verbal learning scores, characterized by an inefficient postoperative response within the remaining ipsilateral posterior medial temporal lobe structures. The correlation at the peak voxel in the left posterior medial temporal lobe is shown. (*Modified from* Bonelli SB, Thompson PJ, Yogarajah M, et al. Memory reorganization following anterior temporal lobe resection: a longitudinal functional MRI study. Brain 2013;136:1896, 1897; with permission.)

Simultaneous Electroencephalography-Functional Magnetic Resonance Imaging in Epilepsy

Scalp electroencephalography-functional magnetic resonance imaging

Interictal scalp EEG-fMRI can map IED-related BOLD changes but has low sensitivity (30%–40%) because of the dependence on scalp EEG to identify IED and suboptimal modeling of the fMRI signal.[108] The sensitivity can be improved by explaining more variance in the fMRI signal[109] or using topographic map correlation between EEGs recorded outside and inside the scanner.[110,111] It shows reproducible IED-related BOLD maps,[112,113] providing more specific localization of the epileptic focus,[114] which may help plan the implantation of intracranial electrodes.[115] The potential clinical value lies in its ability to corroborate negative evidence regarding surgical candidacy, suggesting poor postsurgical outcome, or to suggest reconsideration of surgery after previous rejection as surgical candidates.[116–118]

Scalp EEG-fMRI can also map seizure-related BOLD networks during and before seizures. Seizures were captured either by chance during interictal studies[119–123] or intentionally.[124] The technique can localize the epileptic focus at sublobar level (better than scalp EEG) in ~85% of cases (Fig. 3),[124] and can separate seizure onset–related BOLD changes from propagation-related BOLD changes.[124–126] Scalp EEG-fMRI studies are constrained because seizures are unpredictable in nature and seizure-related motion can affect data quality adversely. Focal or widespread BOLD changes have also been shown before the onset of IED or seizure on scalp EEG, highlighting the low sensitivity of scalp EEG and suggesting that hemodynamic changes start before the seizure onset on scalp EEG.[123,124,127,128] The localization of the seizure focus and IED-related BOLD network provided by scalp EEG-fMRI can be used during presurgical assessment. However, larger studies are required comparing the localization provided by scalp EEG-fMRI with postsurgical outcome.

EEG-fMRI studies have played an important role in evolving the debate from zones to networks.[129] It has strengthened the evidence for the existence of corticosubcortical networks associated with generalized spike wave discharges (GSWDs) in idiopathic generalized epilepsy (IGE), involving BOLD increases in the thalamus and widespread BOLD decreases in medial and lateral frontal, superior parietal, posterior cingulate, precuneus and caudate, and posterior brainstem.[130–134] It has highlighted the role of the default mode network[135] in maintaining awareness in generalized and focal epilepsy,[124,131,136,137] because BOLD networks for attention[138–140] and working memory[141] are altered by the presence of GSWDs during the task performance. It is possible that precuneus (part of the default mode network) may facilitate the occurrence of GSWDs,[142,143] consistent with the cortical focus theory of initiation of absences.[144] BOLD changes in propagation-related networks in refractory focal seizures,[124] visual attention network in children with photoparoxysmal response,[127,145] musicogenic network in musicogenic seizures,[146,147] reading epilepsy-related network,[126,148] and motor network in epilepsia partialis continua of the hand[149] have been shown using scalp EEG-fMRI. Scalp EEG-fMRI has shown different GSWD-related BOLD patterns for patients who are refractory or responsive to valproate treatment,[150,151] and a common area (ie, frontal piriform cortex), ipsilateral to the epileptic focus, has been shown for different types of IED.[152,153] These findings may be helpful in designing new strategies of treatment of focal epilepsy.

It is unclear as yet how the different nodes of interictal and ictal BOLD networks contribute to the epileptogenicity in a particular patient with focal epilepsy. It is possible that 1 node of the network acts as a principal node, removal of which results in seizure freedom. In contrast, in patients who continue to have seizures after surgery, a second node in the widespread epileptic BOLD network becomes epileptogenic.

Intracranial electroencephalography-functional magnetic resonance imaging

Simultaneous recording of intracranial EEG-fMRI has been made possible after extensive feasibility and safety studies.[154–157] Significant IED-related BOLD changes have been seen both close to and remote from the most active intracranial electrode,[158,159] and it has also been suggested that concordance of IED-related BOLD maps, shown by intracranial EEG-fMRI, with the epileptic focus may explain postsurgical outcome better in patients who become seizure free compared with patients who continue having seizures after surgery.[160] Intracranial EEG-fMR imaging has higher electrophysiologic sensitivity and regional specificity and can help to understand the coupling between neurophysiologic and BOLD signal.

APPLICATIONS OF DIFFUSION TENSOR IMAGING IN EPILEPSY

Diffusion tensor imaging (DTI) is sensitive to the diffusion of water molecules. In the brain, relevant quantitative measures are mean diffusivity (MD: also referred to as apparent diffusion

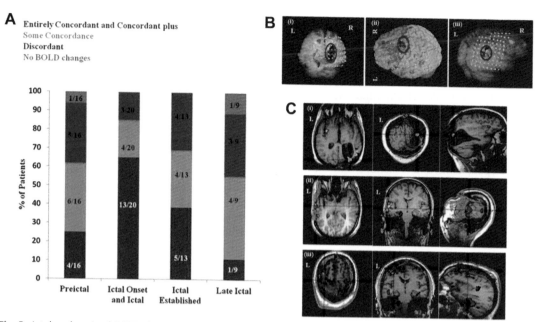

Fig. 3. Ictal and preictal BOLD changes and their comparison with the seizure focus and cortical resection. (*A*) Bar chart showing level of concordance of BOLD changes with the presumed seizure onset zone, during ictal and preictal phases. (*B*) Statistical parametric maps of F-statistics overlaid on three-dimensional rendered brain in individual space, showing the relationship between preictal (*orange*) and ictal onset phase-related BOLD changes (*green*), implanted electrodes, and structural lesion (*red*). (*Bi*) Patient with ischemic damage in right temporo-occipital region: the global-maximum cluster in the right occipitotemporal region for the preictal and ictal phase was within the presumed seizure onset zone and was 2.5 and 1.8 cm, respectively, from the invasively defined seizure onset zone. (*Bii*) Patient with focal cortical dysplasia in left frontal lobe: the global-maximum cluster in the left superior/MFG for the ictal phase was within the presumed seizure onset zone at 1.5 cm from the invasively defined seizure onset zone. For the preictal phase, another cluster in medial superior frontal gyrus was within the presumed seizure onset zone at 2.5 cm from the invasively defined seizure onset zone. (*Biii*) Patient with cortical tubers in right parietal lobe: for the ictal onset phase, the second most statistically significant BOLD cluster in right inferior parietal lobe was within the presumed seizure onset zone at 1.9 cm from the invasively defined seizure onset zone. The global-maximum preictal cluster in the right parietal region was within the presumed seizure onset zone at 3 cm from the invasively defined seizure onset zone. (*C*) Ictal onset phase-related maps overlaid on coregistered postsurgical T_1-volume. Cross-hair shows the BOLD cluster within the presumed seizure onset zone. (*Ci*) Patient had a cortical resection including the right parietal tuber and overlapping ictal onset phase-related cluster (cross-hair; International League Against Epilepsy (ILAE) class I at 1.5 year). (*Cii*) Patient underwent left ATLR, which did not involve the ictal onset phase-related global-maximum cluster in superior temporal gyrus (cross-hair; ILAE class III at 1 year). (*Ciii*) Patient had a resection including right posterior superior frontal gyrus/MFG and part of the supplementary motor area and ictal onset phase-related global-maximum cluster (cross-hair; ILAE class I at 1 year). (*Modified from* Chaudhary UJ, Carmichael DW, Rodionov R, et al. Mapping preictal and ictal haemodynamic networks using video-electroencephalography and functional imaging. Brain 2012;135:3651; with permission.)

coefficient [ADC]) and diffusion anisotropy, and qualitatively, tractography. The most common measure of diffusion anisotropy used is fractional anisotropy (FA).[161] Tractography determines the three-dimensional pathway between distinct brain regions and may be deterministic or probabilistic. Seed regions can be selected anatomically or based on the maximum activation of fMRI map for a particular task involving a particular fiber tract. Structural abnormalities can displace tracts, making anatomically chosen seed regions suboptimal.[162] DTI has been useful in helping to better

understand mechanisms of epilepsy, to detect changes that are not seen using conventional MRI, and to localize critical tracts and cortex in patients undergoing epilepsy surgery.

Detecting Unseen Changes and Understanding the Mechanism of Epilepsy

In patients with TLE, DTI has shown widespread diffusion abnormalities in white matter tracts involving temporal and extratemporal structures, irrespective of the presence of HS.[163] HS results in more extensive diffusion abnormalities involving ipsilateral and contralateral temporal neocortex and medial temporal structures, ipsilateral frontal lobe white matter, corpus callosum, basal ganglia, thalamus, and cerebellum.[163–176] Similarly, significant widespread diffusion abnormalities are found in the white matter tracts adjacent to and distant from lesions (eg, focal cortical dysplasia[177–179]; in frontal lobes in children with drug-resistant focal epilepsy[180]; in corticothalamic network in IGE and its subtypes, JME and childhood absence epilepsy[181–186]). These widespread changes are not detected by conventional structural imaging and may reflect microstructural damage in a network distribution.

Longer duration of epilepsy and an earlier age at onset are associated with diffusion abnormalities in the thalamus[170] in adult patients with TLE. It is possible that because of shorter duration of epilepsy,[187] children with TLE do not show decreased FA in temporal lobe white matter, as is shown for adults. Decreased structural connectivity may result in decreased functional connectivity between the default mode network and temporal lobes,[188] although the connection strength is increased for the remaining connections[189] in TLE. Also, decreased integrity of frontotemporal white matter tracts may affect the cognitive performance in TLE, reflecting degenerative processes.[190]

DTI has shown syndrome-specific white matter changes in patients with IGE. Patients with JME show lower FA in fornix, corpus callosum, uncinate fasciculi, superior longitudinal fasciculi, internal capsule, and corticospinal tracts compared with patients with IGE-GTCS. Focal diffusion abnormalities in the supplementary motor area (SMA), posterior cingulate cortex, and corpus callosum[191–194] suggest reduced structural connectivity of mesial frontal cortex, explaining the frontal lobe dysfunction[192,193,195] in JME. However, structural and functional connectivity between the prefrontal and motor cortex is increased,[196] and increased coactivation of the motor cortex and SMA with increased cognitive load may represent the anatomic basis for cognitive triggering of myoclonic jerks.[196,197]

DTI can detect transient (immediately after seizures), progressive (after resective surgery), and permanent (an effect of epilepsy) diffusion changes in relation to seizures. Widespread postictal diffusion changes around the seizure focus and remote areas (eg, thalamus and basal ganglia) have been shown in patients with focal and generalized epilepsy.[165,184,198–200] Recurrent seizures, earlier age at seizure onset, and longer duration of epilepsy may also lead to microstructural changes along the seizure spread pathways.[167,172,199,201]

Detecting Postoperative Changes

Acute and chronic diffusion abnormalities, ipsilateral and contralateral to the epileptic focus, have also been seen after ATLR.[202–206] In patients undergoing ATLR, increases in FA in ipsilateral ventromedial language network were shown for the first time by Yogarajah and colleagues[203] (Fig. 4i) at 4 months after surgery, and later confirmed by Winston and colleagues.[206] These changes are correlated with postoperative verbal fluency and naming test scores. The larger the increase in parallel diffusivity in ventromedial language network area, the smaller the decrease in language proficiency postsurgically, reflecting plasticity in language networks in response to ATLR (see Fig. 4ii).[203] FA increases are also seen in the contralateral arcuate fasciculus after left ATLR and are correlated with duration after surgery.[205,207] Ipsilateral changes may reflect initial cytotoxic edema, granular disintegration, or inflammatory changes followed by myelin degradation; and contralateral changes may reflect compensatory reorganization.[202,207] Postsurgical seizure-free patients after ATLR show irreversible temporal and extratemporal diffusion abnormalities, suggesting axonal/myelin injury as a result of epilepsy.[208–210]

Localizing Seizure Focus and Propagation

Diffusion abnormalities may be helpful in localizing or lateralizing epileptic focus. The localizing information provided by DTI has been shown to be concordant with other independent techniques, including structural MR imaging, EEG, equivalent current dipole,[211,212] Megnatoencephalography[213,214] and stereo-EEG.[215]

Seizure onset areas show increased diffusivity in the cortical gray matter and white matter in the vicinity of the epileptic focus, whereas healthy cortex has decreased diffusivity in the inner and middle cortical fractions compared with healthy controls.[216] Focal cortical dysplasia (FCD) visible on conventional MR imaging[217] shows diffusion abnormalities concordant with the structural lesion,[213] and abnormal tracts may reflect ictal spread pathways,[218] although there is a lack of proof for this contention. At times, diffusion abnormalities around FCDs are more extensive, involving gray and deep white matter beyond MR imaging visible lesions, which can help to define the epileptogenic zone.[219] Reduced FA or increased MD ipsilateral to the seizure focus has been seen in TLE.[220–225] Similarly, patients with tuberous sclerosis,[226] symptomatic and cryptogenic focal epilepsy[226] and extra-TLE[215] may have diffusion abnormalities in the white matter

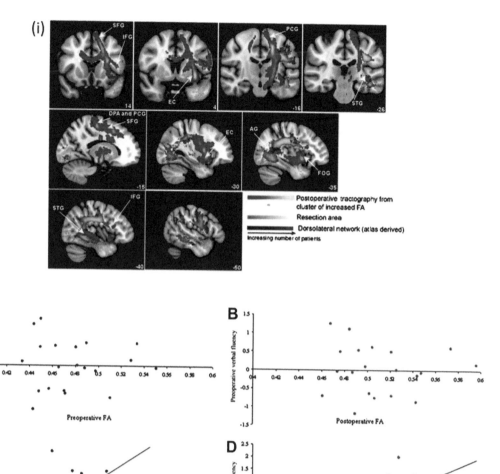

Fig. 4. (*i*) Group variability map of tractography results after seeding from the local maxima of the cluster identified as showing an increase in FA after left ATLR. The group variability map (*yellow-red*, with *yellow* representing voxels identified by the tractography in all patients) visualizes connections from the precentral gyrus via the internal capsule, and connections from the premotor and prefrontal areas, the superior and IFG (including the deep frontal operculum), which pass via the external capsule to the posterior, superior temporal gyrus, and angular gyrus. This network of connections is medial to the traditional dorsolateral language pathway composed of the arcuate fasciculus and inferior longitudinal fasciculus. The latter pathway is shown for reference in blue and is derived from the Johns Hopkins University white matter tractography atlas supplied with FSL software. Also shown is the group variability map for the surgical resection area (*dark pink* to *light pink*) created from the postoperative images. It is evident that after an ATLR, the dorsolateral language connections may be more susceptible to resection and damage than the ventromedial connections. Montreal Neurological Institute coordinates are shown on each slice. AG, angular gyrus; DPA, dorsal premotor area; EC, external capsule; FOG, fronto-orbital gyrus; PCG, precentral gyrus; SFG, superior frontal gyrus; STG, superior temporal gyrus. (*ii*) Scatterplots of verbal fluency scores against the mean FA in left posterior limb internal capsule, external capsule, and corona radiata before (*black dots*) and after (*red dots*) left ATLR. There was a significant correlation between the mean FA in this cluster before and after left ATLR, and postoperative verbal fluency ($r = 0.482$, $P = .009$ and $r = 0.469$, $P = .010$, respectively) (*C* and *D*) but not preoperative verbal fluency scores (*A* and *B*). (*Modified from Yogarajah M, Focke NK, Bonelli SB, et al. The structural plasticity of white matter networks following anterior temporal lobe resection. Brain 2010;133:2357, 2358; with permission.*)

(i)

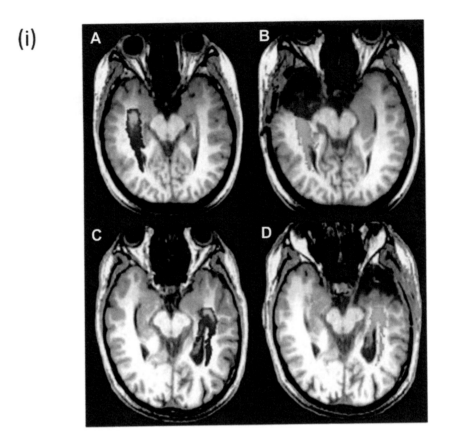

(ii)

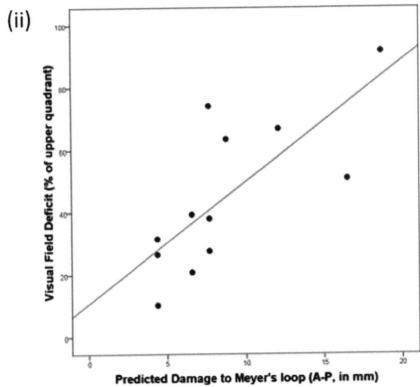

tracts under the epileptogenic tubers and gray matter within the epileptic focus, respectively.

Automated detection of epileptic focus using gray matter segmentation, MD values,[227] and type-specific quantitative neuroimaging analyses[228] has been successful in patients with/without HS and FLE and can also detect occult abnormalities in candidates for epilepsy surgery.[227] A new diffusion sequence (neurite orientation dispersion and density imaging) has promise for showing malformations with increased conspicuity.[229]

Localizing Language Networks

Absence of bilateral arcuate fasciculus and other associated fasciculi has been detected by DTI in children with congenital bilateral perisylvian syndrome, which may result in abnormal and delayed language organization.[230,231] Children with focal epilepsy show regional diffusion abnormalities in bilateral frontal and temporal lobes and right parietal and occipital lobes, which are associated with cognitive performance on language evaluations, reflecting disruption in the connectivity for cortical processing networks.[232] Arcuate fasciculus, as shown by DTI, localizes well with anterior language areas, but less so with posterior language areas and may be sparse in patients with refractory focal epilepsy.[233] Diffusion abnormalities in the left frontal lobe are correlated with category fluency scores in patients with TLE, suggesting that white matter integrity has a role to play in language impairment.[172] LI for asymmetry of arcuate fasciculus have been found to be concordant with Wada test in most patients; however, combining LI with fMRI activity in the Broca area and handedness can lateralize 95% of patients with TLE.[234] Moreover, patients with right TLE with left lateralized fMRI changes show left lateralized arcuate fasciculus, whereas patients with left TLE show decoupling between the functional and structural indices of the arcuate fasciculus, suggesting that language network organization is complex in these patients.[38]

Diffusion Tensor Imaging and Memory Networks

In patients with left TLE, left and right FA values are correlated with verbal and nonverbal memory scores, respectively,[171] and ADC values in the left uncinate fasciculus are negatively correlated with auditory immediate and delayed memory.[235] Increased MD in the left uncinate fasciculus, parahippocampus, cingulum, and inferior fronto-occipital fasciculus are associated with poor verbal memory and associated with cognitive performance.[236] These findings suggest that diffusion abnormalities ipsilateral to the epileptogenic zone may affect the integrity of the memory network, in turn affecting memory performance.[235] Similarly, working memory requires integrity of the frontoparietal network in patients with unilateral HS, suggesting that apparently isolated HS may be associated with widespread diffusion abnormalities affecting working memory performance.[237] Diffusion abnormalities in the medial frontal cortex affect verbal memory in JME and can also predict performance.[191]

Role of Diffusion Tensor Imaging for Localizing Optic Radiation

Tractography can map optic radiation in patients undergoing epilepsy surgery for intraoperative visualization. Disruption in the Meyer loop during TLR produces visual field defect, although it is incomplete quadrantopsia in most patients.[204,238] The extent of damage to the Meyer loop is correlated with degree of postsurgical visual field defect (**Fig. 5**).[239–243] However, optic radiation shows significant anatomic variability,[241] and the distance between the most anterior part of the Meyer loop and the temporal pole ranges from 34 to 51 mm.[244] Mapping optic radiation and its relationship to epileptogenic lesion can help to better customize surgical resection plan and to predict possible risks in each case.[241] After TLR, optic radiation on the contralateral side shows increased FA,[245] and operated/intact side FA ratio decreases and ADC ratio increases,[246] representing plasticity.[245]

Algorithms for visualizing the optic radiation preoperatively and coregistering this with intraoperative images, to be used during surgery and to minimize the risk of visual field defects, have been developed.[240,247] Also, preoperative and intraoperative comparison and estimation of optic

Fig. 5. (*i*) Preoperative structural T1-weighted image and optic radiation (*A*) and postoperative structural T1-weighted image with propagated preoperative tractography (*B*) show that part of the optic radiation was resected (*blue*) in patient 7, who developed a severe visual field deficit (VFD). Corresponding preoperative (*C*) and postoperative images (*D*) are shown in patient 12, who did not develop a VFD. (*ii*) Correlation between measured visual field deficit and the predicted damage to the Meyer loop by image registration. A-P, anterior-posterior. (*Modified from* Winston GP, Daga P, Stretton J, et al. Optic radiation tractography and vision in anterior temporal lobe resection. Ann Neurol 2012;71:337, 338; with permission.)

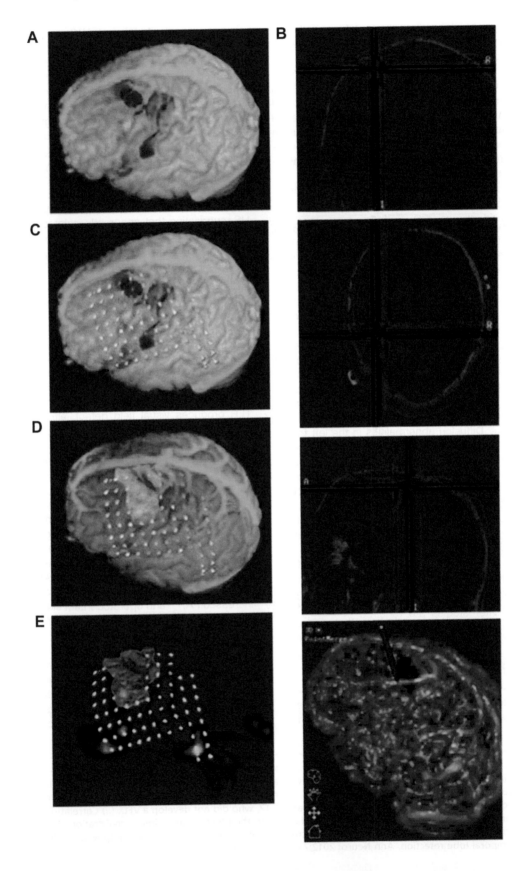

radiation can be used to predict postsurgical visual field defect accurately.[239]

MULTIMODAL IMAGE INTEGRATION

Integration of imaging techniques (such as structural MRI, fMRI, and DTI) acquired and processed preoperatively with intraoperative structural images can be performed successfully. Multimodal image integration has been performed to show structural lesions, surface veins, BOLD activations for hand motor and expressive language areas (mapped using fMRI), IED-related BOLD changes (mapped using EEG-fMRI), and corticospinal tract (mapped using DTI) in 1 common image.[248,249] These integrated images can be shown on three-dimensional, surface-rendered brain of individual patients[248,250] and can be used presurgically/intrasurgically/postsurgically to understand the relationship between different brain structures and functions; for clinical decision making; to implant intracranial electrodes; and to perform surgical resections (**Fig. 6**). They can improve precision and safety during epilepsy surgery, especially for small and deep-seated targets.[251] Image integration is helpful to reduce the risk of damaging eloquent cortex and can assist with completely removing the epileptogenic focus and good postsurgical outcome.[252,253]

SUMMARY

fMRI and DTI have shown great promise in mapping language, memory, and epileptic BOLD networks, and diffusion changes in these networks, respectively. These techniques have been helpful in improving the understanding of mechanisms of seizure generation and cognitive processing in epilepsy and also in predicting the effect of epilepsy and surgery on cognitive and epileptic networks. Multicenter studies are required to standardize the imaging techniques and interpretation of results and to improve the specificity of localization of language, memory, and epileptic networks at individual level so that the techniques can be used as clinical investigation tools in the presurgical assessment of individuals with refractory focal epilepsy.

REFERENCES

1. Ngugi AK, Bottomley C, Kleinschmidt I, et al. Estimation of the burden of active and life-time epilepsy: a meta-analytic approach. Epilepsia 2010;51:883–90.
2. Beleza P. Refractory epilepsy: a clinically oriented review. Eur Neurol 2009;62:65–71.
3. Kwan P, Brodie MJ. Early identification of refractory epilepsy. N Engl J Med 2000;342:314–9.
4. Duncan JS. Selecting patients for epilepsy surgery: synthesis of data. Epilepsy Behav 2011;20:230–2.
5. Chaudhary UJ, Duncan JS, Lemieux L. Mapping hemodynamic correlates of seizures using fMRI: a review. Hum Brain Mapp 2013;34:447–66.
6. Abbott DF, Waites AB, Lillywhite LM, et al. fMRI assessment of language lateralization: an objective approach. Neuroimage 2010;50:1446–55.
7. Anderson DP, Harvey AS, Saling MM, et al. FMRI lateralization of expressive language in children with cerebral lesions. Epilepsia 2006;47:998–1008.
8. Appel S, Duke ES, Martinez AR, et al. Cerebral blood flow and fMRI BOLD auditory language activation in temporal lobe epilepsy. Epilepsia 2012; 53:631–8.
9. Arora J, Pugh K, Westerveld M, et al. Language lateralization in epilepsy patients: fMRI validated with the Wada procedure. Epilepsia 2009;50:2225–41.
10. Ashtari M, Perrine K, Elbaz R, et al. Mapping the functional anatomy of sentence comprehension and application to presurgical evaluation of patients with brain tumor. AJNR Am J Neuroradiol 2005;26: 1461–8.
11. Backes WH, Deblaere K, Vonck K, et al. Language activation distributions revealed by fMRI in postoperative epilepsy patients: differences between left- and right-sided resections. Epilepsy Res 2005;66:1–12.
12. Binder JR, Gross WL, Allendorfer JB, et al. Mapping anterior temporal lobe language areas with fMRI: a multicenter normative study. Neuroimage 2011;54:1465–75.
13. Bonelli SB, Powell R, Thompson PJ, et al. Hippocampal activation correlates with visual confrontation

Fig. 6. Multimodal image integration for a patient undergoing epilepsy surgery for focal cortical dysplasia in left frontal lobe (*left lateral three-dimensional views*). (A) Before implantation; (B) during implantation. The dark blue pointer on (B) shows Stealth navigation probe when it was placed on the large cortical vein; (C) after implantation; (D, E) after resection with highlighted removed cortex. Color codes: red, lesion; green, hand motor cortex; magenta, ictal hyperperfusion from single-photon emission computed tomography; orange, expressive language areas; brown (on A, C), IED-related BOLD signal change; cyan, surface veins; blue (E), corticospinal tract. (*Modified from* Rodionov R, Vollmar C, Nowell M, et al. Feasibility of multimodal 3D neuroimaging to guide implantation of intracranial EEG electrodes. Epilepsy Res 2013;107:94; with permission.)

naming: fMRI findings in controls and patients with temporal lobe epilepsy. Epilepsy Res 2011;95: 246–54.

14. Gartus A, Foki T, Geissler A, et al. Improvement of clinical language localization with an overt semantic and syntactic language functional MR imaging paradigm. AJNR Am J Neuroradiol 2009;30:1977–85.

15. Sanjuan A, Bustamante JC, Forn C, et al. Comparison of two fMRI tasks for the evaluation of the expressive language function. Neuroradiology 2010;52:407–15.

16. Szaflarski JP, Holland SK, Jacola LM, et al. Comprehensive presurgical functional MRI language evaluation in adult patients with epilepsy. Epilepsy Behav 2008;12:74–83.

17. Kesavadas C, Thomas B, Sujesh S, et al. Real-time functional MR imaging (fMRI) for presurgical evaluation of paediatric epilepsy. Pediatr Radiol 2007; 37:964–74.

18. Williams EJ, Stretton J, Centeno M, et al. Clinical language fMRI with real-time monitoring in temporal lobe epilepsy: online processing methods. Epilepsy Behav 2012;25:120–4.

19. Wilke M, Schmithorst VJ. A combined bootstrap/ histogram analysis approach for computing a lateralization index from neuroimaging data. Neuroimage 2006;33:522–30.

20. Wilke M, Lidzba K, Staudt M, et al. An fMRI task battery for assessing hemispheric language dominance in children. Neuroimage 2006;32:400–10.

21. Wilke M, Lidzba K. LI-tool: a new toolbox to assess lateralization in functional MR data. J Neurosci Methods 2007;163:128–36.

22. Seghier ML. Laterality index in functional MRI: methodological issues. Magn Reson Imaging 2008;26:594–601.

23. Jones SE, Mahmoud SY, Phillips MD. A practical clinical method to quantify language lateralization in fMRI using whole-brain analysis. Neuroimage 2011;54:2937–49.

24. Suarez RO, Whalen S, Nelson AP, et al. Threshold-independent functional MRI determination of language dominance: a validation study against clinical gold standards. Epilepsy Behav 2009;16:288–97.

25. Karunanayaka P, Kim KK, Holland SK, et al. The effects of left or right hemispheric epilepsy on language networks investigated with semantic decision fMRI task and independent component analysis. Epilepsy Behav 2011;20:623–32.

26. Mbwana J, Berl MM, Ritzl EK, et al. Limitations to plasticity of language network reorganization in localization related epilepsy. Brain 2009;132:347–56.

27. You X, Guillen M, Bernal B, et al. fMRI activation pattern recognition: a novel application of PCA in language network of pediatric localization related epilepsy. Conf Proc IEEE Eng Med Biol Soc 2009; 2009:5397–400.

28. You X, Adjouadi M, Wang J, et al. A decisional space for fMRI pattern separation using the principal component analysis–a comparative study of language networks in pediatric epilepsy. Hum Brain Mapp 2013;34(9):2330–42.

29. Wang J, You X, Wu W, et al. Classification of fMRI patterns–a study of the language network segregation in pediatric localization related epilepsy. Hum Brain Mapp 2014;35(4):1446–60.

30. You X, Adjouadi M, Guillen MR, et al. Sub-patterns of language network reorganization in pediatric localization related epilepsy: a multisite study. Hum Brain Mapp 2011;32:784–99.

31. Berl MM, Balsamo LM, Xu B, et al. Seizure focus affects regional language networks assessed by fMRI. Neurology 2005;65:1604–11.

32. Thivard L, Hombrouck J, du Montcel ST, et al. Productive and perceptive language reorganization in temporal lobe epilepsy. Neuroimage 2005; 24:841–51.

33. Jensen EJ, Hargreaves IS, Pexman PM, et al. Abnormalities of lexical and semantic processing in left temporal lobe epilepsy: an fMRI study. Epilepsia 2011;52:2013–21.

34. Powell HW, Parker GJ, Alexander DC, et al. Abnormalities of language networks in temporal lobe epilepsy. Neuroimage 2007;36:209–21.

35. Cousin E, Baciu M, Pichat C, et al. Functional MRI evidence for language plasticity in adult epileptic patients: preliminary results. Neuropsychiatr Dis Treat 2008;4:235–46.

36. Voets NL, Adcock JE, Flitney DE, et al. Distinct right frontal lobe activation in language processing following left hemisphere injury. Brain 2006;129: 754–66.

37. Duke ES, Tesfaye M, Berl MM, et al. The effect of seizure focus on regional language processing areas. Epilepsia 2012;53:1044–50.

38. Rodrigo S, Oppenheim C, Chassoux F, et al. Language lateralization in temporal lobe epilepsy using functional MRI and probabilistic tractography. Epilepsia 2008;49:1367–76.

39. Gaillard WD, Berl MM, Moore EN, et al. Atypical language in lesional and nonlesional complex partial epilepsy. Neurology 2007;69:1761–71.

40. Wilke M, Pieper T, Lindner K, et al. Clinical functional MRI of the language domain in children with epilepsy. Hum Brain Mapp 2011;32: 1882–93.

41. Benke T, Koylu B, Visani P, et al. Language lateralization in temporal lobe epilepsy: a comparison between fMRI and the Wada test. Epilepsia 2006; 47:1308–19.

42. Janecek JK, Swanson SJ, Sabsevitz DS, et al. Language lateralization by fMRI and Wada testing in 229 patients with epilepsy: rates and predictors of discordance. Epilepsia 2013;54:314–22.

43. Kim KK, Privitera MD, Szaflarski JP. Lessons learned from a comparison of language localisation using fMRI and electrocortical mapping: case studies of neocortical epilepsy patients. Epileptic Disord 2011;13:368–74.

44. Lee D, Swanson SJ, Sabsevitz DS, et al. Functional MRI and Wada studies in patients with inter-hemispheric dissociation of language functions. Epilepsy Behav 2008;13:350–6.

45. de RS, Fohlen M, Bulteau C, et al. Presurgical language mapping in children with epilepsy: clinical usefulness of functional magnetic resonance imaging for the planning of cortical stimulation. Epilepsia 2012;53:67–78.

46. Wagner K, Hader C, Metternich B, et al. Who needs a Wada test? Present clinical indications for amobarbital procedures. J Neurol Neurosurg Psychiatry 2012;83:503–9.

47. Waites AB, Briellmann RS, Saling MM, et al. Functional connectivity networks are disrupted in left temporal lobe epilepsy. Ann Neurol 2006;59:335–43.

48. Vlooswijk MC, Jansen JF, Majoie HJ, et al. Functional connectivity and language impairment in cryptogenic localization-related epilepsy. Neurology 2010;75:395–402.

49. Pravata E, Sestieri C, Mantini D, et al. Functional connectivity MR imaging of the language network in patients with drug-resistant epilepsy. AJNR Am J Neuroradiol 2011;32:532–40.

50. Protzner AB, McAndrews MP. Network alterations supporting word retrieval in patients with medial temporal lobe epilepsy. J Cogn Neurosci 2011;23: 2605–19.

51. Brazdil M, Chlebus P, Mikl M, et al. Reorganization of language-related neuronal networks in patients with left temporal lobe epilepsy–an fMRI study. Eur J Neurol 2005;12:268–75.

52. Briellmann RS, Labate A, Harvey AS, et al. Is language lateralization in temporal lobe epilepsy patients related to the nature of the epileptogenic lesion? Epilepsia 2006;47:916–20.

53. Fakhri M, Oghabian MA, Vedaei F, et al. Atypical language lateralization: an fMRI study in patients with cerebral lesions. Funct Neurol 2013;28:55–61.

54. Hadac J, Brozova K, Tintera J, et al. Language lateralization in children with pre- and postnatal epileptogenic lesions of the left hemisphere: an fMRI study. Epileptic Disord 2007;9(Suppl 1):S19–27.

55. Wellmer J, Weber B, Urbach H, et al. Cerebral lesions can impair fMRI-based language lateralization. Epilepsia 2009;50:2213–24.

56. Sanjuan A, Bustamante JC, Garcia-Porcar M, et al. Bilateral inferior frontal language-related activation correlates with verbal recall in patients with left temporal lobe epilepsy and typical language distribution. Epilepsy Res 2013;104:118–24.

57. Everts R, Harvey AS, Lillywhite L, et al. Language lateralization correlates with verbal memory performance in children with focal epilepsy. Epilepsia 2010;51:627–38.

58. Labudda K, Mertens M, Janszky J, et al. Atypical language lateralisation associated with right fronto-temporal grey matter increases–a combined fMRI and VBM study in left-sided mesial temporal lobe epilepsy patients. Neuroimage 2012;59:728–37.

59. Kunii N, Kamada K, Ota T, et al. Characteristic profiles of high gamma activity and blood oxygenation level-dependent responses in various language areas. Neuroimage 2013;65:242–9.

60. Araujo D, de Araujo DB, Pontes-Neto OM, et al. Language and motor FMRI activation in polymicrogyric cortex. Epilepsia 2006;47:589–92.

61. Gauffin H, van Ettinger-Veenstra H, Landtblom AM, et al. Impaired language function in generalized epilepsy: inadequate suppression of the default mode network. Epilepsy Behav 2013;28:26–35.

62. Datta AN, Oser N, Bauder F, et al. Cognitive impairment and cortical reorganization in children with benign epilepsy with centrotemporal spikes. Epilepsia 2013;54:487–94.

63. Yuan W, Szaflarski JP, Schmithorst VJ, et al. fMRI shows atypical language lateralization in pediatric epilepsy patients. Epilepsia 2006;47:593–600.

64. Lillywhite LM, Saling MM, Harvey AS, et al. Neuropsychological and functional MRI studies provide converging evidence of anterior language dysfunction in BECTS. Epilepsia 2009;50:2276–84.

65. Janecek JK, Swanson SJ, Sabsevitz DS, et al. Naming outcome prediction in patients with discordant Wada and fMRI language lateralization. Epilepsy Behav 2013;27:399–403.

66. Bonelli SB, Thompson PJ, Yogarajah M, et al. Imaging language networks before and after anterior temporal lobe resection: results of a longitudinal fMRI study. Epilepsia 2012;53:639–50.

67. Rosazza C, Ghielmetti F, Minati L, et al. Preoperative language lateralization in temporal lobe epilepsy (TLE) predicts peri-ictal, pre- and post-operative language performance: an fMRI study. Neuroimage Clin 2013;3:73–83.

68. Noppeney U, Price CJ, Duncan JS, et al. Reading skills after left anterior temporal lobe resection: an fMRI study. Brain 2005;128:1377–85.

69. Szaflarski JP, Allendorfer JB. Topiramate and its effect on fMRI of language in patients with right or left temporal lobe epilepsy. Epilepsy Behav 2012;24:74–80.

70. Yasuda CL, Centeno M, Vollmar C, et al. The effect of topiramate on cognitive fMRI. Epilepsy Res 2013;105:250–5.

71. Janszky J, Mertens M, Janszky I, et al. Left-sided interictal epileptic activity induces shift of language lateralization in temporal lobe epilepsy: an fMRI study. Epilepsia 2006;47:921–7.

72. Yu A, Wang X, Xu G, et al. A functional MRI study of language networks in left medial temporal lobe epilepsy. Eur J Radiol 2011;80:441–4.

73. Helmstaedter C, Fritz NE, Gonzalez Perez PA, et al. Shift-back of right into left hemisphere language dominance after control of epileptic seizures: evidence for epilepsy driven functional cerebral organization. Epilepsy Res 2006;70:257–62.

74. Stretton J, Thompson PJ. Frontal lobe function in temporal lobe epilepsy. Epilepsy Res 2012;98:1–13.

75. Hoppe C, Elger CE, Helmstaedter C. Long-term memory impairment in patients with focal epilepsy. Epilepsia 2007;48(Suppl 9):26–9.

76. Centeno M, Thompson PJ, Koepp MJ, et al. Memory in frontal lobe epilepsy. Epilepsy Res 2010;91:123–32.

77. Binder JR, Sabsevitz DS, Swanson SJ, et al. Use of preoperative functional MRI to predict verbal memory decline after temporal lobe epilepsy surgery. Epilepsia 2008;49:1377–94.

78. Bonelli SB, Thompson PJ, Yogarajah M, et al. Memory reorganization following anterior temporal lobe resection: a longitudinal functional MRI study. Brain 2013;136:1889–900.

79. Branco DM, Suarez RO, Whalen S, et al. Functional MRI of memory in the hippocampus: laterality indices may be more meaningful if calculated from whole voxel distributions. Neuroimage 2006; 32:592–602.

80. Addis DR, Moscovitch M, McAndrews MP. Consequences of hippocampal damage across the autobiographical memory network in left temporal lobe epilepsy. Brain 2007;130:2327–42.

81. Milton F, Butler CR, Benattayallah A, et al. The neural basis of autobiographical memory deficits in transient epileptic amnesia. Neuropsychologia 2012;50:3528–41.

82. Alessio A, Pereira FR, Sercheli MS, et al. Brain plasticity for verbal and visual memories in patients with mesial temporal lobe epilepsy and hippocampal sclerosis: an fMRI study. Hum Brain Mapp 2013;34:186–99.

83. Koylu B, Trinka E, Ischebeck A, et al. Neural correlates of verbal semantic memory in patients with temporal lobe epilepsy. Epilepsy Res 2006;72:178–91.

84. Bonelli SB, Powell RH, Yogarajah M, et al. Imaging memory in temporal lobe epilepsy: predicting the effects of temporal lobe resection. Brain 2010; 133:1186–99.

85. Koylu B, Walser G, Ischebeck A, et al. Functional imaging of semantic memory predicts postoperative episodic memory functions in chronic temporal lobe epilepsy. Brain Res 2008;1223:73–81.

86. Powell HW, Richardson MP, Symms MR, et al. Reorganization of verbal and nonverbal memory in temporal lobe epilepsy due to unilateral hippocampal sclerosis. Epilepsia 2007;48:1512–25.

87. Maccotta L, Buckner RL, Gilliam FG, et al. Changing frontal contributions to memory before and after medial temporal lobectomy. Cereb Cortex 2007;17: 443–56.

88. Bigras C, Shear PK, Vannest J, et al. The effects of temporal lobe epilepsy on scene encoding. Epilepsy Behav 2013;26:11–21.

89. Figueiredo P, Santana I, Teixeira J, et al. Adaptive visual memory reorganization in right medial temporal lobe epilepsy. Epilepsia 2008;49:1395–408.

90. McCormick C, Quraan M, Cohn M, et al. Default mode network connectivity indicates episodic memory capacity in mesial temporal lobe epilepsy. Epilepsia 2013;54:809–18.

91. Pereira FR, Alessio A, Sercheli MS, et al. Asymmetrical hippocampal connectivity in mesial temporal lobe epilepsy: evidence from resting state fMRI. BMC Neurosci 2010;11:66.

92. Banks SJ, Sziklas V, Sodums DJ, et al. fMRI of verbal and nonverbal memory processes in healthy and epileptogenic medial temporal lobes. Epilepsy Behav 2012;25:42–9.

93. Guedj E, Bettus G, Barbeau EJ, et al. Hyperactivation of parahippocampal region and fusiform gyrus associated with successful encoding in medial temporal lobe epilepsy. Epilepsia 2011;52:1100–9.

94. Sidhu MK, Stretton J, Winston GP, et al. A functional magnetic resonance imaging study mapping the episodic memory encoding network in temporal lobe epilepsy. Brain 2013;136:1868–88.

95. Doucet G, Osipowicz K, Sharan A, et al. Hippocampal functional connectivity patterns during spatial working memory differ in right versus left temporal lobe epilepsy. Brain Connect 2013;3(4): 398–406.

96. Stretton J, Winston GP, Sidhu M, et al. Disrupted segregation of working memory networks in temporal lobe epilepsy. Neuroimage Clin 2013;2: 273–81.

97. Stretton J, Winston G, Sidhu M, et al. Neural correlates of working memory in temporal lobe epilepsy— an fMRI study. Neuroimage 2012;60:1696–703.

98. Braakman HM, Vaessen MJ, Jansen JF, et al. Frontal lobe connectivity and cognitive impairment in pediatric frontal lobe epilepsy. Epilepsia 2013; 54:446–54.

99. Vlooswijk MC, Jansen JF, Reijs RP, et al. Cognitive fMRI and neuropsychological assessment in patients with secondarily generalized seizures. Clin Neurol Neurosurg 2008;110:441–50.

100. Vlooswijk MC, Jansen JF, Jeukens CR, et al. Memory processes and prefrontal network dysfunction in cryptogenic epilepsy. Epilepsia 2011;52:1467–75.

101. Roebling R, Scheerer N, Uttner I, et al. Evaluation of cognition, structural, and functional MRI in juvenile myoclonic epilepsy. Epilepsia 2009;50:2456–65.

102. Protzner AB, Kovacevic N, Cohn M, et al. Characterizing functional integrity: intraindividual brain signal variability predicts memory performance in patients with medial temporal lobe epilepsy. J Neurosci 2013;33:9855–65.

103. Frings L, Wagner K, Halsband U, et al. Lateralization of hippocampal activation differs between left and right temporal lobe epilepsy patients and correlates with postsurgical verbal learning decrement. Epilepsy Res 2008;78:161–70.

104. Powell HW, Richardson MP, Symms MR, et al. Preoperative fMRI predicts memory decline following anterior temporal lobe resection. J Neurol Neurosurg Psychiatry 2008;79:686–93.

105. Richardson MP, Strange BA, Duncan JS, et al. Memory fMRI in left hippocampal sclerosis: optimizing the approach to predicting postsurgical memory. Neurology 2006;66:699–705.

106. Janszky J, Jokeit H, Kontopoulou K, et al. Functional MRI predicts memory performance after right mesiotemporal epilepsy surgery. Epilepsia 2005;46:244–50.

107. Cheung MC, Chan AS, Lam JM, et al. Pre- and postoperative fMRI and clinical memory performance in temporal lobe epilepsy. J Neurol Neurosurg Psychiatry 2009;80:1099–106.

108. Salek-Haddadi A, Diehl B, Hamandi K, et al. Hemodynamic correlates of epileptiform discharges: an EEG-fMRI study of 63 patients with focal epilepsy. Brain Res 2006;1088:148–66.

109. Chaudhary UJ, Rodionov R, Carmichael DW, et al. Improving the sensitivity of EEG-fMRI studies of epileptic activity by modelling eye blinks, swallowing and other video-EEG detected physiological confounds. Neuroimage 2012;61:1383–93.

110. Grouiller F, Thornton RC, Groening K, et al. With or without spikes: localization of focal epileptic activity by simultaneous electroencephalography and functional magnetic resonance imaging. Brain 2011;134:2867–86.

111. Elshoff L, Groening K, Grouiller F, et al. The value of EEG-fMRI and EEG source analysis in the presurgical setup of children with refractory focal epilepsy. Epilepsia 2012;53:1597–606.

112. Gholipour T, Moeller F, Pittau F, et al. Reproducibility of interictal EEG-fMRI results in patients with epilepsy. Epilepsia 2011;52:433–42.

113. Pesaresi I, Cosottini M, Belmonte G, et al. Reproducibility of BOLD localization of interictal activity in patients with focal epilepsy: intrasession and intersession comparisons. MAGMA 2011;24:285–96.

114. Pittau F, Dubeau F, Gotman J. Contribution of EEG/fMRI to the definition of the epileptic focus. Neurology 2012;78:1479–87.

115. van Houdt PJ, De Munck JC, Leijten FS, et al. EEG-fMRI correlation patterns in the presurgical evaluation of focal epilepsy: a comparison with electrocorticographic data and surgical outcome measures. Neuroimage 2013;75:246–56.

116. Zijlmans M, Huiskamp G, Hersevoort M, et al. EEG-fMRI in the preoperative work-up for epilepsy surgery. Brain 2007;130:2343–53.

117. Zijlmans M, Buskens E, Hersevoort M, et al. Should we reconsider epilepsy surgery? The motivation of patients once rejected. Seizure 2008;17:374–7.

118. Thornton R, Vulliemoz S, Rodionov R, et al. Epileptic networks in focal cortical dysplasia revealed using electroencephalography-functional magnetic resonance imaging. Ann Neurol 2011;70:822–37.

119. LeVan P, Tyvaert L, Moeller F, et al. Independent component analysis reveals dynamic ictal BOLD responses in EEG-fMRI data from focal epilepsy patients. Neuroimage 2010;49:366–78.

120. Thornton RC, Rodionov R, Laufs H, et al. Imaging haemodynamic changes related to seizures: comparison of EEG-based general linear model, independent component analysis of fMRI and intracranial EEG. Neuroimage 2010;53:196–205.

121. Tyvaert L, Hawco C, Kobayashi E, et al. Different structures involved during ictal and interictal epileptic activity in malformations of cortical development: an EEG-fMRI study. Brain 2008;131:2042–60.

122. Tyvaert L, LeVan P, Dubeau F, et al. Noninvasive dynamic imaging of seizures in epileptic patients. Hum Brain Mapp 2009;30:3993–4011.

123. Donaire A, Bargallo N, Falcon C, et al. Identifying the structures involved in seizure generation using sequential analysis of ictal-fMRI data. Neuroimage 2009;47:173–83.

124. Chaudhary UJ, Carmichael DW, Rodionov R, et al. Mapping preictal and ictal haemodynamic networks using video-electroencephalography and functional imaging. Brain 2012;135:3645–63.

125. Meletti S, Vignoli A, Benuzzi F, et al. Ictal involvement of the nigrostriatal system in subtle seizures of ring chromosome 20 epilepsy. Epilepsia 2012;53:e156–60.

126. Vaudano AE, Carmichael DW, Salek-Haddadi A, et al. Networks involved in seizure initiation. A reading epilepsy case studied with EEG-fMRI and MEG. Neurology 2012;79:249–53.

127. Jacobs J, LeVan P, Moeller F, et al. Hemodynamic changes preceding the interictal EEG spike in patients with focal epilepsy investigated using simultaneous EEG-fMRI. Neuroimage 2009;45:1220–31.

128. Federico P, Abbott DF, Briellmann RS, et al. Functional MRI of the pre-ictal state. Brain 2005;128:1811–7.

129. Laufs H. Functional imaging of seizures and epilepsy: evolution from zones to networks. Curr Opin Neurol 2012;25:194–200.

130. Salek-Haddadi A, Lemieux L, Merschhemke M, et al. Functional magnetic resonance imaging of human absence seizures. Ann Neurol 2003;53:663–7.

131. Gotman J, Grova C, Bagshaw A, et al. Generalized epileptic discharges show thalamocortical activation and suspension of the default state of the brain. Proc Natl Acad Sci U S A 2005;102:15236–40.

132. Archer JS, Abbott DF, Waites AB, et al. fMRI "deactivation" of the posterior cingulate during generalized spike and wave. Neuroimage 2003;20:1915–22.

133. Moeller F, Siebner HR, Wolff S, et al. Changes in activity of striato-thalamo-cortical network precede generalized spike wave discharges. Neuroimage 2008;39:1839–49.

134. Carney PW, Masterton RA, Harvey AS, et al. The core network in absence epilepsy. Differences in cortical and thalamic BOLD response. Neurology 2010;75:904–11.

135. Raichle ME, MacLeod AM, Snyder AZ, et al. A default mode of brain function. Proc Natl Acad Sci U S A 2001;98:676–82.

136. Laufs H, Hamandi K, Salek-Haddadi A, et al. Temporal lobe interictal epileptic discharges affect cerebral activity in "default mode" brain regions. Hum Brain Mapp 2007;28:1023–32.

137. Fahoum F, Zelmann R, Tyvaert L, et al. Epileptic discharges affect the default mode network–fMRI and intracerebral EEG evidence. PLoS One 2013; 8:e68038.

138. Bai X, Vestal M, Berman R, et al. Dynamic time course of typical childhood absence seizures: EEG, behavior, and functional magnetic resonance imaging. J Neurosci 2010;30:5884–93.

139. Berman R, Negishi M, Vestal M, et al. Simultaneous EEG, fMRI, and behavior in typical childhood absence seizures. Epilepsia 2010;51:2011–22.

140. Killory BD, Bai X, Negishi M, et al. Impaired attention and network connectivity in childhood absence epilepsy. Neuroimage 2011;56:2209–17.

141. Chaudhary UJ, Centeno M, Carmichael DW, et al. Imaging the interaction: epileptic discharges, working memory, and behavior. Hum Brain Mapp 2013;34(11):2910–7.

142. Vaudano AE, Laufs H, Kiebel SJ, et al. Causal hierarchy within the thalamo-cortical network in spike and wave discharges. PLoS One 2009;4:e6475.

143. Benuzzi F, Mirandola L, Pugnaghi M, et al. Increased cortical BOLD signal anticipates generalized spike and wave discharges in adolescents and adults with idiopathic generalized epilepsies. Epilepsia 2012;53:622–30.

144. Meeren H, van LG, Lopes da SF, et al. Evolving concepts on the pathophysiology of absence seizures: the cortical focus theory. Arch Neurol 2005; 62:371–6.

145. Moeller F, Siebner HR, Ahlgrimm N, et al. fMRI activation during spike and wave discharges evoked by photic stimulation. Neuroimage 2009; 48:682–95.

146. Morocz IA, Karni A, Haut S, et al. fMRI of triggerable aurae in musicogenic epilepsy. Neurology 2003;60:705–9.

147. Marrosu F, Barberini L, Puligheddu M, et al. Combined EEG/fMRI recording in musicogenic epilepsy. Epilepsy Res 2009;84:77–81.

148. Salek-Haddadi A, Mayer T, Hamandi K, et al. Imaging seizure activity: a combined EEG/EMG-fMRI study in reading epilepsy. Epilepsia 2009;50:256–64.

149. Vaudano AE, Di BC, Carni M, et al. Ictal haemodynamic changes in a patient affected by "subtle" epilepsia partialis continua. Seizure 2012;21:65–9.

150. Szaflarski JP, Lindsell CJ, Zakaria T, et al. Seizure control in patients with idiopathic generalized epilepsies: EEG determinants of medication response. Epilepsy Behav 2010;17:525–30.

151. Szaflarski JP, Kay B, Gotman J, et al. The relationship between the localization of the generalized spike and wave discharge generators and the response to valproate. Epilepsia 2013;54:471–80.

152. Laufs H, Richardson MP, Salek-Haddadi A, et al. Converging PET and fMRI evidence for a common area involved in human focal epilepsies. Neurology 2011;77:904–10.

153. Flanagan D, Badawy RA, Jackson GD. EEG-fMRI in focal epilepsy: local activation and regional networks. Clin Neurophysiol 2014;125:21–31.

154. Boucousis SM, Beers CA, Cunningham CJ, et al. Feasibility of an intracranial EEG-fMRI protocol at 3T: risk assessment and image quality. Neuroimage 2012;63:1237–48.

155. Carmichael DW, Thornton JS, Rodionov R, et al. Safety of localizing epilepsy monitoring intracranial electroencephalograph electrodes using MRI: radiofrequency-induced heating. J Magn Reson Imaging 2008;28:1233–44.

156. Carmichael DW, Thornton JS, Rodionov R, et al. Feasibility of simultaneous intracranial EEG-fMRI in humans: a safety study. Neuroimage 2010;49: 379–90.

157. Carmichael DW, Vulliemoz S, Rodionov R, et al. Simultaneous intracranial EEG-fMRI in humans: protocol considerations and data quality. Neuroimage 2012;63:301–9.

158. Vulliemoz S, Carmichael DW, Rosenkranz K, et al. Simultaneous intracranial EEG and fMRI of interictal epileptic discharges in humans. Neuroimage 2011; 54:182–90.

159. Cunningham CB, Goodyear BG, Badawy R, et al. Intracranial EEG-fMRI analysis of focal epileptiform discharges in humans. Epilepsia 2012;53:1636–48.

160. Chaudhary UJ, Carmichael DW, Rodionov R, et al. Mapping the irritative zone using simultaneous intracranial EEG-fMRI and comparison with postsurgical outcome. Epilepsia 2012;53(Suppl 5):14.

161. Alexander AL, Lee JE, Lazar M, et al. Diffusion tensor imaging of the brain. Neurotherapeutics 2007;4:316–29.

162. Schonberg T, Pianka P, Hendler T, et al. Characterization of displaced white matter by brain tumors using combined DTI and fMRI. Neuroimage 2006; 30:1100–11.

163. Bonilha L, Edwards JC, Kinsman SL, et al. Extrahippocampal gray matter loss and hippocampal deafferentation in patients with temporal lobe epilepsy. Epilepsia 2010;51:519–28.

164. Concha L, Beaulieu C, Gross DW. Bilateral limbic diffusion abnormalities in unilateral temporal lobe epilepsy. Ann Neurol 2005;57:188–96.

165. Keller SS, Ahrens T, Mohammadi S, et al. Voxel-based statistical analysis of fractional anisotropy and mean diffusivity in patients with unilateral temporal lobe epilepsy of unknown cause. J Neuroimaging 2013;23:352–9.

166. Kim CH, Koo BB, Chung CK, et al. Thalamic changes in temporal lobe epilepsy with and without hippocampal sclerosis: a diffusion tensor imaging study. Epilepsy Res 2010;90:21–7.

167. Kim H, Piao Z, Liu P, et al. Secondary white matter degeneration of the corpus callosum in patients with intractable temporal lobe epilepsy: a diffusion tensor imaging study. Epilepsy Res 2008;81:136–42.

168. Knake S, Salat DH, Halgren E, et al. Changes in white matter microstructure in patients with TLE and hippocampal sclerosis. Epileptic Disord 2009;11:244–50.

169. Riley JD, Franklin DL, Choi V, et al. Altered white matter integrity in temporal lobe epilepsy: association with cognitive and clinical profiles. Epilepsia 2010;51:536–45.

170. Wang XQ, Iang SY, Lu H, et al. Executive function impairment in patients with temporal lobe epilepsy: neuropsychological and diffusion-tensor imaging study. Zhonghua Yi Xue Za Zhi 2007;87:3183–7 [in Chinese].

171. Yogarajah M, Powell HW, Parker GJ, et al. Tractography of the parahippocampal gyrus and material specific memory impairment in unilateral temporal lobe epilepsy. Neuroimage 2008;40: 1755–64.

172. Wang XQ, Lang SY, Hong LU, et al. Changes in extratemporal integrity and cognition in temporal lobe epilepsy: a diffusion tensor imaging study. Neurol India 2010;58:891–9.

173. Focke NK, Yogarajah M, Bonelli SB, et al. Voxel-based diffusion tensor imaging in patients with mesial temporal lobe epilepsy and hippocampal sclerosis. Neuroimage 2008;40:728–37.

174. Lin JJ, Riley JD, Juranek J, et al. Vulnerability of the frontal-temporal connections in temporal lobe epilepsy. Epilepsy Res 2008;82:162–70.

175. Concha L, Beaulieu C, Collins DL, et al. White-matter diffusion abnormalities in temporal-lobe epilepsy with and without mesial temporal sclerosis. J Neurol Neurosurg Psychiatry 2009;80:312–9.

176. Concha L, Livy DJ, Beaulieu C, et al. In vivo diffusion tensor imaging and histopathology of the fimbria-fornix in temporal lobe epilepsy. J Neurosci 2010; 30:996–1002.

177. Dumas de la Roque A, Oppenheim C, Chassoux F, et al. Diffusion tensor imaging of partial intractable epilepsy. Eur Radiol 2005;15:279–85.

178. Fonseca VC, Yasuda CL, Tedeschi GG, et al. White matter abnormalities in patients with focal cortical dysplasia revealed by diffusion tensor imaging analysis in a voxelwise approach. Front Neurol 2012;3:121.

179. Isik U, Dincer A, Ozek MM. Surgical treatment of polymicrogyria with advanced radiologic and neurophysiologic techniques. Childs Nerv Syst 2007;23:443–8.

180. Holt RL, Provenzale JM, Veerapandiyan A, et al. Structural connectivity of the frontal lobe in children with drug-resistant partial epilepsy. Epilepsy Behav 2011;21:65–70.

181. Hutchinson E, Pulsipher D, Dabbs K, et al. Children with new-onset epilepsy exhibit diffusion abnormalities in cerebral white matter in the absence of volumetric differences. Epilepsy Res 2010;88:208–14.

182. Li Y, Du H, Xie B, et al. Cerebellum abnormalities in idiopathic generalized epilepsy with generalized tonic-clonic seizures revealed by diffusion tensor imaging. PLoS One 2010;5:e15219.

183. Deppe M, Kellinghaus C, Duning T, et al. Nerve fiber impairment of anterior thalamocortical circuitry in juvenile myoclonic epilepsy. Neurology 2008;71:1981–5.

184. Keller SS, Ahrens T, Mohammadi S, et al. Microstructural and volumetric abnormalities of the putamen in juvenile myoclonic epilepsy. Epilepsia 2011; 52:1715–24.

185. Kim H, Harrison A, Kankirawatana P, et al. Major white matter fiber changes in medically intractable neocortical epilepsy in children: a diffusion tensor imaging study. Epilepsy Res 2013;103:211–20.

186. Yang T, Guo Z, Luo C, et al. White matter impairment in the basal ganglia-thalamocortical circuit of drug-naive childhood absence epilepsy. Epilepsy Res 2012;99:267–73.

187. Nilsson D, Go C, Rutka JT, et al. Bilateral diffusion tensor abnormalities of temporal lobe and cingulate gyrus white matter in children with temporal lobe epilepsy. Epilepsy Res 2008;81:128–35.

188. Liao W, Zhang Z, Pan Z, et al. Default mode network abnormalities in mesial temporal lobe epilepsy: a study combining fMRI and DTI. Hum Brain Mapp 2011;32:883–95.

189. Ellmore TM, Pieters TA, Tandon N. Dissociation between diffusion MR tractography density and strength in epilepsy patients with hippocampal sclerosis. Epilepsy Res 2011;93:197–203.

190. Kucukboyaci NE, Girard HM, Hagler DJ Jr, et al. Role of frontotemporal fiber tract integrity in task-switching performance of healthy controls and patients with temporal lobe epilepsy. J Int Neuropsychol Soc 2012;18:57–67.

191. O'Muircheartaigh J, Vollmar C, Barker GJ, et al. Focal structural changes and cognitive dysfunction in juvenile myoclonic epilepsy. Neurology 2011;76: 34–40.

192. Vulliemoz S, Vollmar C, Koepp MJ, et al. Connectivity of the supplementary motor area in juvenile myoclonic epilepsy and frontal lobe epilepsy. Epilepsia 2011;52:507–14.

193. Kim JH, Suh SI, Park SY, et al. Microstructural white matter abnormality and frontal cognitive dysfunctions in juvenile myoclonic epilepsy. Epilepsia 2012;53:1371–8.

194. Liu M, Concha L, Beaulieu C, et al. Distinct white matter abnormalities in different idiopathic generalized epilepsy syndromes. Epilepsia 2011;52:2267–75.

195. O'Muircheartaigh J, Vollmar C, Barker GJ, et al. Abnormal thalamocortical structural and functional connectivity in juvenile myoclonic epilepsy. Brain 2012;135:3635–44.

196. Vollmar C, O'Muircheartaigh J, Symms MR, et al. Altered microstructural connectivity in juvenile myoclonic epilepsy: the missing link. Neurology 2012;78:1555–9.

197. Vollmar C, O'Muircheartaigh J, Barker GJ, et al. Motor system hyperconnectivity in juvenile myoclonic epilepsy: a cognitive functional magnetic resonance imaging study. Brain 2011;134:1710–9.

198. Diehl B, Symms MR, Boulby PA, et al. Postictal diffusion tensor imaging. Epilepsy Res 2005;65: 137–46.

199. Gerdes JS, Keller SS, Schwindt W, et al. Progression of microstructural putamen alterations in a case of symptomatic recurrent seizures using diffusion tensor imaging. Seizure 2012;21:478–81.

200. Luo C, Xia Y, Li Q, et al. Diffusion and volumetry abnormalities in subcortical nuclei of patients with absence seizures. Epilepsia 2011;52:1092–9.

201. Keller SS, Schoene-Bake JC, Gerdes JS, et al. Concomitant fractional anisotropy and volumetric abnormalities in temporal lobe epilepsy: cross-sectional evidence for progressive neurologic injury. PLoS One 2012;7:e46791.

202. Liu M, Gross DW, Wheatley BM, et al. The acute phase of Wallerian degeneration: longitudinal diffusion tensor imaging of the fornix following temporal lobe surgery. Neuroimage 2013;74:128–39.

203. Yogarajah M, Focke NK, Bonelli SB, et al. The structural plasticity of white matter networks following anterior temporal lobe resection. Brain 2010;133:2348–64.

204. McDonald CR, Hagler DJ Jr, Girard HM, et al. Changes in fiber tract integrity and visual fields after anterior temporal lobectomy. Neurology 2010;75:1631–8.

205. Nguyen D, Vargas MI, Khaw N, et al. Diffusion tensor imaging analysis with tract-based spatial statistics of the white matter abnormalities after epilepsy surgery. Epilepsy Res 2011;94(3):189–97.

206. Winston GP, Stretton J, Sidhu MK, et al. Progressive white matter changes following anterior temporal lobe resection for epilepsy. Neuroimage Clin 2013;4:190–200.

207. Goradia D, Chugani HT, Govindan RM, et al. Reorganization of the right arcuate fasciculus following left arcuate fasciculus resection in children with intractable epilepsy. J Child Neurol 2011;26:1246–51.

208. Concha L, Gross DW, Wheatley BM, et al. Diffusion tensor imaging of time-dependent axonal and myelin degradation after corpus callosotomy in epilepsy patients. Neuroimage 2006;32:1090–9.

209. Concha L, Beaulieu C, Wheatley BM, et al. Bilateral white matter diffusion changes persist after epilepsy surgery. Epilepsia 2007;48:931–40.

210. Schoene-Bake JC, Faber J, Trautner P, et al. Widespread affections of large fiber tracts in postoperative temporal lobe epilepsy. Neuroimage 2009;46: 569–76.

211. Cho YW, Yi SD, Motamedi GK. Frontal lobe epilepsy may present as myoclonic seizures. Epilepsy Behav 2010;17:561–4.

212. Seifer G, Blenkmann A, Princich JP, et al. Noninvasive approach to focal cortical dysplasias: clinical, EEG, and neuroimaging features. Epilepsy Res Treat 2012;2012:736784.

213. Widjaja E, Geibprasert S, Otsubo H, et al. Diffusion tensor imaging assessment of the epileptogenic zone in children with localization-related epilepsy. AJNR Am J Neuroradiol 2011;32:1789–94.

214. Bhardwaj RD, Mahmoodabadi SZ, Otsubo H, et al. Diffusion tensor tractography detection of functional pathway for the spread of epileptiform activity between temporal lobe and Rolandic region. Childs Nerv Syst 2010;26:185–90.

215. Thivard L, Bouilleret V, Chassoux F, et al. Diffusion tensor imaging can localize the epileptogenic zone in nonlesional extra-temporal refractory epilepsies when [(18)F]FDG-PET is not contributive. Epilepsy Res 2011;97:170–82.

216. Govindan RM, Asano E, Juhasz C, et al. Surface-based laminar analysis of diffusion abnormalities in cortical and white matter layers in neocortical epilepsy. Epilepsia 2013;54:667–77.

217. Gross DW, Bastos A, Beaulieu C. Diffusion tensor imaging abnormalities in focal cortical dysplasia. Can J Neurol Sci 2005;32:477–82.

218. Diehl B, Tkach J, Piao Z, et al. Diffusion tensor imaging in patients with focal epilepsy due to cortical dysplasia in the temporo-occipital region: electro-clinico-pathological correlations. Epilepsy Res 2010;90:178–87.

219. Widjaja E, Zarei MS, Otsubo H, et al. Subcortical alterations in tissue microstructure adjacent to focal cortical dysplasia: detection at diffusion-tensor MR imaging by using magnetoencephalographic dipole cluster localization. Radiology 2009;251:206–15.

220. Ahmadi ME, Hagler DJ Jr, McDonald CR, et al. Side matters: diffusion tensor imaging tractography in left and right temporal lobe epilepsy. AJNR Am J Neuroradiol 2009;30:1740–7.

221. Concha L, Kim H, Bernasconi A, et al. Spatial patterns of water diffusion along white matter tracts in temporal lobe epilepsy. Neurology 2012;79:455–62.

222. Duning T, Kellinghaus C, Mohammadi S, et al. Individual white matter fractional anisotropy analysis on patients with MRI negative partial epilepsy. J Neurol Neurosurg Psychiatry 2010;81:136–9.

223. Kimiwada T, Juhasz C, Makki M, et al. Hippocampal and thalamic diffusion abnormalities in children with temporal lobe epilepsy. Epilepsia 2006;47:167–75.

224. Rodrigo S, Oppenheim C, Chassoux F, et al. Uncinate fasciculus fiber tracking in mesial temporal lobe epilepsy. Initial findings. Eur Radiol 2007;17:1663–8.

225. Salmenpera TM, Simister RJ, Bartlett P, et al. High-resolution diffusion tensor imaging of the hippocampus in temporal lobe epilepsy. Epilepsy Res 2006;71:102–6.

226. Lippe S, Poupon C, Cachia A, et al. White matter abnormalities revealed by DTI correlate with interictal grey matter FDG-PET metabolism in focal childhood epilepsies. Epileptic Disord 2012;14:404–13.

227. Focke NK, Yogarajah M, Symms MR, et al. Automated MR image classification in temporal lobe epilepsy. Neuroimage 2012;59:356–62.

228. Mueller SG, Young K, Hartig M, et al. A two-level multimodality imaging Bayesian network approach for classification of partial epilepsy: preliminary data. Neuroimage 2013;71:224–32.

229. Winston GP, Micallef C, Symms MR, et al. Advanced diffusion imaging sequences could aid assessing patients with focal cortical dysplasia and epilepsy. Epilepsy Res 2014;108(2):336–9.

230. Saporta AS, Kumar A, Govindan RM, et al. Arcuate fasciculus and speech in congenital bilateral perisylvian syndrome. Pediatr Neurol 2011;44:270–4.

231. Bernal B, Rey G, Dunoyer C, et al. Agenesis of the arcuate fasciculi in congenital bilateral perisylvian syndrome: a diffusion tensor imaging and tractography study. Arch Neurol 2010;67:501–5.

232. Widjaja E, Skocic J, Go C, et al. Abnormal white matter correlates with neuropsychological impairment in children with localization-related epilepsy. Epilepsia 2013;54:1065–73.

233. Diehl B, Piao Z, Tkach J, et al. Cortical stimulation for language mapping in focal epilepsy: correlations with tractography of the arcuate fasciculus. Epilepsia 2010;51:639–46.

234. Ellmore TM, Beauchamp MS, Breier JI, et al. Temporal lobe white matter asymmetry and language laterality in epilepsy patients. Neuroimage 2010;49:2033–44.

235. Diehl B, Busch RM, Duncan JS, et al. Abnormalities in diffusion tensor imaging of the uncinate fasciculus relate to reduced memory in temporal lobe epilepsy. Epilepsia 2008;49:1409–18.

236. McDonald CR, Ahmadi ME, Hagler DJ, et al. Diffusion tensor imaging correlates of memory and language impairments in temporal lobe epilepsy. Neurology 2008;71:1869–76.

237. Winston GP, Stretton J, Sidhu MK, et al. Structural correlates of impaired working memory in hippocampal sclerosis. Epilepsia 2013;54:1143–53.

238. Powell HW, Parker GJ, Alexander DC, et al. MR tractography predicts visual field defects following temporal lobe resection. Neurology 2005;65:596–9.

239. Chen X, Weigel D, Ganslandt O, et al. Prediction of visual field deficits by diffusion tensor imaging in temporal lobe epilepsy surgery. Neuroimage 2009;45:286–97.

240. Daga P, Winston G, Modat M, et al. Accurate localization of optic radiation during neurosurgery in an interventional MRI suite. IEEE Trans Med Imaging 2012;31:882–91.

241. Winston GP, Yogarajah M, Symms MR, et al. Diffusion tensor imaging tractography to visualize the relationship of the optic radiation to epileptogenic lesions prior to neurosurgery. Epilepsia 2011;52:1430–8.

242. Winston GP, Daga P, Stretton J, et al. Optic radiation tractography and vision in anterior temporal lobe resection. Ann Neurol 2012;71:334–41.

243. Yogarajah M, Focke NK, Bonelli S, et al. Defining Meyer's loop-temporal lobe resections, visual field deficits and diffusion tensor tractography. Brain 2009;132:1656–68.

244. Nilsson D, Starck G, Ljungberg M, et al. Intersubject variability in the anterior extent of the optic radiation assessed by tractography. Epilepsy Res 2007;77:11–6.

245. Govindan RM, Chugani HT, Makki MI, et al. Diffusion tensor imaging of brain plasticity after occipital lobectomy. Pediatr Neurol 2008;38:27–33.

246. Taoka T, Sakamoto M, Iwasaki S, et al. Diffusion tensor imaging in cases with visual field defect

after anterior temporal lobectomy. AJNR Am J Neuroradiol 2005;26:797–803.

247. Stefan H, Nimsky C, Scheler G, et al. Periventricular nodular heterotopia: a challenge for epilepsy surgery. Seizure 2007;16:81–6.

248. Rodionov R, Vollmar C, Nowell M, et al. Feasibility of multimodal 3D neuroimaging to guide implantation of intracranial EEG electrodes. Epilepsy Res 2013;107:91–100.

249. Gonzalez-Darder JM, Gonzalez-Lopez P, Talamantes F, et al. Multimodal navigation in the functional microsurgical resection of intrinsic brain tumors located in eloquent motor areas: role of tractography. Neurosurg Focus 2010;28:E5.

250. Holowka SA, Otsubo H, Iida K, et al. Three-dimensionally reconstructed magnetic source imaging and neuronavigation in pediatric epilepsy: technical note. Neurosurgery 2004;55: 1226.

251. Wurm G, Ringler H, Knogler F, et al. Evaluation of neuronavigation in lesional and non-lesional epilepsy surgery. Comput Aided Surg 2003;8:204–14.

252. Sommer B, Grummich P, Hamer H, et al. Frameless stereotactic functional neuronavigation combined with intraoperative magnetic resonance imaging as a strategy in highly eloquent located tumors causing epilepsy. Stereotact Funct Neurosurg 2013;92:59–67.

253. Ortler M, Trinka E, Dobesberger J, et al. Integration of multimodality imaging and surgical navigation in the management of patients with refractory epilepsy. A pilot study using a new minimally invasive reference and head-fixation system. Acta Neurochir (Wien) 2010;152:365–78.

Technical Considerations for Functional Magnetic Resonance Imaging Analysis

Chris J. Conklin, MS[a], Scott H. Faro, MD[b],
Feroze B. Mohamed, PhD[c],*

KEYWORDS

• fMRI • BOLD • Realignment • Normalization • Smoothing • Statistical inference

KEY POINTS

- Blood oxygenation level–dependent (BOLD) functional magnetic resonance imaging has gained clinical relevance in the past decade. However, acquiring BOLD data is straightforward, there are numerous considerations with regard to experimental design and analysis.
- Analysis has 2 distinct sections: preprocessing and postprocessing.
- The preprocessing steps relate to the spatial transformations and operations that ensure the data are properly aligned and in the same coordinate space.
- With the data properly rendered, postprocessing techniques are applied to infer statistically significant physiologic changes.
- As the field continues to evolve at a rapid pace and newer algorithms are developed it is inevitable that measurement and analysis of BOLD will improve in the years to come.

LEARNING OBJECTIVES

1. Discuss the preprocessing pipeline typically used in clinical blood oxygenation level–dependent (BOLD) functional magnetic resonance imaging (fMRI).
2. Highlight the importance of preprocessing BOLD fMRI data before statistical inference.
3. Discuss the significance of quality assurance of clinical BOLD fMRI data.
4. Understanding different statistical tests and algorithms to increase the confidence of fMRI results.

INTRODUCTION

fMRI has become ubiquitous in modern cognitive research and clinical imaging communities. Not only is fMRI being used by neuroscientists, psychologists, economists, marketers, and others to enhance clinicians' understanding of the brain, it has also progressed into several clinicians' protocols; for example, presurgical brain mappings of language and sensorimotor cortex. The statistical activation maps generated after analysis of functional data can help decrease patient morbidity while facilitating the neurosurgeon's surgical

[a] Department of Electrical Engineering and Radiology, Temple University Magnetic Resonance Imaging Center, Temple University, Philadelphia, PA 19140, USA; [b] Department of Radiology, Bioengineering and Electrical Engineering, Temple University Magnetic Resonance Imaging Center, Temple University, Philadelphia, PA 19140, USA; [c] Department of Radiology, Neuroscience, Bioengineering and Electrical Engineering, Temple University Magnetic Resonance Imaging Center, Temple University, Philadelphia, PA 19140, USA
* Corresponding author. Department of Radiology, Neuroscience, Bioengineering and Electrical Engineering, Temple University, 3401 N. Broad St, Philadelphia, PA 19140.
E-mail address: feroze@temple.edu

Neuroimag Clin N Am 24 (2014) 695–704
http://dx.doi.org/10.1016/j.nic.2014.07.005
1052-5149/14/$ – see front matter © 2014 Elsevier Inc. All rights reserved.

planning for tumor resection in an effort to improve patient outcome. Acquisition of BOLD fMRI data relies heavily on the T2* changes in blood oxygenation levels, as initially observed by Thulborn and colleagues[1] in test tube samples and later called BOLD by Ogawa and colleagues[2] through in-vivo demonstration with rats. Later it was Kwong and colleagues[3] who showed this effect in human brains. The BOLD effect can be summarized as follows: given the paramagnetic nature of deoxyhemoglobin it is possible to quantify the decrease in MR signal caused by a deficiency in oxygen. In essence, the susceptibility differences between deoxyhemoglobin and surrounding tissue lead to a rapid dephasing of regional spins, thereby decreasing the overall MR imaging signal. In contrast, an increase in oxyhemoglobin or decrease in deoxyhemoglobin leads to an increase in MR imaging signal. This process is the seminal principle involved with BOLD fMRI, and it can be detected using a fast susceptibility sensitivity MR imaging pulse sequence such as a gradient echo (GRE) echoplanar imaging sequence. However, the relative change in signal is only between 3% and 5% on scanners with a field strength of 1.5 T, which makes it difficult to distinguish between brain activation and noise (physiologic and scanner). The implication of this result necessitates the construction of higher field strength scanners (to increase signal) and the use of novel statistical techniques to parse out real signals of interest that represent signals that are different enough from background noise to be classified as significant.

This article focuses on the analysis of BOLD fMRI data. Once acquired, there are many preprocessing steps to temper the data in preparation for statistical testing. The processing procedure includes motion correction, coregistration of functional images to structural, segmentation, normalization to a standard space, and smoothing to increase signal/noise ratio (SNR) and decrease the number of multiple comparisons. The combination of all these steps yields a data set ready for statistical estimation and presentation of the maps of brain activations. **Fig. 1** shows an overall work flow chart describing the various steps involved in the BOLD image analysis. In the rest of the article these various steps are explained in detail.

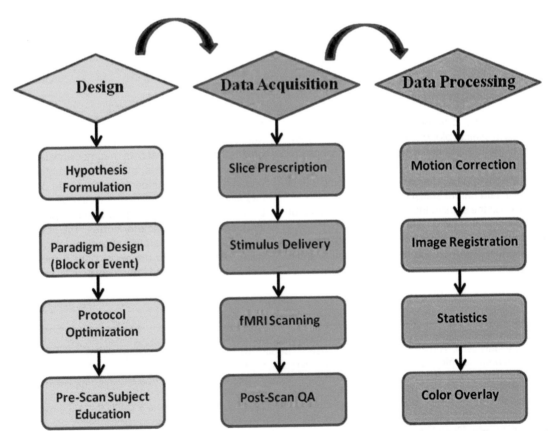

Fig. 1. Workflow pipeline outlining the key steps in the postprocessing of BOLD fMRI data. QA, quality assurance.

DATA ACQUISITION

fMRI data is typically acquired through the use of echo planar imaging (EPI) with a GRE excitation scheme. By using a single excitation pulse and rapidly cycling the frequency encoding gradient, an echo can be generated. Coupled with the blip-ped phase encoding gradient typical for EPI se-quences, fMRI data can be acquired very rapidly. Because GRE sequences are heavily $T2^*$ weighted, it is the logical choice for exploitation of the BOLD effect.

Of equal or potentially greater importance to GRE EPI acquisition schemes is the experimental paradigm design. Before data collection it is crit-ical to define the anticipated result explicitly. To design a study that is exploratory rather than hy-pothesis driven is to invite confusion and lack of confidence; the hypothesis ultimately dictates the statistical parameters used to threshold and display the results. For example, consider a study dealing with the cognitive requisites for decision making, which involves the executive function net-works. In such an experiment, clinicians would expect to see activation in the orbital frontal cortex (OFC). If the results show OFC activation after analysis, that provides an additional level of confi-dence because it coincides with the anticipated response. However, the hypothesis also influ-ences the choice of acquisition parameters. Continuing with the previous example, if activation in the OFC is expected certain parameters need to be altered. The OFC is a high-susceptibility region and it would be advantageous to reduce the echo time of the EPI acquisition to collect the signal before spin dephasing attenuates the local signal. The choice of hypothesis and acquisition protocol is study dependent and both are important to opti-mize the results of a BOLD fMRI study.

Optimization of the acquisition protocol is of paramount importance because of the inherent ar-tifacts associated with EPI sequences. Ghosting, chemical shift, and blurring from $T2^*$ decay are the primary sources for EPI image degradation. Using parallel imaging techniques and/or restrict-ing the k-space window by reducing the echo train length or interecho spacing can substantially miti-gate artifact generation. The acquisition field of view (FOV) prescription assignment can also be altered to avoid motion-related effects. In the past the FOV has been prescribed tangential to the plane connecting the anterior commissure and posterior commissure to help facilitate the ef-ficiency of image registration algorithms to routine T1-weighted or T2-weighted structural images. However, given the advances in algorithm design, more flexibility now exists. For example,

prescribing the FOV at a 20° to 30° tilt to avoid the orbit can prevent the wrapping of eye-related motion to the cerebellum and avoid high-susceptibility regions.

In terms of the functional paradigm design and optimization there are 2 primary modalities: block-related and event-related designs. Block designs are the clear choice from a clinical perspective because of the ease of development and simplicity of analysis. A block design is characterized by a periodic boxcar function (**Fig. 2**) that alternates between cycles of activity and rest. Given the repetitive nature of block-related designs, stronger signals can be obtained because of averaging of signals arising from similar trials during a block. Block designs are more forgiving in that the inherent averaging that occurs tends to have less impact when stimuli are missed. However, excessive repetition and/or trial duration can cause habituation. In contradis-tinction with the simplicity of block designs are event-related paradigms.

The event-related paradigms are popular among research-oriented groups because stron-ger correlations tend to exist. The implementation of event-related designs involves the delivery and presentation of stimuli at either specific or random time points. Although these designs are capable of parsing and isolating neural activity caused by a focused task, they are substantially more tedious to analyze and more sensitive to timing issues. Each paradigm design has its advantages and the choice is up to the end user based on the study/acquisition goal.

Another consideration when setting up func-tional protocols is the incorporation of a GRE acquisition to map field inhomogeneities. Field mappings can generate both phase and magni-tude images that can be used to correct or visu-alize distortions caused by susceptibility and inhomogeneous fields. An additional BOLD scan

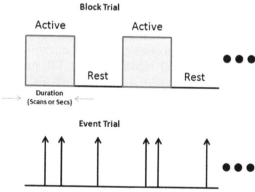

Fig. 2. Commonly used block-related (*top*) versus event-related (*bottom*) paradigms.

that is relevant in a clinical setting is to challenge the brain using breath holding, thereby causing a transient increase in blood carbon dioxide levels. This process induces vasodilation and a subsequent increase in cerebral blood flow, which can be used to map the cerebral vascular reserve. This scan can also be used for screening patients because these maps may also provide additional information regarding the neurovascular uncoupling in patients with brain tumors.

NEUROVASCULAR UNCOUPLING

The physiologic underpinning of BOLD functional imaging relates to cerebral blood flow (CBF). It has been shown that in response to stimulus an increase in CBF manifests locally to regions of neuronal activation.[4] Typical brain functioning relies on cerebrovascular autoregulation; the process by which normal blood flow is maintained despite dynamic physiologic stressors. This autoregulation modulates blood flow by varying vascular resistance, which is a function of the cerebrovascular reserve. If blood flow augmentation is altered because of a tumor, diseased/occluded vascular networks, or a steal phenomenon from an arteriovascular malformation, then neuronal activation is adversely affected. This outcome has the undesirable consequence of yielding false-negative results with the potential for gross underestimation of cortical activation. In a clinical setting this could be detrimental to neurosurgical patients because proper surgical planning is contingent on accurate localization of the eloquent cortex containing language and sensorimotor regions. Neurovascular uncoupling is highly prevalent for patients with low-grade gliomas and can provide a more comprehensive evaluation of presurgical mappings.[5]

BOLD DATA PREPROCESSING STEPS BEFORE STATISTICAL ANALYSIS

With an understanding of the physiologic basis for fMRI signal generation as well as optimized considerations for acquisition, the next step is to extract the BOLD signal from the T2* images. Although it is possible simply to begin statistical testing on the raw functional data, the results would lack confidence and statistical validity. Subject motion, time discrepancies between multislice acquisitions, misregistration of anatomic overlays, and low SNR are potential sources of significant error and require attention before the statistical analysis. These corrections are referred to as preprocessing steps and are essential to obtain reliable BOLD data. The various postprocessing

steps and methods currently used in BOLD imaging are discussed later.

DISTORTION CORRECTION

As mentioned earlier, it helps to acquire GRE field maps characterizing both the magnitude and phase information associated with local field inhomogeneities. This information can be used to review potential areas in the BOLD image that may be susceptible to inhomogeneities and potentially correct for signal attenuation as a result of susceptibility differences created by B_0 inhomogeneities if present in the acquired T2* images.

REALIGNMENT

The BOLD signal is analyzed at a voxel level and intrascan or interslice motion is detrimental to the accuracy of the generated results in fMRI because of the small signal changes that are of interest as a result of the BOLD effect. Although single-shot EPI sequences are less sensitive to motion given the rapid acquisition time for whole-brain coverage, subject motion of more than the smallest voxel dimension over time can significantly alter the interpreted results and decrease detection sensitivity. The hemodynamic response precipitating signal change is typically insignificant relative to perceived changes in signal caused by motion. Single-shot acquisition offers reasonable temporal resolution but typically has low spatial resolution. All of this mandates the implementation of realignment algorithms when analyzing functional MR data. As the names suggests, realignment is used to ensure that a slice of a chosen volume is aligned to each acquired volume during a specific trial, which is most commonly achieved by applying a rigid-body (6 parameter affine) transformation that minimizes the mean squared error between images.[6] For rigid-body registration the 6 parameters are in 2 classes: rotations and translations. Corrections need to be applied in the x, y, z directions, which are representative of subject-induced translations as well as rotations. **Fig. 3** shows a typical realignment plot that details any motion-related changes in head positioning. Realignment is classified as within-modality registration because all the data being mapped and transformed are within the same acquisition and therefore the same contrast mechanism.

Excessive subject motion can manifest as false-positive activation while also decreasing the sensitivity of statistical testing. The *t*-test that is typically used assesses BOLD signal changes relative to the residual variance, which is derived from differences between the data

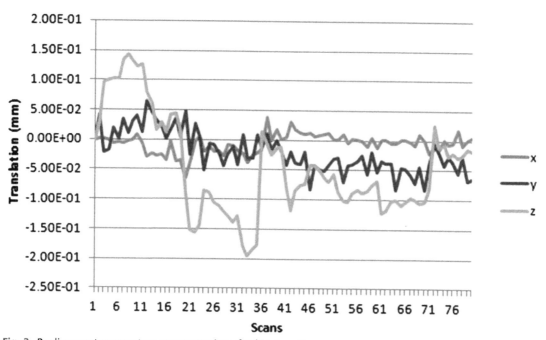

Fig. 3. Realignment parameters representative of subject motion.

and its fitted linear model.[6] As motion-related artifacts increase the residual variance, the sensitivity of the *t*-test is reduced. This process is discussed in greater detail later. With this in mind, investigation of the realignment parameters is an essential quality assurance (QA) step. Often overlooked during analysis, it behooves clinicians and researchers to be diligent about QA evaluation and documentation because potential problems and outliers can be found early in the data analysis without dealing with the uncertainty in interpreting results that are incongruent with the initial hypotheses. The transformation information used during the realignment stage to match the source to the reference images can be plotted and investigated with various software applications. This information can also be used as a potential regressor in the general linear model to supplement and enhance statistical testing. If the plot shows movement at a particular time point in excess of the smallest voxel dimension then care must be taken. Either the data set can be discarded or just the affected volume. If the latter option is chosen then artifact detection/removal techniques (ART) such as ART repair must be used to account for the loss of data.[7]

SLICE TIMING CORRECTION

Of particular importance in event-related paradigm designs is slice timing correction. EPI sequences are acquired slicewise and therefore the last slice is acquired 1 repetition time later than the first. This is particularly pronounced in interleaved acquisitions. In the event of using a single basis function to model the stimulus response with onset times relative to the first acquired slice, the last acquired slice is delayed by repetition time (TR) compared with the model, which has the adverse effect of yielding biased parameter estimates. Solutions to this problem include interpolation of the data to make the slices seem to have been acquired simultaneously or the use of a temporal basis set.[8] Timing corrections are also prevalent and important to consider in resting-state fMRI, which seeks to map and understand the default mode network.

COREGISTRATION

In contradistinction with the realignment step, in which registration is performed within a modality (same contrast), coregistration is the technique to map functional EPI volumes to a high-resolution anatomic reference scan (T1/T1-gadolinum/T2/fluid-attenuated inversion recovery). The choice of anatomic image is based on the pathology of the lesion. Additional refinement is needed because no linear relationship exists between the different signal intensities generated from the unique contrast mechanisms. This between-modality registration is critical from a clinical perspective because it allows the most accurate overlay of the functional activation map onto a high-resolution image. A secondary advantage to coregistration is a more accurate spatial normalization. It is intuitive that an image with more SNR and higher in-plane resolution can be normalized more accurately because voxels are easily discernible. Rather than minimizing the sum of squared error, coregistration seeks to maximize mutual information.

Similar to realignment, coregistration offers another opportunity for QA checking. It is important to qualitatively, and preferably quantitatively, assess the accuracy of the registration algorithm. By linking the newly registered functional volume to the structural volume it is possible to check well-defined and easily identifiable landmarks in the brain based on anatomy. It is recommended to check all 3 planes (axial, sagittal, coronal). If there is good visual anatomic correspondence between the linked images confidence is gained with the implementation of the algorithm. Having the most accurate activation overlay on a high-resolution, subject-specific image is paramount, especially in neurosurgical planning. This process can be further enhanced by segmentation models that use probability maps for tissue classification to further facilitate accurate correlation between images of different contrasts.

SEGMENTATION

There are many types of segmentation technique. Statistical parametric mapping (SPM) involves a unified segmentation model whereby tissue classification, image registration, and bias correction may all occur within the framework of the algorithm.[9] This approach uses a mixed gaussian model to probabilistically classify different tissue types (gray matter, white matter, cerebrospinal fluid) based on signal intensity. By first registering the source image to a standard template space, voxels with a high probability of belonging to a given tissue type can be assigned. An additional refinement relates to the modeling of intensity distributions and using tissue probability maps to appropriately weight tissue classification using conditional probability. A less sophisticated approach to segmentation is to warp the template image to match the image of interest. By overlaying the template image, in which different tissues and structures are already identified, onto the image to be segmented, automatic detection of the tissue classifications can be obtained.

A common artifact prevalent in MR images that affects segmentation is bias. Bias manifests as a smooth, spatially varying artifact that generates nonuniformity across image intensity. Many factors can create bias in an image, but magnetic field inhomogeneities possibly caused by improper shimming as well as nonuniformity in the radiofrequency coils tends to be the predominant cause.[10,11] To correct for said bias before segmentation and to help facilitate automatic classification, parametric techniques are used, as opposed to the classic nonparametric analysis of image histograms.[12–15] When using parametric techniques it is essential to specify how the bias interacts with noise. A variety of common approaches exist that involve scaling the signal with bias and noise, adding the noise before bias scaling, log transforming the data so that the multiplicative bias can be simply additive in log space, and parameterizing the bias as the exponential of the linear combination of low-frequency basis functions. The last technique uses a small number of basis functions to accurately model the smoothness of bias artifacts.[6]

NORMALIZATION

As noted earlier with regard to realignment and coregistration, normalization is a nonlinear registration technique. Although using rigid-body transformations is sufficient for mapping and transforming brains from an intrasubject perspective, it is ineffective for intersubject comparisons because standard rigid-body algorithms assume that brain shapes remain the same. This assumption fails when considering a larger sample size than a single individual. Because of this, normalization becomes of paramount importance when doing clinical trials or large research studies as results need to be extrapolated or generalized to a larger population. This technique is also one of the few ways to make comparisons between studies. If the same normalization template is used among research sites then regions of activations found at one site can be compared with results found at another. These comparisons are only possible if each subject is spatially normalized to a standard space so that conclusions for larger populations can be made. If necessary, in clinical cases this procedure is typically performed onto the patient's high-resolution structural data as an additional refinement.

Nonlinear registration can be classified into 2 distinct categories: label based and intensity based. Label-based methods seek homologous features between a reference and source image to generate a best-fit mapping from one image space to another. A classic example of this type of registration is manual identification of the line tangential to the anterior commissure and posterior commissure. Landmarking in this manner is subjective. In comparison, intensity-based techniques determine a transformation that is a function of voxel similarity, which is often achieved by maximizing correlations between images or minimizing the mean squared error. However, successful implementation is contingent on warping the reference images to the space of the source. Regardless of the methodology, objective functions are the metric used to quantify the quality of fit between images.[6]

SMOOTHING

With the functional data realigned and normalized, the final preprocessing step involves smoothing the images. Smoothing is an essential step because it effectively increases the SNR and spatial correlation and decreases the number of multiple comparisons needed during the statistical testing of the large BOLD data sets. As discussed later, random field theory is a branch of mathematics specifically created to deal with and analyze smoothed data sets. By blending similar intensity valued voxels the number of distinctly unique regions is reduced; therefore, when doing the t statistics, fewer comparisons need to be made and consequently a reduction in type I (false-positive) error results.

Smoothing occurs by averaging the signal intensities of neighboring voxels, which is achieved by convolving a gaussian kernel of predefined width with the image. Several schools of thoughts are prevalent as it pertains to the smoothing kernel size. The simplest choice is to make the full width half maximum (FWHM) of the kernel twice the imaging voxel size. Other techniques include sizing the FWHM to the expected width of the hemodynamic response or the expected width of the BOLD activation. These last two techniques require much a priori investigation to achieve the optimal kernel. Choosing the right size is essential because excessive smoothing can lead to a decrease in SNR and can also force smaller activation to extinction. Too little smoothing can merge distinct activations into a single region. **Fig. 4** shows the effect of smoothing. Note that because of the low pass nature of the smoothing kernel the edges and other fine details of the image are lost. Despite this, smoothing has the beneficial effect of increasing SNR and reducing the number of multiple comparisons, provided it is applied properly.

STATISTICAL TESTING

Once the imaging data have been rendered through the requisite preprocessing steps, the final step is to determine whether the observed signal

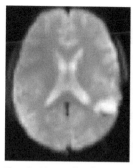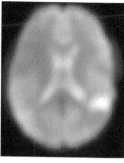

Fig. 4. Normalized EPI image of patient with a left temporal-parietal neoplasm shown against the smoothed image (*right*). Smoothing is done to reduce multiple comparisons while increasing SNR.

changes relative to some baseline condition are statistically significant. The results generated from the statistical testing provide both the qualitative and quantitative activation mappings that clinicians and researchers use to make claims about the functionality of the brain in response to certain stimuli. There are 2 traditional schools of thought for dealing with the statistical analysis of functional data. There are classical statistics, which involve the use of a general linear model (GLM) and t-testing with the corresponding P value and bayesian statistics. Cross-correlation methods can also be used and are seminal in connectivity studies.[16] Bayesian statistics infer that the activation effect is greater than some threshold with valid neurophysiologic underpinnings. In essence, bayesian statistics analyze the posterior probability of activation within each imaging voxel. Stated simply, classical inference calculates the probability of the activation given no effect, whereas bayesian inference determines the probability of seeing the activation given the effect. This notion of posterior probability through bayesian analysis is probably the more desirable of results.

From a classical perspective the GLM method for statistical inference is the most common. The end result of GLM definition and estimation is an SPM. These maps are spatially dependent statistical metrics containing relevant information regarding a given hypothesis. Although hypothesis testing can be done using a variety of techniques, SPMs can model comparisons ranging from t-tests to correlation coefficients to analysis of covariance. This flexibility and portability makes GLMs ideal for analysis of functional BOLD data as long as the experimental design matrix is manipulated to fit within the GLM framework.[17] Modeling the data appropriately is often the biggest challenge when calculating germane statistics. SPMs are typically treated as mass-univariate problems, meaning that the same model is applied to each voxel to garner the data of interest. The same holds true for statistical testing. The GLM has the following mathematical form:

$$Y = X\beta + \mathcal{E}$$

where Y is the data matrix containing the observed, or response variables (such as regional BOLD), X is the design matrix containing explanatory variables, β are the parameters to be estimated such that the explanatory variables explain the observed data set, and $\mathcal{E}$ is the error term. This equation is an example of a standard linear regression problem. As an example, assume that the observed data set contains the acquired functional data, specifically BOLD quantification at a voxel level. A simple block design is typically used for neuronal stimulus delivery, alternating between active (condition of interest) and rest. The design matrix would then consist of information that can be used to explain or model the observed effect. In this case active and rest conditions would be coded into the matrix such that the observed effect at a given scan or voxel corresponds with the appropriate condition. Other factors, such as confounds or realignment parameters, can also be inserted into the design matrix to account for other effects that may affect the observed results. The regression model is then solved, typically by implementation of ordinary least squares methods.

STATISTICAL INFERENCE

On completion of the statistical inference an important issue remains when interpreting the results; namely the difference between statistical significance and clinical relevance. Statistical significance is a measure of the likelihood that a difference does exist between 2 groups, samples, and so forth regardless of the type or size of difference. Statistical significance does not address the magnitude, or importance, of the observed difference. Clinical relevance centers on the importance of the difference and is a judgment by the clinician, but statistical significance is a necessary precondition for clinical relevance.

When establishing a method for the interpretation of results in a clinical setting the topic of thresholding must be addressed. It is still common practice to use a threshold based strictly on P values. Given that this relies solely on the null distribution, only false-positive rates are factored into the thresholding decision. For clinical work, it is often ideal to balance false-positives and false-negatives (because they are inversely related) and subsequently a more thorough understanding of the distribution of the subject/patient's data is required. Recent studies have shown the benefit of incorporating mixture models into the postprocessing framework. This model clusters the data (activations, deactivations, and so forth) and creates probability distributions to compare with the null conditions thus enabling detection of false-negative rates. Using this information the statistical threshold is adapted for each individual as each mixture model is fitted based on the quality of the acquired data.[18] This technique eliminates the subjectivity often associated with determining an appropriate threshold for display of the calculated statistical maps.[19] Another method for removing ambiguity and increasing reproducibility from the statistical interpretation is activation mapping as percentage of local excitation (AMPLE) normalization, which is achieved by normalizing each cluster of activation as a function of local peak signal amplitude.[20] More such methods are required for choosing the appropriate thresholds in BOLD analysis.

If more power is needed during the analysis, there are several methods to increase statistical confidence when dealing with the generated parametric maps. Masking is one such technique that allows the definition of a region of interest (ROI). By ignoring or nulling the statistical metrics of areas outside the defined region the number of multiple comparisons is further reduced, thereby reducing type I error propagation and increasing confidence. ROIs can be either user defined and developed or incorporated into the thresholding procedure from atlases. The use of masks also facilitates the confidence factor as it applies to acceptance or rejection of the underlying hypothesis. There is both a qualitative and quantitative element to the interpretation of functional data. Inspection of the activation mappings can yield qualitative visual confirmation of neuronal activity, an example of which is shown in **Fig. 5**. However, if a more quantitative approach is desired, as is typical for neurosurgical applications, there are other metrics that are being used: extent of activation, center of activation mass, and laterality index. The extent of activation is a distance measure from the tumor or lesion of interest, whereas the center of activation mass corresponds with the isocenter of a certain activation cluster. Laterality index is used to ascertain hemispherical dominance for specific tasks such as those related to motor or language.

In terms of attempting to control for false-positives, clinicians can compare the percentage of anticipated false-positives with the number of voxels found to be positive. This technique is

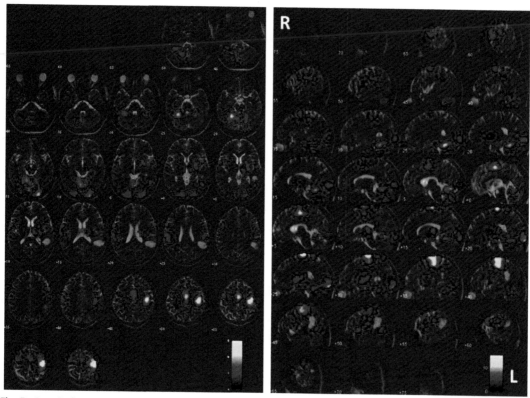

Fig. 5. A typical presentation of a right hand squeeze BOLD activation map overlaid on subject-specific anatomic acquisition in axial (*left*) and sagittal (*right*) planes.

called false discovery rate.[21,22] Another method examines the family of voxel statistics and the likelihood that familywise error came about by chance.[6] Both methods increase statistical confidence as the conditions for significance become more stringent.

SUMMARY

BOLD fMRI has gained significant relevance in the clinical realm over the past decade. However, although acquiring BOLD data is straightforward, numerous considerations need to be made with regard to experimental design and analysis. Hypotheses must be formulated, paradigms and protocols optimized, and analysis pipelines constructed. Analysis can be classified into 2 distinct sections: preprocessing and postprocessing. The preprocessing steps relate to the spatial transformations and operations that ensure the data are properly aligned and in the same coordinate space. Smoothing is also performed to reduce the number of multiple comparisons while increasing SNR. With the data properly rendered, postprocessing techniques are applied to infer statistically significant physiologic changes. These techniques may include

GLM estimation and testing, correlation coefficients, and adaptive thresholding on a voxelwise basis. Clinicians are then provided with an additional diagnostic tool to supplement functional testing. This article provides a proper framework to facilitate and guide these decisions. As the field continues to evolve at a rapid pace and newer algorithms are developed it is inevitable that measurement and analysis of BOLD will improve in the years to come.

REFERENCES

1. Thulborn KR, Waterton JC, Matthews PM, et al. Oxygenation dependence of the transverse relaxation time of water protons in whole blood at high field. Biochim Biophys Acta 1982;714:265–70.
2. Ogawa S, Lee TM, Kay AR, et al. Brain magnetic resonance imaging with contrast dependent on blood oxygenation. Proc Natl Acad Sci U S A 1990;87:9868–72.
3. Kwong KK, Belliveau JW, Chesler DA, et al. Dynamic magnetic resonance imaging of human brain activity during primary sensory stimulation. Proc Natl Acad Sci U S A 1992;89:5675–9.

4. Ye FQ, Yang Y, Duyn J, et al. Quantitation of regional cerebral blood flow increases during motor activation: a multislice, steady-state, arterial spin tagging study. Magn Reson Med 1999;42:404–7.

5. Pillai JJ, Zaca D. Clinical utility of cerebrovascular reactivity mapping in patients with low grade gliomas. World J Clin Oncol 2011;12:397–403.

6. Friston KJ, Ashburner JT, Kiebel SJ, et al. Statistical parametric mapping: the analysis of functional brain images. New York: Elsevier; 2007.

7. Mazaika PK, Whitfield-Gabrieli S, Reiss A, et al. Artifact repair of fMRI data from high motion clinical subjects (with new results from 3-D large motion correction). Annual meeting of the Organization for Human Brain Mapping. Chicago, 2007.

8. Henson RN, Buechel C, Josephs O, et al. The slice-timing problem in event-related fMRI. Neuroimage 1999;9:125.

9. Asburner J, Friston KJ. Unified segmentation. Neuroimage 2005;26:839–51.

10. Sled JG, Zijdenbos AP, Evans AC. A non-parametric method for automatic correction of intensity non-uniformity in MRI data. IEEE Trans Med Imaging 1998;17:87–97.

11. Belaroussi B, Milles J, Carme S, et al. Intensity non-uniformity correction in MRI: existing methods and their validation. Med Image Anal 2006;10:234–46.

12. Pham DL, Prince JL. Adaptive fuzzy segmentation of magnetic resonance images. IEEE Trans Med Imaging 1999;18:737–52.

13. Shattuck DW, Sandor-Leahy SR, Schaper KA, et al. Magnetic resonance image tissue classification using a partial volume model. Neuroimage 2001; 13:856–76.

14. Wells WM III, Viola P, Atsumi H, et al. Multi-modal volume registration by maximization of mutual information. Med Image Anal 1996;1:35–51.

15. Styner M. Parametric estimate of intensity inhomogeneities applied to MRI. IEEE Trans Med Imaging 2000;19:153–65.

16. Hyde JS, Jesmanowicz A. Cross-correlation: an fMRI signal-processing strategy. Neuroimage 2012; 15:848–51.

17. Friston KJ, Holmes AP, Worsley KJ, et al. Statistical parametric maps in functional imaging: a general linear approach. Hum Brain Mapp 1995;2:189–210.

18. Woolrich MW, Behrens TE, Beckmann CF, et al. Mixture models with adaptive spatial regularization for segmentation with an application to fMRI data. IEEE Trans Med Imaging 2005;24:1–11.

19. Gorgolewski KJ, Storkey AJ, Bastin ME, et al. Adaptive thresholding for reliable topological inference in single subject fMRI analysis. Front Hum Neurosci 2012;6:245.

20. Voyvodic JT. Reproducibility of single-shot fMRI language mapping with AMPLE normalization. J Magn Reson Imaging 2012;36:569–80.

21. Benjamini Y, Hochberg Y. Controlling the false discovery rate: a practical and powerful approach to multiple testing. J R Stat Soc Series B Stat Methodol 1995;57:289–300.

22. Genovese CR, Lazar NA, Nichols TE. Thresholding of statistical maps in functional neuroimaging using the false discovery rate. Neuroimage 2002;15:772–86.

Special Considerations/ Technical Limitations of Blood-Oxygen-Level-Dependent Functional Magnetic Resonance Imaging

Domenico Zacà, PhD[a,b], Shruti Agarwal, PhD[b], Sachin K. Gujar, MBBS[b], Haris I. Sair, MD[b], Jay J. Pillai, MD[b,*]

KEYWORDS

- Blood-oxygen-level-dependent • Functional magnetic resonance imaging • Special considerations
- Technical limitations

KEY POINTS

- Blood-oxygen-level-dependent (BOLD) functional magnetic resonance imaging (fMRI) has the potential to become a more universal standard of care in presurgical planning for localization of eloquent cortex at risk during surgical resection.
- BOLD imaging is affected by a series of technical issues limiting the widespread clinical use of BOLD fMRI.
- Extensive and standardized quality control tools need to be established for appropriate interpretation of both clinical and research fMRI studies.
- Newly developed methods can overcome current BOLD imaging issues and enhance future research and clinical application of BOLD fMRI.

INTRODUCTION

Over the last 20 years, blood-oxygen-level-dependent (BOLD) functional magnetic resonance imaging (fMRI) has been effectively used for clinical presurgical mapping.[1,2] However, there are important technical limitations and special considerations that one must be aware of to avoid pitfalls in both clinical and research applications of BOLD fMRI.

IMAGE ACQUISITION
Susceptibility Artifacts

Most clinical and research fMRI studies are performed by using a two-dimensional T2*-weighted gradient recalled echo (GRE) sequence with echo planar imaging (EPI) readout.[3] The rationale behind this choice is the high sensitivity of this pulse sequence to BOLD-related susceptibility changes and its ability to scan the whole brain with adequate spatial (2–3 mm) and temporal (2–3 seconds) resolution to monitor brain activation over time.[4] However, T2* GRE EPI shows high sensitivity as well to intravoxel dephasing caused by macroscopic magnetic field gradients generated by the difference in magnetic susceptibility of multiple tissues contained in 1 voxel.[5] The different magnetic fields experienced by the spins make them precess at different frequencies and,

[a] Center for Mind/Brain Sciences, University of Trento, Via delle Regole 101, Mattarello (TN) 38121, Italy; [b] Division of Neuroradiology, Russell H. Morgan Department of Radiology and Radiological Science, The Johns Hopkins Hospital, Johns Hopkins University School of Medicine, 1800 Orleans Street, Baltimore, MD 21287, USA
* Corresponding author.
E-mail address: jpillai1@jhmi.edu

Neuroimag Clin N Am 24 (2014) 705–715
http://dx.doi.org/10.1016/j.nic.2014.07.006
1052-5149/14/$ – see front matter © 2014 Elsevier Inc. All rights reserved.

over time, dephasing leads to signal loss. This effect is strong and results in signal loss in regions of the brain characterized by strong susceptibility differences at the junctions between air and tissues such as the orbitofrontal cortex (from the paranasal sinuses) or the medial temporal and the inferior temporal lobes (from the petrous apices and mastoid air complexes),[6] as shown in **Fig. 1**. These regions are important in visual and cognitive processing, including language and memory function.[7–9] The effect of this signal loss is a reduced sensitivity to brain activation in these regions, which may not be recognized when the statistical maps are overlaid on less distorted high-resolution T1-weighted anatomic images. Such susceptibility-related signal loss may result in regional false-negative activation on BOLD presurgical mapping studies. The amount of signal loss has been shown to be dependent on the image orientation, echo time (TE), and spatial resolution.[10] Because the magnetic field gradients are generated along the slice selection, phase encoding, and readout directions, in-plane dispersion is experienced as well as through-plane dispersion of the voxel magnetization.[11] Spatial resolution also counts, because the larger the voxel size,

the larger the difference in Larmor frequencies among the spins contained in the voxel and, in turn, the faster the signal dispersion.[12] Reducing voxel size reduces the effects of susceptibility artifacts but at the cost of temporal resolution or reduced brain coverage. The spin dephasing increases along time; therefore, the strength of signal loss depends also on the TE.[13] In principle, one could reduce the TE, but this is at the expense of reducing BOLD sensitivity in other regions of the brain less affected by susceptibility artifacts. In current clinical studies, a tradeoff between spatial/temporal resolution and BOLD sensitivity needs to be achieved.

In clinical functional imaging, additional potential sources of susceptibility artifacts include vascular clips, stent grafts, or craniotomy hardware related to previous surgery. These devices can induce strong macroscopic field gradients and generate dramatic signal loss, as shown in **Fig. 2** for a patient who underwent presurgical

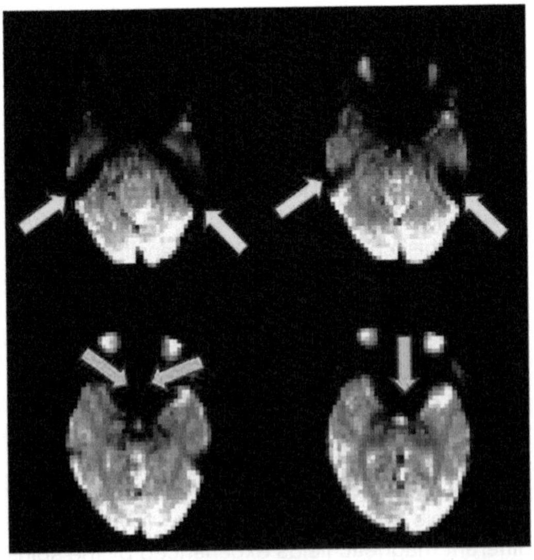

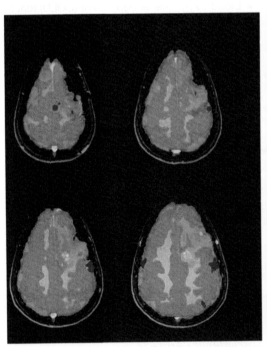

Fig. 2. Susceptibility artifact related to a left fronto-parietal craniotomy that obscures activation in the dorsolateral prefrontal cortex/middle frontal gyrus on a silent word-generation verbal fluency task. Notice that the BH CVR map that has been overlaid on the raw EPI image shows loss of regional vascular reactivity, but this is caused by surgical hardware–related susceptibility artifact rather than neurovascular uncoupling (NVU). Note also that the degree of susceptibility-related anatomic distortion is greater on the EPI images than on the underlay of postcontrast T1 three-dimensional magnetization prepared rapid acquisition gradient echo images.

Fig. 1. Example of areas commonly affected by susceptibility artifacts in single-shot T2*-weighted EPI images (repetition time/echo time = 2000/30 milliseconds) acquired in a 37-year-old patient with grade II fibrillary astrocytoma referred for fMRI presurgical mapping at our institution. (*Top row*) Right and left inferior temporal lobes (*yellow arrows*) obscured by artifact from the petrous apices; (*bottom row*) susceptibility artifact from the sphenoid sinus, which may affect visualization of orbitofrontal activation (*orange arrows*).

mapping after previous surgery.[14] Furthermore, tumor-related or surgery-related hemorrhages can also cause susceptibility artifacts.[15] Adequate presurgical mapping may still be possible in most of these cases, as reported by Peck and colleagues.[16] However, statistically significant decreased volume of motor activation in the tumor hemisphere was reported in their group of patients with previous surgery compared with another group of patients who had no previous surgery. The investigators explained this difference in volume of activation as a consequence of the loss of BOLD signal and sensitivity to neural activation caused by the artifacts as a result of previous surgery. It is therefore advisable as a general quality control step in clinical functional imaging studies to visually inspect the raw EPI images to assess areas potentially affected by susceptibility artifacts, which may be areas prone to false-negative activation.

Susceptibility artifacts represent one of the major limitations of BOLD functional imaging performed using T2* EPI sequences. In the past, other sequences, such as spin echo EPI or fast low-angle shot or T1-weighted sequences have been explored to overcome this problem.[17–19] However, they have been plagued by reduced sensitivity to neural activation, inadequate temporal resolution, or the need for exogenous contrast media. Multiple variants of the T2*-weighted BOLD sequences have been proposed in the last few years that attempt to reduce susceptibility artifacts and maintain sensitivity throughout the brain. From a clinical functional imaging standpoint, multiecho EPI and slice-dependent TE sequences with parallel imaging acquisition are promising.[6,20] With the increasing availability of multichannel coils at high field (3 T), they can be easily implemented on clinical scanners, because they are slightly modified versions of the standard product GRE sequences. In addition, postprocessing requires only minor changes from standard streamlined processing pipelines.

Geometric Distortions

EPI sequences provide the great advantage of acquiring an entire image in a fraction of a second. It is mainly for this reason that they have been the chosen sequences for most research and clinical brain functional imaging studies.[21] One of the main drawbacks for these sequences is the high sensitivity of EPI to geometric distortions, which manifest as mislocalization of the signal in the phase encoding direction and signal intensity loss.[22] The most prominent source of distortion

for EPI sequences is the effect of magnetic field inhomogeneities.[23] The low bandwidth in the phase encoding direction (~20 Hz/pixel) compared with the larger bandwidth in the readout direction (>1000 Hz/pixel) makes EPI signal sensitive to small variations of the main magnetic field. A field inhomogeneity of 100 HZ can then lead to a 5-pixel displacement (~15 mm in a typical fMRI experiment with 3-mm voxel size). Regions of the brain close to air–soft tissue interfaces, such as the paranasal sinuses, are the most prone to distortions because of strong magnetic susceptibility variation.[24] A minor source of distortions is the imperfect linearity of the gradient waveforms.[25] The most critical consequence of geometric distortions is the suboptimal coregistration of the fMRI data with the structural images acquired in the same session, especially if simple rigid body or even affine algorithms are used, as shown in **Fig. 3**.[26] When activation maps are overlaid on structural images, the localization of neuronal activation can be inaccurate in some areas of the brain, if proper algorithms with local linear and nonlinear warping are not used for coregistration. Two strategies are commonly used to reduce and correct for image distortions: one consists of acquiring field maps by using a gradient echo sequence with 2 echoes. The field value is calculated voxelwise by the difference in phase between 2 gradient echo images acquired at the 2 different echoes. The local field variation can then be used to estimate the amount of shift to

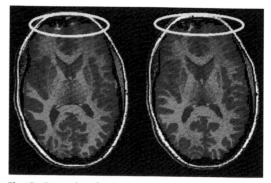

Fig. 3. Example of suboptimal coregistration caused by magnetic field distortion in 25-year-old healthy individual participating in a control language mapping study. The variations of the main magnetic field in the inferior frontal cortex (areas within the *yellow circle*) cause distortion of the BOLD signal, preventing accurate overlap between the functional and the structural data, even when a 12° of freedom affine registration algorithm was applied. (*Data from* Zacà D, Jarso S, Pillai JJ. Role of semantic paradigms for optimization of language mapping in clinical FMRI studies. AJNR Am J Neuroradiol 2013;34(10):1966–71.)

apply to each pixel to correct for distortion.[27] As shown in **Fig. 4**, the correction of geometric distortion results in more accurate coregistration with the structural images and consequently, more accurate activation localization. The point spread function (PSF) is another popular technique to correct geometric distortions. It uses acquisitions with additional phase encoding gradients applied in the x, y, or z directions to map the one-dimensional, two-dimensional, or three-dimensional PSF of each voxel.[28] These PSFs encode the spatial information about the distortion and the overall distribution of intensities from a single voxel. The measured image is the convolution of the undistorted density and the PSF. Measuring the PSF allows the distortion in geometry and intensity to be corrected. Both these techniques require additional scan time and processing time, and, for this reason, they are not routinely applied in presurgical clinical functional imaging examinations.[29] For this reason, a manual coregistration approach has been suggested by Nennig and colleagues[30] in their proposed pipeline for standardized clinical fMRI data processing. This approach has been shown to provide reliable results but is still operator dependent and requires dedicated personnel. In current and future generations of clinical scanners with the increasing availability of multiple channel coils (16–32 channels), parallel imaging can play a crucial role as a tool for reduction of geometric distortions.[31] Reducing by half or more the number of acquired k-space lines reduces the rate of k-space transversal that is proportional to the magnitude of susceptibility-induced distortions.[32]

IMAGE ANALYSIS AND INTERPRETATION: FALSE-POSITIVE AND FALSE-NEGATIVE ACTIVATION
Venous Effects

Brain mapping with BOLD fMRI detects transient changes in blood flow, blood volume, and blood oxygenation after the onset of neuronal activation.[33] Although the whole brain coverage and noninvasive nature of BOLD fMRI are advantages, the associated hemodynamic changes can propagate from the capillary beds adjacent to the site of neuronal activation downstream into large draining veins far from the areas of activated neurons, resulting in uncertainty of localization of neural activity by BOLD fMRI.[34,35] The BOLD contrast arises from a complex interplay between cerebral blood flow, cerebral blood volume, and cerebral metabolic rate of oxygen consumption on a spatial scale that lumps together hundreds of thousands of neurons in each MR imaging voxel. For this reason, the BOLD baseline signal and its increase on neuronal activity have been shown to be highly dependent on the characteristics of the local vasculature.[36,37] At 1.5 T and 3 T, BOLD activation is predominantly located in veins and venules in spatial proximity to activated neurons, and since the earliest days of BOLD fMRI, it became clear that the strongest BOLD signal change was generated in draining veins.[38,39] BOLD activation maps then lack spatial specificity because of these so-called venous effects. Venous effects increase the probability of type I error (false-positive or spurious activation), particularly in areas of high vascular density or in close spatial proximity to large draining veins, such as the sagittal sinus and adjacent cortical veins (**Fig. 5**). Likewise, the attempt to improve spatial specificity by increasing the statistical threshold may increase the chance of type II error (false-negatives), because the weaker parenchyma signal may wash out. Multiple solutions have been suggested in the literature to reduce or suppress the venous BOLD signal. Some methods attempt to discriminate the venous signal by exploiting the differences between BOLD percentage signal change and response latency between voxels with low and high vascular density.[40] Other methods use venous vascular masks generated from different sequences, such as susceptibility weighted imaging to remove BOLD venous signal.[41] With the introduction of ultrahigh field magnets (≥7 T fields), activation

Fig. 4. Coregistration of structural (*red contours*) and functional images before and after the application of a distortion correction technique based on field mapping for EPI images acquired on a 4-T scanner. Note how the misalignment of ventricles and brain edges (*yellow arrows*) was substantially reduced when registration was performed on FM corrected EPI images. (*Courtesy of* Dr Jorge Jovicich, Center for Mind/Brain Sciences, University of Trento, Italy.)

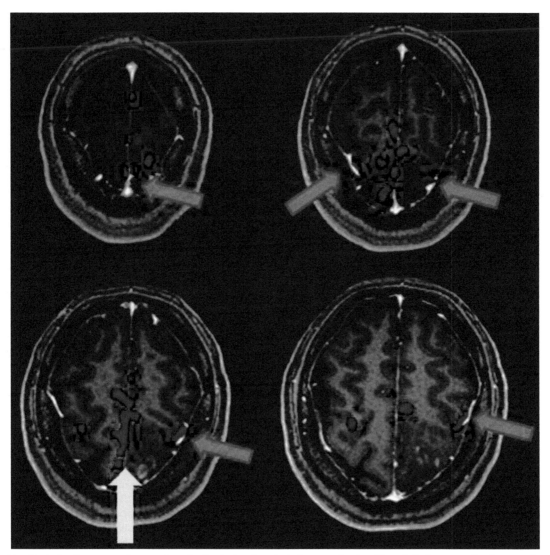

Fig. 5. Activation map from a toe flexion/extension task in a patient with a left frontoparietal convexity intermediate-grade glioma referred for presurgical mapping at our institution. The significant BOLD signal change along the superior sagittal sinus and superior convexity cortical veins (*blue arrows*) represents false-positive activation, whereas the more medial activation depicted by the yellow arrow represents true positive activation in the foot representation area of the primary motor cortex.

maps are expected to be less affected by the venous effect. Multiple studies suggest an improvement not only in sensitivity but also in specificity for BOLD signal at 7 T and higher field, because the increase of BOLD signal change in the parenchyma is predicted to be higher in microvasculature than macrovasculature, because the BOLD contrast is proportional to B0 for large vessels and proportional to $B0^2$ for small vessels and capillaries.[18,42] However, in a recent study aimed to quantitatively compare BOLD activation at 3 and 7 T,[43] a statistically significant higher increase of specificity compared with sensitivity was not found.

Physiologic Noise and Motion

Physiologic noise and head motion are 2 sources of subject-dependent artifacts that contribute to the BOLD signal and potentially affect the sensitivity and specificity of fMRI in detecting sensorimotor, visual, and cognitive activation. All fMRI studies are potentially affected by this kind of artifact, which generally affects studies involving aging and patient groups more than those involving young or healthy control groups.[44,45] Estimating and removing physiologic noise and head motion in fMRI data preprocessing are critical. The increase in BOLD signal associated with neuronal activation is only approximately 2% to 5%.[46] Thus, BOLD signal is sensitive to any sources of artifact. This issue becomes even more important in resting state BOLD signal analysis, in which there is no stimulus paradigm, and functional networks are detected by investigating the correlation of subtly fluctuating signals throughout the whole brain.[47] Physiologic noise comes from the metabolic and other fluctuations associated with cardiac and respiratory activity. Techniques for physiologic noise correction are applied prospectively during the data acquisition through gating and synchronization techniques or retrospectively while preprocessing fMRI data.[48–50] The retrospective techniques correct for physiologic noise by determining patterns of the BOLD signal related to physiologic fluctuations and removing them from the signal itself as regressors of no interest.[50,51] These regressors can be determined by the phase of respiration or cardiac cycle during each acquisition reconstructed by continuously measuring the chest motion and the end-tidal pressure in the individual undergoing the scan. Some groups have suggested also to add as regressors the variations in heart beat and respiration, because they have been shown to be significantly correlated with fMRI signal changes in task activation and resting state analysis in gray matter and near large vessels.[52] When it is not possible to directly monitor the individual's physiologic parameters, the regressors of no interest can still be generated by calculating the average time series in regions of interest (such as the white matter or cerebrospinal fluid), in which the BOLD signal fluctuations are not expected to have a neuronal origin.[53] A major limitation of measuring and removing physiologic noise from the BOLD signal is that cardiac and respiratory fluctuations occur at a frequency that is not adequately sampled by the fMRI data acquisition rate (circa 0.5 Hz). These fluctuations are aliased into the frequency of the BOLD signal, and if there are physiologic fluctuation frequencies overlapping with frequency of BOLD activation, then removing the physiologic noise also decreases the BOLD signal.[54,55] For this reason, multiple studies have also investigated the effectiveness of decomposition techniques such as principal component analysis and independent component analysis in separating signal from noise sharing the same frequency bands.[56,57] Physiologic noise correction has been shown to improve fMRI signal detection; however, there is no clear consensus regarding which technique is optimal for removal of this nonneuronal-related source of variance.[50] However, because most of the commercial scanners are equipped with devices for recording of chest wall movements related to respiration and end-tidal pressure, retrospective correction algorithms for physiologic noise could be implemented in a streamlined processing pipeline suitable for clinical fMRI examinations.

Head motion is a critical issue for any MR imaging study, because it limits accurate localization and introduces artifacts in the reconstructed images.[58] A peculiarity of head motion in BOLD fMRI is that it can decrease the signal detection power, because it can induce BOLD signal changes not related to neuronal activation or decrease the BOLD contrast in eloquent areas elicited by the performed tasks. Likewise, resting state fMRI data also can be motion degraded. Head motion correction in fMRI data preprocessing is usually performed by aligning the multiple acquired EPI volumes through a rigid body registration algorithm and by removing from the signal as regressors of no interest the motion parameters for translation and rotation estimated by the rigid body registration algorithm. The first approach is usually sufficient to improve signal detection for block design studies using univariate statistical analysis to detect strong and spatially localized functional activation.[59,60] On the other hand, the regression of motion parameters has become routinely used for analyses of weaker BOLD signals and correlation analysis performed with multivariate statistical technique,[61,62] and it has also been shown to be an important denoising step in instances of task-correlated motion.[63,64] Head motion has been identified as one of the earliest sources of spurious variance of fMRI signal.[65] Motion correction has become a routinely applied preprocessing step in fMRI data analysis, and multiple studies have reported the importance of standard motion correction.[66,67] However, studies have reported that rigid body motion correction algorithms can introduce artifacts, especially with minimal subject movement,[68,69] and some investigators choose to not perform it in such cases.[70] Overall, detection and correction for head motion are among the most important quality control analysis steps in both research and clinical fMRI studies, because motion-corrupted data can lead to incorrect inferences in research analyses and nondiagnostic data in patients. **Fig. 6** gives an example of prominent motion artifact in a patient with a left periorolandic low-grade glioma. To this regard, it is advisable to routinely use fast and reliable real-time fMRI analysis software packages in addition to patient monitoring tools to assess whether or not the ongoing acquired fMRI data are motion corrupted.[71]

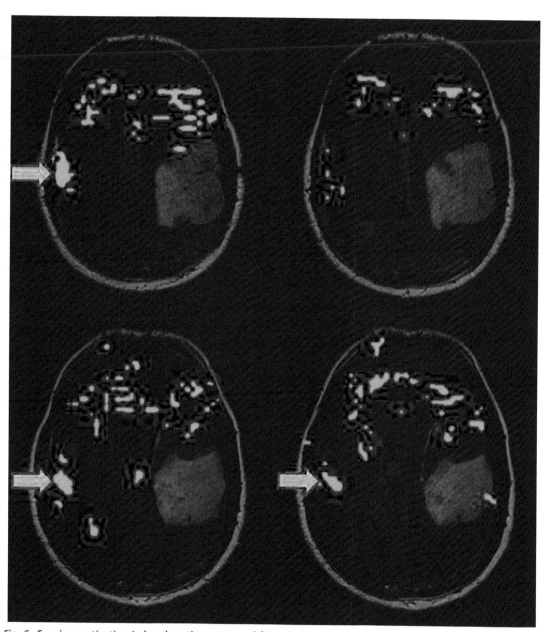

Fig. 6. Spurious activation in head motion corrupted fMRI dataset. On this vertical tongue movement task, note that in addition to expected activation in the face representation area of the right primary motor cortex, excessive false-positive activation is seen throughout the anterior frontal lobes as well as in the extracranial structures, including the right frontal sinus and calvarial diploic space with a typical arclike configuration. The gold arrows depict the expected motor cortical activation, whereas the rest of the activation represents motion-related artifact.

Neurovascular Uncoupling

Another potential pitfall in clinical BOLD fMRI is the issue of neurovascular decoupling or neurovascular uncoupling (NVU). Although in normal volunteers, NVU is not a concern, because normal hemodynamics are encountered in these individuals, in patients with structural brain lesions such as brain tumors or arteriovenous malformations, in whom regional hemodynamics are abnormally altered, this can be a major cause of potential false-negative activation. The normal neurovascular coupling cascade involves many steps from initial neuronal firing to neurotransmitter release at synapses to chemical mediator release from both interneurons and astrocytes to final arteriolar smooth muscle contraction or relaxation, resulting in vasoconstriction or vasodilatation, respectively.[72,73] When any step in this neurovascular coupling cascade is impaired, it results in abnormally decreased or even absent BOLD response. Such false-negative activation within electrically active eloquent cortex can be a major problem for interpretation and usefulness of clinical fMRI, because it may result in inadvertent resection of eloquent cortex and resultant permanent postoperative neurologic deficits.

There are different methods for detection of NVU, such as T2* dynamic susceptibility contrast perfusion MR imaging, breath-hold cerebrovascular reactivity mapping (BH CVR), cerebrovascular reactivity mapping using exogenous carbon dioxide administration or administration of acetazolamide for assessment of cerebrovascular reserve. Some of these approaches, such as exogenous CO_2 administration, may be difficult to use in a standard clinical setting with neurologically debilitated patients, and others (such as

acetazolamide challenges) interfere with BOLD fMRI that is performed during the same scan session or is more invasive. BH CVR mapping, on the other hand, is a and safe and well-tolerated approach that is simple to implement and that can be performed by almost all patients, in our experience, and also has been documented to be an effective method of NVU detection.[74] Furthermore, although MR perfusion imaging may be able to detect NVU potential by detecting angiogenesis in high-grade brain tumors, we have shown this to be less effective overall than BH CVR mapping in detecting NVU across all grades of primary gliomas.[75] **Fig. 7** gives an example of a BH CVR map showing abnormally decreased CVR in a patient with a left perirolandic low-grade glioma; this area of regionally decreased CVR corresponds to an area of abnormally decreased sensorimotor activation adjacent to the tumor.

In cases in which NVU is suspected based on results of BH CVR mapping or other methods, complementary electrophysiologic methods (ie,

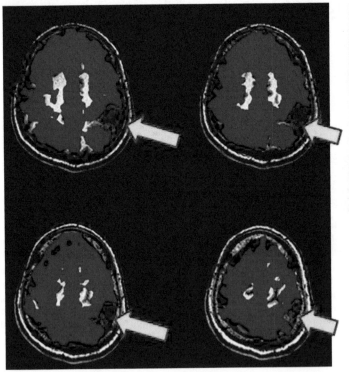
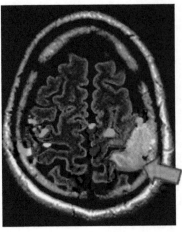

Fig. 7. BOLD BH CVR map shows regional loss of normal CVR (*yellow arrows*) in the cortex along the lateral margin of a left perirolandic glioma, which corresponds to absent left primary somatosensory cortical (PSC) activation (*blue arrow*) on a corresponding BOLD activation map obtained during performance of multiple individually color-coded hand (*cyan, green, yellow* and *red*) and foot (*magenta*) motor tasks. Note the presence of expected ipsilesional primary motor cortical (PMC) activation just anterior to the infiltrative expansile left postcentral gyral mass, as well as the presence of both contralesional PMC and PSC activation on the right. This is an example of NVU, because the patient did not show any sensory or motor deficit, and thus this represents false-negative activation in expected eloquent cortex.

intraoperative cortical stimulation mapping) should be performed in addition to presurgical BOLD fMRI to correctly identify eloquent cortex in the vicinity of brain lesions and thus avoid inadvertent resection of BOLD-silent but electrically active essential functional cortex. This same problem applies to research applications of BOLD fMRI involving patients with focal brain lesions, such as tumors, stroke, or arteriovenous malformation, or in patients with cerebrovascular disease in whom cerebrovascular reserve may be compromised. In general, NVU is an underrecognized problem with BOLD fMRI, and CVR mapping, either using BH techniques or exogenous CO_2 administration, may be an effective method of coping with this potential pitfall. It is important that those who use fMRI for clinical or research purposes are aware of this limitation.

SUMMARY

In this review, a list of limitations affecting the results of presurgical mapping with BOLD fMRI are discussed. There is a great need to standardize fMRI acquisition and analysis methods and establish guidelines to effectively address many of the quality control issues described in this article. Several national and international organizations are formulating such guidelines and standards for both clinical and research applications of BOLD fMRI. In the near future, consensus regarding management of these issues will likely both improve the clinical standard of care and enhance future research applications of fMRI.

REFERENCES

1. Pillai JJ. The evolution of clinical functional imaging during the past 2 decades and its current impact on neurosurgical planning. AJNR Am J Neuroradiol 2010;31(2):219–25.
2. Petrella JR, Shah LM, Harris KM, et al. Preoperative functional MR imaging localization of language and motor areas: effect on therapeutic decision making in patients with potentially resectable brain tumors. Radiology 2006;240(3):793–802.
3. Norris DG. Principles of magnetic resonance assessment of brain function. J Magn Reson Imaging 2006;23(6):794–807.
4. Turner R, Howseman A, Rees GE, et al. Functional magnetic resonance imaging of the human brain: data acquisition and analysis. Exp Brain Res 1998;123(1–2):5–12.
5. Czervionke LF, Daniels DL, Wehrli FW, et al. Magnetic susceptibility artifacts in gradient-recalled echo MR imaging. AJNR Am J Neuroradiol 1988; 9(6):1149–55.
6. Domsch S, Linke J, Heiler PM, et al. Increased BOLD sensitivity in the orbitofrontal cortex using slice-dependent echo times at 3 T. Magn Reson Imaging 2013;31(2):201–11.
7. Luders H, Lesser RP, Hahn J, et al. Basal temporal language area. Brain 1991;114(Pt 2):743–54.
8. Nobre AC, Allison T, McCarthy G. Word recognition in the human inferior temporal lobe. Nature 1994; 372(6503):260–3.
9. Haxby JV, Horwitz B, Ungerleider LG, et al. The functional organization of human extrastriate cortex: a PET-rCBF study of selective attention to faces and locations. J Neurosci 1994;14(11 Pt 1):6336–53.
10. Ojemann JG, Akbudak E, Snyder AZ, et al. Anatomic localization and quantitative analysis of gradient refocused echo-planar fMRI susceptibility artifacts. Neuroimage 1997;6(3):156–67.
11. Olman CA, Davachi L, Inati S. Distortion and signal loss in medial temporal lobe. PLoS One 2009; 4(12):e8160.
12. Gesierich B, Jovicich J, Riello M, et al. Distinct neural substrates for semantic knowledge and naming in the temporoparietal network. Cereb Cortex 2012; 22(10):2217–26.
13. Gorno-Tempini ML, Hutton C, Josephs O, et al. Echo time dependence of BOLD contrast and susceptibility artifacts. Neuroimage 2002;15(1): 136–42.
14. Belyaev AS, Peck KK, Brennan NM, et al. Clinical applications of functional MR imaging. Magn Reson Imaging Clin N Am 2013;21(2):269–78.
15. Kim MJ, Holodny AI, Hou BL, et al. The effect of prior surgery on blood oxygen level-dependent functional MR imaging in the preoperative assessment of brain tumors. AJNR Am J Neuroradiol 2005;26(8):1980–5.
16. Peck KK, Bradbury M, Petrovich N, et al. Presurgical evaluation of language using functional magnetic resonance imaging in brain tumor patients with previous surgery. Neurosurgery 2009;64(4): 644–52 [discussion: 652–3].
17. Parkes LM, Schwarzbach JV, Bouts AA, et al. Quantifying the spatial resolution of the gradient echo and spin echo BOLD response at 3 Tesla. Magn Reson Med 2005;54(6):1465–72.
18. Gati JS, Menon RS, Ugurbil K, et al. Experimental determination of the BOLD field strength dependence in vessels and tissue. Magn Reson Med 1997;38(2):296–302.
19. Ben Bashat D, Sivan I, Ziv M, et al. T1-weighted functional imaging based on a contrast agent in presurgical mapping. J Magn Reson Imaging 2008;28(5):1245–50.
20. Poser BA, Versluis MJ, Hoogduin JM, et al. BOLD contrast sensitivity enhancement and artifact

reduction with multiecho EPI: parallel-acquired in-homogeneity-desensitized fMRI. Magn Reson Med 2006;55(6):1227–35.

21. Bandettini PA. Seven topics in functional magnetic resonance imaging. J Integr Neurosci 2009;8(3): 371–403.

22. Weisskoff RM, Davis TL. Correcting gross distortion on echo planar images. Proceedings of the SMRM, 4515, Berlin, 1992.

23. Jezzard P. Correction of geometric distortion in fMRI data. Neuroimage 2012;62(2):648–51.

24. Hutton C, Bork A, Josephs O, et al. Image distortion correction in fMRI: a quantitative evaluation. Neuroimage 2002;16(1):217–40.

25. Jezzard P, Balaban RS. Correction for geometric distortion in echo planar images from B0 field variations. Magn Reson Med 1995;34(1):65–73.

26. Zacà D, Jarso S, Pillai JJ. Role of semantic paradigms for optimization of language mapping in clinical FMRI studies. AJNR Am J Neuroradiol 2013;34(10):1966–71.

27. Robinson S, Jovicich J. B0 mapping with multichannel RF coils at high field. Magn Reson Med 2011;66(4):976–88.

28. Zaitsev M, Hennig J, Speck O. Point spread function mapping with parallel imaging techniques and high acceleration factors: fast, robust, and flexible method for echo-planar imaging distortion correction. Magn Reson Med 2004;52(5):1156–66.

29. Pillai JJ. The significance of streamlined postprocessing approaches for clinical FMRI. AJNR Am J Neuroradiol 2013;34(6):1194–6.

30. Nennig E, Heiland S, Rasche D, et al. Functional magnetic resonance imaging for cranial neuronavigation: methods for automated and standardized data processing and management. a technical note. Neuroradiol J 2007;20(2):159–68.

31. Wiggins GC, Polimeni JR, Potthast A, et al. 96-Channel receive-only head coil for 3 Tesla: design optimization and evaluation. Magn Reson Med 2009;62(3):754–62.

32. Wald LL. The future of acquisition speed, coverage, sensitivity, and resolution. Neuroimage 2012;62(2):1221–9.

33. Ogawa S, Tank DW, Menon R, et al. Intrinsic signal changes accompanying sensory stimulation: functional brain mapping with magnetic resonance imaging. Proc Natl Acad Sci U S A 1992;89(13):5951–5.

34. Duong TQ, Kim DS, Ugurbil K, et al. Localized cerebral blood flow response at submillimeter columnar resolution. Proc Natl Acad Sci U S A 2001;98(19):10904–9.

35. Duong TQ, Kim DS, Ugurbil K, et al. Spatiotemporal dynamics of the BOLD fMRI signals: toward mapping submillimeter cortical columns using the early negative response. Magn Reson Med 2000; 44(2):231–42.

36. Kim SG, Ogawa S. Biophysical and physiological origins of blood oxygenation level-dependent fMRI signals. J Cereb Blood Flow Metab 2012; 32(7):1188–206.

37. Moon CH, Fukuda M, Kim SG. Spatiotemporal characteristics and vascular sources of neural-specific and -nonspecific fMRI signals at submillimeter columnar resolution. Neuroimage 2013;64: 91–103.

38. Menon RS, Ogawa S, Tank DW, et al. Tesla gradient recalled echo characteristics of photic stimulation-induced signal changes in the human primary visual cortex. Magn Reson Med 1993; 30(3):380–6.

39. Bianciardi M, Fukunaga M, van Gelderen P, et al. Negative BOLD-fMRI signals in large cerebral veins. J Cereb Blood Flow Metab 2011;31(2): 401–12.

40. Krings T, Erberich SG, Roessler F, et al. MR blood oxygenation level-dependent signal differences in parenchymal and large draining vessels: implications for functional MR imaging. AJNR Am J Neuroradiol 1999;20(10):1907–14.

41. Casciaro S, Bianco R, Distante A. Quantification of venous blood signal contribution to BOLD functional activation in the auditory cortex at 3 T. Magn Reson Imaging 2008;26(9):1221–31.

42. Yacoub E, Shmuel A, Pfeuffer J, et al. Imaging brain function in humans at 7 Tesla. Magn Reson Med 2001;45(4):588–94.

43. Geissler A, Fischmeister FP, Grabner G, et al. Comparing the microvascular specificity of the 3- and 7-T BOLD response using ICA and susceptibility-weighted imaging. Front Hum Neurosci 2013;7:474.

44. D'Esposito M, Deouell LY, Gazzaley A. Alterations in the BOLD fMRI signal with ageing and disease: a challenge for neuroimaging. Nat Rev Neurosci 2003;4(11):863–72.

45. Seto E, Sela G, McIlroy WE, et al. Quantifying head motion associated with motor tasks used in fMRI. Neuroimage 2001;14(2):284–97.

46. Menon RS, Ogawa S, Hu X, et al. BOLD based functional MRI at 4 Tesla includes a capillary bed contribution: echo-planar imaging correlates with previous optical imaging using intrinsic signals. Magn Reson Med 1995;33(3):453–9.

47. Fox MD, Raichle ME. Spontaneous fluctuations in brain activity observed with functional magnetic resonance imaging. Nat Rev Neurosci 2007;8(9): 700–11.

48. Stenger VA, Peltier S, Boada FE, et al. 3D spiral cardiac/respiratory ordered fMRI data acquisition at 3 Tesla. Magn Reson Med 1999;41(5):983–91.

49. Hu X, Kim SG. Reduction of signal fluctuation in functional MRI using navigator echoes. Magn Reson Med 1994;31(5):495–503.

50. Glover GH, Li TQ, Ress D. Image-based method for retrospective correction of physiological motion effects in fMRI: RETROICOR. Magn Reson Med 2000;44(1):162–7.

51. Hu X, Le TH, Parrish T, Erhard P. Retrospective estimation and correction of physiological fluctuation in functional MRI. Magn Reson Med 1995;34(2):201–12.

52. Birn RM, Diamond JB, Smith MA, et al. Separating respiratory-variation-related fluctuations from neuronal-activity-related fluctuations in fMRI. Neuroimage 2006;31(4):1536–48.

53. Greicius MD, Srivastava G, Reiss AL, et al. Default-mode network activity distinguishes Alzheimer's disease from healthy aging: evidence from functional MRI. Proc Natl Acad Sci U S A 2004; 101(13):4637–42.

54. Beall EB. Adaptive cyclic physiologic noise modeling and correction in functional MRI. J Neurosci Methods 2010;187(2):216–28.

55. Harvey AK, Pattinson KT, Brooks JC, et al. Brainstem functional magnetic resonance imaging: disentangling signal from physiological noise. J Magn Reson Imaging 2008;28(6):1337–44.

56. McKeown MJ, Makeig S, Brown GG, et al. Analysis of fMRI data by blind separation into independent spatial components. Hum Brain Mapp 1998;6(3): 160–88.

57. Thomas CG, Harshman RA, Menon RS. Noise reduction in BOLD-based fMRI using component analysis. Neuroimage 2002;17(3):1521–37.

58. Iwama T, Andoh T, Sakai N, et al. Artifacts in magnetic resonance imaging of the head. Neurol Med Chir (Tokyo) 1989;29(8):701–6.

59. Schwartz S, Maquet P, Frith C. Neural correlates of perceptual learning: a functional MRI study of visual texture discrimination. Proc Natl Acad Sci U S A 2002;99(26):17137–42.

60. Kastner S, De Weerd P, Ungerleider LG. Texture segregation in the human visual cortex: a functional MRI study. J Neurophysiol 2000;83(4):2453–7.

61. Biswal BB, Ulmer JL. Blind source separation of multiple signal sources of fMRI data sets using independent component analysis. J Comput Assist Tomogr 1999;23(2):265–71.

62. Beckmann CF, DeLuca M, Devlin JT, et al. Investigations into resting-state connectivity using independent component analysis. Philos Trans R Soc Lond B Biol Sci 2005;360(1457):1001–13.

63. Bullmore ET, Brammer MJ, Rabe-Hesketh S, et al. Methods for diagnosis and treatment of stimulus-correlated motion in generic brain activation studies using fMRI. Hum Brain Mapp 1999;7(1): 38–48.

64. Johnstone T, Ores Walsh KS, Greischar LL, et al. Motion correction and the use of motion covariates in multiple-subject fMRI analysis. Hum Brain Mapp 2006;27(10):779–88.

65. Friston KJ, Holmes AP, Poline JB, et al. Analysis of fMRI time-series revisited. Neuroimage 1995;2(1): 45–53.

66. Morgan VL, Dawant BM, Li Y, et al. Comparison of fMRI statistical software packages and strategies for analysis of images containing random and stimulus-correlated motion. Comput Med Imaging Graph 2007;31(6):436–46.

67. Oakes TR, Johnstone T, Ores Walsh KS, et al. Comparison of fMRI motion correction software tools. Neuroimage 2005;28(3):529–43.

68. Bannister PR, Jenkinson M. TIGER–a new model for spatio-temporal realignment of fMRI data. Berlin; Heidelberg (Germany): Springer-Verlag; 2004.

69. Orchard JA. Iterating registration and activation detection to overcome activation bias. fMRI motion estimates. Berlin; Heidelberg (Germany): Springer-Verlag; 2003.

70. Voyvodic JT. Reproducibility of single-subject fMRI language mapping with AMPLE normalization. J Magn Reson Imaging 2012;36(3):569–80.

71. Soldati N, Calhoun VD, Bruzzone L, et al. ICA analysis of fMRI with real-time constraints: an evaluation of fast detection performance as function of algorithms, parameters and a priori conditions. Front Hum Neurosci 2013;7:19.

72. Koehler RC, Roman RJ, Harder DR. Astrocytes and the regulation of cerebral blood flow (review). Trends in Neurosci 2009;32(3):160–9.

73. Attwell D, Buchan AM, Charpak S, et al. Glial and neuronal control of brain blood flow (review). Nature 2010;468(7321):232–43.

74. Zacà D, Jovicich J, Nadar SR, et al. Cerebrovascular reactivity mapping in patients with low grade gliomas undergoing presurgical sensorimotor mapping with BOLD fMRI. J Magn Reson Imaging 2014;40(2):383–90.

75. Pillai JJ, Zacà D. Comparison of BOLD cerebrovascular reactivity mapping and DSC MR perfusion imaging for prediction of neurovascular uncoupling potential in brain tumors. Technol Cancer Res Treat 2012;11(4):361–74.

The Economics of Functional Magnetic Resonance Imaging
Clinical and Research

David M. Yousem, MD, MBA

KEYWORDS

- Functional magnetic resonance imaging • Economics • Equipment • Functional imaging • BOLD
- Revenue • Costs • Expenses

KEY POINTS

- Given the time commitment and hardware and software costs of performing high-quality functional magnetic resonance imaging (fMRI) studies, reimbursement by insurers is unlikely to recoup costs.
- The sophistication of the fMRI setup and paradigms used may vary widely, as will costs of equipment to perform and analyze fMRI studies.
- Performing fMRI studies is "valued" based on its benefits for patient care and outcomes related to neurosurgery.
- Research fMRI programs may fund the resources needed through large/shared instrumentation grants.

INTRODUCTION

Creating a viable functional magnetic resonance imaging (fMRI) service requires a significant investment in infrastructure, hardware, and software, whether for a clinical service or for a research enterprise. Because of the duration of the overall examination needed to create the necessary anatomic and functional studies, devising a service that yields sufficient revenue to create a profitable endeavor is often challenging. Put into the context of a brain tumor surgery service line, however, it is a valuable commodity. Many patient customers are now savvy enough to ask for, and possibly even demand, functional imaging as part of their preoperative paradigm, particularly for parenchymal masses in the frontal, temporal, and parietal lobes.

To understand the financials associated with a clinical fMRI service, one must understand the process by which relative value units (RVUs) were assigned to fMRI, the expected reimbursement for patient care cases, and the expenses required to create a comprehensive clinical service. A research service may be supported by grants that help to offset the initial and maintenance costs. The payment for time on a research magnet may be adjusted based on the need to offset these expenses and National Institutes of Health guidelines.

VALUATION OF FUNCTIONAL MRI: THE RESOURCE-BASED RELATIVE VALUE SCALE SYSTEM

The resource-based relative value scale system was implemented by the Centers for Medicare and Medicaid Services in 1992 and replaced the system previously utilized based on usual, customary and reasonable charge system.[1–3] Each imaging procedure is assigned a Current Procedure Terminology (CPT) code that eventually is allotted a relative value unit (RVU), which leads to monetary reimbursement. CPT codes are

Disclosure: The author has nothing to disclose.
The Russell H. Morgan Department of Radiology and Radiological Science, Johns Hopkins Medical Institution, 600 North Wolfe Street Phipps B100F, Baltimore, MD 21287, USA
E-mail address: dyousem1@jhu.edu

Neuroimag Clin N Am 24 (2014) 717–724
http://dx.doi.org/10.1016/j.nic.2014.07.007
1052-5149/14/$ – see front matter © 2014 Elsevier Inc. All rights reserved.

neuroimaging.theclinics.com

assigned by the American Medical Association (AMA) through its CPT Editorial Panel and CPT Advisory Committee. The CPT Editorial Panel consists of 17 members who are nominated by the National Medical Specialty Societies, Blue Cross and Blue Shield Association, the America's Health Insurance Plans, the American Hospital Association, and the Centers for Medicare and Medicaid Services and approved by the AMA Board of Trustees. The panel is responsible for maintaining, revising, updating, and modifying the CPT code set. The CPT Advisory Committee comprises physicians associated with AMA House of Delegate societies and advises the CPT Editorial Panel on correct procedural descriptions for coding and RVU valuations.[1–3]

The AMA staff first review coding suggestions proposed by its members (**Box 1**). The request is referred to the CPT Advisory Committee, which may rule that a new code is not needed because the procedure is similar to another or it may pass the proposal on to the CPT Editorial Panel.

The AMA formed the AMA/Specialty Society Relative Value Scale Update Committee (commonly known as the "RUC") to act as an expert panel to provide consultation to Centers for Medicare and Medicaid Services for assigning RVUs to CPT codes that the Editorial Panel creates. The RUC represents the entire medical profession with 21 of its 31 members appointed by specialties recognized by the American Board of Medical Specialties, more heavily weighted toward those specialties engaging in patient care, and those specialties with higher percentages of Medicare expenditures. The RUC process is outlined in **Box 2** and **Fig. 1**.

Professional Fees

The resource-based relative value scale system bases the physician professional RVUs on:

1	Physician work	55% of overall value on average
2	Practice expense	42% of overall value on average
3	Malpractice expense	3% of overall value on average

Physician work encompasses professional costs related to the time, training, skill, and intensity or stress of the particular service provision experienced by the physician. When considering the time aspect of the physician work, it includes the preservice, intraservice, and postservice time

---

Box 1
CPT code development workflow

1. A new procedure, technology, or performance measurement is introduced.
2. The new item does not fit into an existing code.
3. A coding request form is submitted.
4. AMA staff review the coding suggestion.
5. If it is a new request the CPT Advisory Committee reviews it.
6. If the CPT Advisory Committee decides a new code is not needed the AMA staff inform the requestor and inform them on how to use existing codes to report the procedure.
7. If the CPT Advisory Committee agrees a change should be made it is then referred to the CPT Editorial Panel.
8. The CPT Editorial Panel can result in 3 outcomes:
   i. Add new code or revise existing nomenclature,
   ii. Postpone/table an item to obtain further information, or
   iii. Reject an item.
9. If the request is rejected the requestor could appeal the rule.
10. To appeal, the AMA must receive a written request that contains the reasons why the CPT Editorial Panel's decision was incorrect. This must be done within 1 year of the initial request.
11. When the appeal is submitted, it goes to the CPT executive committee for review.

Derived from Donovan WD. The resource-based relative value scale and neuroradiology: ASNR's history at the RUC. Neuroimaging Clin N Am 2012;22(3):425; with permission.

---

and effort. In the case of fMRI the preservice work as far as teaching the patients the paradigms and training them to perform appropriately in the scanner may be substantial. In the same vein, the post processing and creation of the functional maps can exact a huge time commitment. This is all part of physician work.

Office supplies, utilities, labor, and expenses associated with billing and collections, as well as rent are examples of practice expenses. As implied by its name, the malpractice expense reflects the payment made to help offset professional liability expenses.

(see below).

Box 2
Process of RUC review

1. The CPT Editorial Panel's new or revised codes and CMS requests to review existing codes are sent to the RUC staff.

2. Members of the RUC Advisory Committee and specialty society staff review the summary and indicate their societies' level of interest in developing a relative value recommendation.

3. Subspecialty societies choose to (1) survey their members to obtain data on the amount of work involved in a service and develop recommendations based on the survey results, (2) comment in writing on recommendations developed by other societies, or (3) take no action.

4. AMA staff distributes survey instruments for the specialty societies.

5. Subspecialty societies survey at least 30 practicing physicians. Physicians receiving the survey are asked to evaluate the work involved in the new or revised code relative to the reference as the Harvard resource-based relative value scale study.

6. The specialty RVS committees conduct the surveys, review the results, and prepare their recommendations to the RUC.

7. The written recommendations are disseminated to the RUC before the meeting and consist of physician work, time, and practice expense recommendations.

8. The specialty advisors present and defend the recommendations at the RUC meeting.

9. The RUC may decide to adopt a specialty society's recommendation, refer it back to the specialty society, or modify it before submitting it to CMS. Final recommendations to CMS must be adopted by a two-thirds majority of the RUC members.

10. The RUC's recommendations are forwarded to CMS in May of each year.

11. The Medicare Physician Payment Schedule, which includes CMS's review of the RUC recommendations, is published in the late fall. CMS's acceptance rate for the RUC's recommendations is typically more than 90% annually

Abbreviation: CMS, Centers for Medicare and Medicaid Services.
  Data from Refs.[1–4]

Thus, for fMRI there is considerable time and effort expended by the physician for preparation of the patient before the fMRI study, and post processing of the study after completion. These were

calculated in the effort assigned to the physician work for fMRI (see below).

Technical Fees

The technical portion of a global RVU (global = professional plus technical RVU) constitutes payment for the expenses in the technical performance of the procedure. Technical reimbursement is intended to cover costs attributed to the facility where the care is provided, equipment for the imaging study, and the technical staff associated with producing the diagnostic and/or therapeutic image. Thus, costs for personnel including business support, front desk personnel, technologists, nurses, secretaries, equipment maintenance workers, post processing computer specialists (in the case of fMRI), and IT support. The nonlabor expenses include the scanners, contrast agents, IV lines, computer programs, supplies, paradigm presentation devices, analysis programs, office supplies, linen, and uniforms.

FUNCTIONAL MRI CPT CODES AND RVUS

The CPT codes that have been assigned to fMRI studies were approved in 2004 by the AMA. The description of the 3 codes are listed below.

70554
  Magnetic resonance imaging, brain, fMRI, including test selection and administration of repetitive body part movement and/or visual stimulation, not requiring physician or psychologist administration. Code 70554 is not to be reported in conjunction with 96020 or 70555 (see below). It is assigned 13.71 RVUs for the technical component and 2.81 RVUs for the professional component (2.11 RVUs for physician work) from the Medicare code key. In Maryland, it has been assigned 10 RVUs for the technical component.[5]

70555
  Magnetic resonance imaging, brain, fMRI; requiring physician or psychologist administration of entire neurofunctional testing. Code 70555 can only be reported when 96020 is performed. It is assigned 13.71 RVUs for the technical component and 3.37 RVUs for the professional component (2.54 RVUs for physician work). (Note: A 0.56-RVU increase in professional RVU from 70554 where the physician does not participate). In Maryland, it has been assigned 18 RVUs for the technical component.[5]

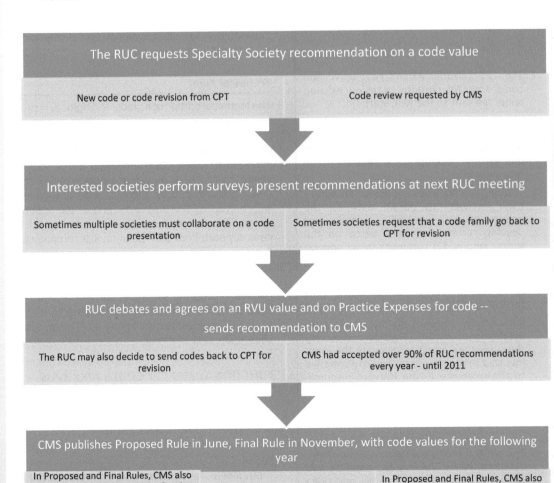

Fig. 1. The CPT–RUC process cycle. (*From* Donovan WD. The resource-based relative value scale and neuroradiology: ASNR's history at the RUC. Neuroimaging Clin N Am 2012;22(3):427; with permission by Elsevier and the author William Donovan.)

96020

Neurofunctional testing selection and administration during noninvasive imaging functional brain mapping, with test administered entirely by a physician or psychologist, with review of test results and report. Codes 70554 and 70555 cannot be reported in conjunction with 70551 (MR imaging brain without contrast), 70552 (MR imaging brain with contrast), or 70553 (MR imaging brain with and without contrast) unless a separate diagnostic MR imaging is performed. It is assigned only a professional RVU allotment because the technical fee is always bundled into the 70555 CPT code. That professional value is 4.46 RVUs (3.43 RVUs for physician work).[5]

Thus, if one combines 70555 and 96020 for a physician-assisted fMRI, the technical RVU component is 13.71 and the professional RVU component is 7.83 (**Table 1**).

By comparison, an unenhanced MRI of the brain, CPT code 70551, finds a technical component of 9.94 to 10.74 and a professional component of 2.02 RVUs.[5]

FUNCTIONAL MRI CHARGES AND PAYMENTS

At our institution, the mean professional fee charge (not payment) for the 70555 code in 2013 was $509.11. For the 96020 professional fee, the charge was $730 in 2013. This is not necessarily what the physicians are paid, of course, except for the exceptional individual who is paying out of pocket the full fare. By comparison, the professional fee charge for the 70554 code was $151.10 on average. The payments for the 70554, 70555, and 96020 in 2013 averaged $57.22, $145.06,

Table 1
Outpatient imaging center reimbursement rates 2007

CPT Code	Technical Fee (RVU)	Professional Fee (RVU)	Total	Inpatient Study (Total)
70554	$348.80 (13.71)	$98.53 (2.81)	$447.33	DRG + $98.53
70555	$348.80 (13.71)	$117.86 (3.37)	$466.66	DRG + $117.86
96020	$108.69	$155.76 (4.46)	$264.45	DRG + $155.76
70551 (unenhanced brain MR imaging)	9.94 RVU	2.04 RVU		

and $193.01, respectively. At our institution payments for 70554, 70555, and 96020 were 37.9%, 28.5%, and 26.4% of charges. Therefore, the per-study professional fee reimbursement for fMRI at Johns Hopkins averaged $338 in 2013 (70555 and 96020 revenue). At 2 other major institutions, the average professional fee reimbursements were $342 and approximately $400 for the same 2 combined 70555 and 96020 CPT codes (Ron Wolf and Jeffrey Petrella, personal communication, 2013).

Most of the payments for fMRI at our institution were from Blue Shield (Carefirst), representing 36% of the volume followed by Medicare. When studies were rejected for payment, it was exclusively for using the 70555 code and the reasons cited were "not enough documentation to support the charges" (n = 4 in 2013), a "medical necessity issue" (n = 2 in 2013), or a "noncovered service." After resubmission, we were paid 100% of cases in calendar 2013 (Bonnie Gillum, Baltimore, Maryland, personal communication, 2013).

If one assumes that, between performing and analyzing fMRI studies, one could complete 4 cases per day and that the professional fee reimbursement was $400 per study, it would suggest that one could garner $1600 per day in professional fees. If one ran the service 46 weeks a year, 5 days a week the service would garner $368,000. The technical fees for the 70555 are 4 times that of the professional fees, but must be used to pay for the expenses of performing the scans. If the rate of reimbursement for the technical fees was the same as the professional fees, the technical revenue given the service would be 4 × $368,000 = $1,472,000.

The realities are that 1 institution rarely has the volume to do 4 fMRI cases a day. The data from the 2012 American Society of Functional Neuroradiology survey of fMRI volume and referrals is displayed in **Table 2** (Jeffrey Petrella, Duke University, Durham, North Carolina, personal communication, 2013). Average cases per year were 71.6

for all institutions responding, yielding 71.6 × $400 = $28,640 in revenue.

The values quoted suggest that even with running a scanner full time for performing fMRI studies for an 8-hour day averaging 4 cases per day may not be able to support the physicians' salaries in toto with benefits (usually computed at 37%), but may cover the annual costs of maintenance contracts, technologists, information technology, and equipment costs of the service.[6] The purchase of the equipment is addressed subsequently.

A word on other "functional Imaging" techniques: Although in concept physicians may consider diffusion-weighted imaging, diffusion tensor imaging, first-pass gadolinium dynamic susceptibility perfusion imaging, arterial spin labeled perfusion imaging, and kurtosis analysis forms of "functional imaging," these techniques do not have separate

Table 2
Data from the 2012 American Society of Functional Neuroradiology survey

Field	Average
Clinical cases/year	71.6
Ordering physician	
Neuroradiologist	—
Neurologist	26.1%
Neurosurgeon	73.3%
Psychologist	—
Neurointerventionalist	0.4%
Other	0.2%
Ordered for	
Tumor	61.3%
Epilepsy	26.2%
Arteriovenous malformation	10.1%
Neurodevelopmental surgery	0.8%
Other	1.7%

CPT codes assigned to them. If they are Food and Drug Administration (FDA)-approved techniques and employ 3-dimensional (3D) post processing on FDA-approved devices with FDA-approved software programs, one might be able to add one of two 3D post processing CPT codes.

76376

3D rendering with interpretation and reporting of CT, MR imaging, ultrasound, or other tomographic modality; not requiring image postprocessing on an independent workstation. This is assigned 0.52 technical RVUs and 0.07 professional RVUs (0.20 physician work RVUs). Global payments from Medicare average $29.02.[5]

76377

3D rendering with interpretation and reporting of CT, MR imaging, ultrasound, or other tomographic modality; requiring image postprocessing on an independent workstation. This is assigned 1.22 technical RVUs and 0.29 professional RVUs (0.79 physician work RVUs). Typical global fees paid are $84.18.[5]

It is most useful to have the requesting physicians specifically order 3D post processing so that claims of self-referral can be eliminated when radiologists perform and charge for these 3D image sets. It is also imperative to store on the Picture Archiving and Communication System the evidence of these 3D images permanently in case of audits. Finally, it must be directly stated in the report whether or not the 3D image sets were generated on an independent workstation or not. If possible, having a separate paragraph documenting what the 3D dataset showed is useful in guaranteeing unencumbered reimbursement.

The 76376 and 76377 codes, like with computed tomography angiography and magnetic resonance angiography, cannot be added to the fMRI CPT codes because their values are "bundled" into the fMRI valuation. These codes can be added to standard MR imaging examinations however.

Expenses

One of the major issues in creating a lucrative clinical fMRI service is the high initial setup expense for a top-of-the-line system that allows functional imaging with cortical and white matter mapping. It is useful to look at the systems from most expensive to least expensive items.

3T scanner purchase

For most high end fMRI programs, a 3T scanner is the minimum field strength recommended. Prices

vary from manufacturer to manufacturer for scanner pricing and certainly academic programs and large private practice groups may be able to negotiate bulk purchases at a discount. However, conventionally the magnet costs between $2 and $3 million. If one includes the highest end gradients for performing diffusion tensor imaging and a 32 or greater channel head coil ($100K–$150K), the price quickly reaches at least $2.5 to $3.5 million. To have an optimized, shielded room in an outpatient or hospital setting may lead to a site preparation fee of as high as $0.5 to 1 million (Angel Molina, Washington, DC, personal communication, 2013).

The annual maintenance contact on a high-end MR imaging machine may cost between $150,000 and 200,000.

Display and paradigm packages

This usually includes the hardware and its associated software. These pieces allow finger tapping sensing, tactile stimulation, high-quality auditory stimuli with head phones, eye tracker, and visual projection systems. The probable cost is a conservative $150,000 to $200,000. A presentation software program such as e-prime has prices quoted on the Internet (for 1–4 licenses) of $2100.

Analysis packages

The next most expensive startup expense is the fMRI analysis software. If one does not use a home grown system (which has some issues if using a non–FDA-approved analysis program in a clinical setting), one must purchase analysis software packages from the MR vendor or a third-party vendor (FDA approved for clinical use) (Table 3). With this package, one will be able to achieve real-time monitoring of motion and interim image analysis, simultaneous diffusion tensor imaging/fMRI data processing, transfer of data to the Picture Archiving and Communication System,

Table 3
Customer prices—United States of America (BrainVoyager QX [BVQX] software package; valid through March 31, 2014)

Quantity	1 License	2–4 per License	5–9 per License
BVQX Standard (BM+SM)	$7854	$7461	$7069
BVQX BM	$4774	$4535	$4297
BVQX SM	$3080	$2926	$2772

Abbreviations: BM, base module; SM, surface module.
Data from http://www.brainvoyager.com/USA_Prices_2014_1Q.pdf.

and conversion of data for use and harmony with surgical navigation systems. The more sites that one includes for software licenses, the more expensive it is.

Brain Voyager, an fMRI analysis package, provides a quote on the Internet as seen in Table 4. It is integrated into an FDA-approved package called Integrated Functional Imaging System. Statistical parametric mapping and software supplied by The Oxford Centre for Functional Magnetic Resonance Imaging of the Brain Software Library may be obtained without a purchase price.

The 2012 American Society of Functional Neuroradiology survey suggests that there is no dominant software being employed (Jeffrey Petrella, Duke University, Durham, North Carolina, personal communication, 2013) (Table 4). Prices can be obtained from vendors.

MR injector

For performing perfusion imaging, one needs a high-quality injector for first-pass gadolinium

performance. The injector usually costs between $40,000 and $60,000. If one had to reduce expenses as much as possible, one can perform fMRI without presentation hardware using the microphone in the scanner to instruct the patient and without using a patient monitoring system. Software available through the National Institutes of Health or other academic programs can be garnered for free.

As far as the personnel expense, this depends on who is doing the training of the patients, the performance of the scan, and the post processing of scan data. The 2012 American Society of Functional Neuroradiology survey suggests that consensus has not been reached in this regard (Table 5) (Jeffrey Petrella, Duke University, Durham, North Carolina, personal communication, 2013).

Research Scanner Considerations

fMRI is frequently employed in imaging research schemes submitted by neuroradiologists, neurologists, neurosurgeons, psychiatrists, psychologists, behavioral scientists, rehabilitation medicine physicians, and cognitive scientists. The billing of these examinations for research will be predicated on whether the payors are governmental agencies (eg, the National Institutes of Health, Department of Defense, National Science Foundation), industry (eg, device manufacturers or pharmaceutical companies), foundations (eg, Dana, Goldhirsch), societies (eg, American Society of Neuroradiology, Brain Tumor Society), or other funding bodies. Although the prices may be regulated in cases of governmental funding, those same prices may be negotiated either at a per hour scanner use rate or by the study.

Table 4
Software programs being utilized

Acquisition software	%
BrainWave	9.1
InVivo/Philips	27.3
MRIx	18.2
NNL	—
Prism	9.1
Siemens	18.2
Other	18.2
Post processing software	
BrainWave	8.3
FSL	12.5
InVivo/Philips	12.5
MRIx	16.7
NNL	8.3
Prism	8.3
Siemens	8.3
SPM	8.3
Other	16.7
Clinical review software	
BrainWave	11.1
FSL	5.6
InVivo/Philips	16.7
MRIx	22.2
NNL	2.8
Prism	11.1
Siemens	11.1
Other	19.4

Table 5
American Society of Functional Neuroradiology 2012 data: personnel

Personnel	%
Patient training by	
Technologist	22.5
Psychologist	8.3
Physicist	6.3
Neuroradiologist	54.6
Neurologist	8.3
Post processing by	
Technologist	27.5
Psychologist	—
Physicist	29.2
Neuroradiologist	35.0
Vendor	8.3

In those instances where the post processing is performed as a service by the research scanner team, there is typically a standardized charge applied for that service. This may be on a per-study basis or by the number of paradigms performed in an fMRI experiment. Storage of data and IT support also tend to incur a charge. These charges are often adjusted based on the annual expenses of the research program, which include the overhead and personnel costs as well as maintenance and upgrade expenses for all components of the fMRI hardware and software.

Purchase of research scanners may be an investment an academic institution feels is justified given their neurosciences program. However, shared instrumentation grants, high-end instrumentation grants, Defense University Research Instrumentation Program, National Science Foundation Major Research Instrumentation Program, or regional resource grants can collectively or seperately help to fund fMRI equipment.

SUMMARY

It is difficult to justify maintaining a clinical fMRI program based solely on revenue generation. The use of fMRI is, therefore, based mostly in patient care considerations, leading to better outcomes. The high costs of the top-of-the-line equipment, hardware, and software needed for state of the art fMRI and the time commitment by multiple professionals are not adequately reimbursed at a representative rate by current payor schemes for the CPT codes assigned. Research programs may adjust charges based on expenses and services provided, but the cost of purchasing the state-of-the-art setup is often borne through philanthropy or equipment/resource grants by governmental agencies.

REFERENCES

1. Lam DL, Medverd JR. How radiologists get paid: resource-based relative value scale and the revenue cycle [review]. AJR Am J Roentgenol 2013; 201(5):947–58. http://dx.doi.org/10.2214/AJR.12. 9715.
2. Donovan WD. The resource-based relative value scale and neuroradiology: ASNR's History at the RUC. Neuroimaging Clin N Am 2012;22(3):421–36.
3. Bledsoe M, Hunt RA, Langdon JC. The resource-based relative value scale. Chapter 8. In: Yousem DM, Beauchamp NJ, editors. Radiology business practice: how to succeed. Philadelphia: Elsevier; 2008. p. 99–117.
4. Available at: http://www.ama-assn.org/resources/doc/rbrvs/ruc-update-booklet.pdf.
5. Available at: http://www.cms.gov/apps/physician-fee-schedule/search/search-criteria.aspx.
6. Medverd JR, Prabhu SJ, Lam DL. Business of radiology: financial fundamentals for radiologists. AJR Am J Roentgenol 2013;201(5):W683–90. http://dx. doi.org/10.2214/AJR.13.10838.

Index

Note: Page numbers of article titles are in **boldface** type.

Neuroimag Clin N Am 24 (2014) 725–727
http://dx.doi.org/10.1016/S1052-5149(14)00097-5
1052-5149/14/$ – see front matter © 2014 Elsevier Inc. All rights reserved.

neuroimaging.theclinics.com

United States Postal Service
Statement of Ownership, Management, and Circulation
(All Periodicals Publications Except Requestor Publications)

1. Publication Title
Neuroimaging Clinics of North America

2. Publication Number
0 1 0 - 5 4 8

3. Filing Date
9/14/14

4. Issue Frequency
Feb, May, Aug, Nov

5. Number of Issues Published Annually
4

6. Annual Subscription Price
$360.00

7. Complete Mailing Address of Known Office of Publication *(Not printer) (Street, city, county, state, and ZIP+4®)*
Elsevier Inc.
360 Park Avenue South
New York, NY 10010-1710

Contact Person
Stephen R. Bushing

Telephone *(Include area code)*
215-239-3688

8. Complete Mailing Address of Headquarters or General Business Office of Publisher *(Not printer)*
Elsevier Inc., 360 Park Avenue South, New York, NY 10010-1710

9. Full Names and Complete Mailing Addresses of Publisher, Editor, and Managing Editor *(Do not leave blank)*

Publisher *(Name and complete mailing address)*
Linda Belfus, Elsevier Inc., 1600 John F. Kennedy Blvd., Suite 1800, Philadelphia, PA 19103-2899

Editor *(Name and complete mailing address)*
John Vassallo, Elsevier Inc., 1600 John F. Kennedy Blvd., Suite 1800, Philadelphia, PA 19103-2899

Managing Editor *(Name and complete mailing address)*
Adrianne Brigido, Elsevier Inc., 1600 John F. Kennedy Blvd., Suite 1800, Philadelphia, PA 19103-2899

10. Owner *(Do not leave blank. If the publication is owned by a corporation, give the name and address of the corporation immediately followed by the names and addresses of all stockholders owning or holding 1 percent or more of the total amount of stock. If not owned by a corporation, give the names and addresses of the individual owners. If owned by a partnership or other unincorporated firm, give its name and address as well as those of each individual owner. If the publication is published by a nonprofit organization, give its name and address.)*

Full Name	Complete Mailing Address
Wholly owned subsidiary of	1600 John F. Kennedy Blvd., Ste. 1800
Reed/Elsevier, US holdings	Philadelphia, PA 19103-2899

11. Known Bondholders, Mortgagees, and Other Security Holders Owning or Holding 1 Percent or More of Total Amount of Bonds, Mortgages, or Other Securities. If none, check box ☐ None

Full Name	Complete Mailing Address
N/A	

12. Tax Status *(For completion by nonprofit organizations authorized to mail at nonprofit rates) (Check one)*
The purpose, function, and nonprofit status of this organization and the exempt status for federal income tax purposes:
☐ Has Not Changed During Preceding 12 Months
☐ Has Changed During Preceding 12 Months *(Publisher must submit explanation of change with this statement)*

PS Form **3526**, August 2012 (Page 1 of 3 (Instructions Page 3)) PSN 7530-01-000-9931 PRIVACY NOTICE: See our Privacy policy in www.usps.com

---

13. Publication Title
Neuroimaging Clinics of North America

14. Issue Date for Circulation Data Below
August 2014

15. Extent and Nature of Circulation

		Average No. Copies Each Issue During Preceding 12 Months	No. Copies of Single Issue Published Nearest to Filing Date
a. Total Number of Copies *(Net press run)*		1,059	1,009
b. Paid Circulation (By Mail and Outside the Mail)	(1) Mailed Outside-County Paid Subscriptions Stated on PS Form 3541 *(Include paid distribution above nominal rate, advertiser's proof copies, and exchange copies)*	746	712
	(2) Mailed In-County Paid Subscriptions Stated on PS Form 3541 *(Include paid distribution above nominal rate, advertiser's proof copies, and exchange copies)*		
	(3) Paid Distribution Outside the Mails Including Sales Through Dealers and Carriers, Street Vendors, Counter Sales, and Other Paid Distribution Outside USPS®	123	120
	(4) Paid Distribution by Other Classes Mailed Through the USPS (e.g. First-Class Mail®)		
c. Total Paid Distribution *(Sum of 15b (1), (2), (3), and (4))*	▲	869	832
d. Free or Nominal Rate Distribution (By Mail and Outside the Mail)	(1) Free or Nominal Rate Outside-County Copies Included on PS Form 3541	26	37
	(2) Free or Nominal Rate In-County Copies Included on PS Form 3541		
	(3) Free or Nominal Rate Copies Mailed at Other Classes Through the USPS (e.g. First-Class Mail)		
	(4) Free or Nominal Rate Distribution Outside the Mail (Carriers or other means)		
e. Total Free or Nominal Rate Distribution *(Sum of 15d (1), (2), (3) and (4))*	▲	26	37
f. Total Distribution *(Sum of 15c and 15e)*	▲	895	869
g. Copies not Distributed *(See instructions to publishers #4 (page #3))*	▲	164	140
h. Total *(Sum of 15f and g)*	▲	1,059	1,009
i. Percent Paid *(15c divided by 15f times 100)*	▲	97.09%	95.74%

16. Total circulation includes electronic copies. Report circulation on PS Form 3526-X worksheet.

17. Publication of Statement of Ownership
If the publication is a general publication, publication of this statement is required. Will be printed in the November 2014 issue of this publication.

18. Signature and Title of Editor, Publisher, Business Manager, or Owner

[signature]
Stephen R. Bushing – Inventory Distribution Coordinator

Date
September 14, 2014

I certify that all information furnished on this form is true and complete. I understand that anyone who furnishes false or misleading information on this form or who omits material or information requested on the form may be subject to criminal sanctions (including fines and imprisonment) and/or civil sanctions (including civil penalties).

PS Form **3526**, August 2012 (Page 2 of 3)

Printed and bound by CPI Group (UK) Ltd, Croydon, CR0 4YY

03/10/2024

01040379-0019